from the
hips

a comprehensive,
open-minded,
uncensored,
totally
honest
guide to
pregnancy,
birth, and
becoming
a parent

from the hips

rebecca odes
ceridwen morris

THREE RIVERS PRESS • NEW YORK

Copyright © 2007 by Rebecca Odes and Ceridwen Morris

All rights reserved.
Published in the United States by Three Rivers Press,
an imprint of the Crown Publishing Group, a division
of Random House, Inc., New York.
www.crownpublishing.com

THREE RIVERS PRESS and the Tugboat design are registered
trademarks of Random House, Inc.

Library of Congress Cataloging-in-Publication Data
Odes, Rebecca.
   From the hips: a comprehensive, open-minded,
uncensored, totally honest guide to pregnancy, birth, and
becoming a parent / Rebecca Odes and Ceridwen Morris.
— 1st ed.
   Includes bibliographical references.
   1. Pregnancy.   I. Morris, Ceridwen.   II. Title.
RG551.O34 2007
618.2—dc22   2006028846

ISBN 978-0-307-23708-8

Printed in China

Design by Georgia Rucker
Illustrations by Rebecca Odes

10 9 8 7 6 5 4

To our families,
for making it all possible

acknowledgments

thanks first to the people who helped make this book happen: Lydia Wills, Georgia Rucker, Shaye Areheart, and Julia Pastore at Crown/Three Rivers Press, and our excellent advisory board.

And thank you . . .

to everyone who lent their eyes, ears, and voices to us during the years of gestation this project demanded: including Esther Drill, Heather McDonald, Mac Chambers, Ruth Root, Rene Steinke, Sharon Gelman, Helen MacInnes, Sofia Ahlberg, Lely Constantinople, Gaia Schemmerhorn, Iain and Annie York, Katrina Onstad, Justine Leguizamo, Steven Johnson, Alexa Robinson, Elizabeth Mitchell, Stefanie Syman, Deborah Horowitz, Michelle Pearlman, Alex Abramovich, Catrin Morris Miller, Chris Miller, Betsy Finston, Susannah Lipsyte, Courtenay and Alexandra Valenti, Ingrid Bernstein, Clora Kelly, Ian Rogers, Julie Jacobs, Dan Sharp, Dana Menussi, Fifi Simon, Amy Hanson, Anna Peterson, Naomi Odes, Emi Guner, Amy Scheibe, Kate Sharp, Jada Shapiro, Terry Richmond, Karrie Adamany, Sara Goodman, Drew McCloud, Julie Farris, David Brendel, David Feuer, Dayana Padilla, the Wine and Whine moms, the Moths, and the many parents who told their stories at thenewmom.com.

to Hedy and Arnold Kanarick, Robert Lipsyte, Lois B. Morris, Fiona and Alun Morris, and Joan and Stuart Odes for supporting us throughout.

to Sensho Wagg and Angela Lopis for giving us the freedom to pursue our work, knowing that our children were in exceptionally good hands.

to our amazing husbands, Craig Kanarick and Sam Lipsyte, for their insight and patience (and for taking the early shift, the afternoon shift, the late shift, and the weekend shift when deadlines required).

and to Ezra, Alfred, and Odessa for teaching us how to be mothers.

contents

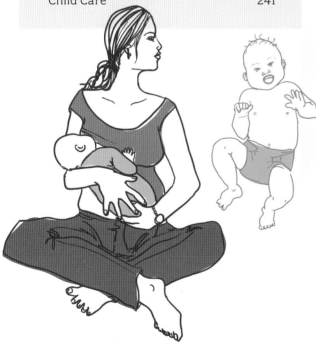

introduction

We have a confession to make. We didn't know what a doula was when we got pregnant. We thought genetic counseling was some kind of science fiction procedure for choosing your baby's eye color in advance. We thought twelve hours of labor was a long time. Little did we know.

Soon enough, we were swept up in a tidal wave of information. The medical establishment, the alternative birth movement, the baby feeding, clothing, and products industries, endless experts touting conflicting theories, and ever-changing research made us feel bombarded, cornered, and forced to make decisions we never thought we'd have to make. *Should I have an amniocentesis? Should I eat this tuna sandwich? Should I circumcise? Will my baby be more comfortable in a $37 organic cotton onesie? Seriously, will this tuna really hurt the fetus? And what the hell is a doula anyway?*

Like most women, we found ourselves braving the road to motherhood without a decent map. We were shocked to discover that every piece of media we encountered on the subject of having a baby made us feel pressured to act in one way or another, rather than encouraging us to find our own voices as parents. There we were, newly pregnant, giddy with excitement as we browsed the bookshelves. To the right, the old-school medical advisory manual, bursting with what to freak out about when you're expecting. To the left, the wise-cracking Hollywood mom, wagging a manicured finger at us all the way to the hospital. Who else? The rustic midwife? The Belgian nun? The more we read, the more lost and intimidated we felt.

Please, we thought, *please somebody help!* We'd have shouted it if we could, but we weren't even supposed to tell anyone for two more months, when it's "cool" to announce that you're pregnant.

Once you're out of the closet, your private life is suddenly subject to public scrutiny. It can be easy to find yourself unearthing insecurities you thought you'd buried in your teens. *Am I fat? Is this normal? What's happening to me?* Body changes, identity issues, social anxieties—pregnancy can give puberty a serious run for its money.

Then when the baby arrives, the shit really hits the fan (and the diaper, and that $37 organic cotton onesie), making a further mess of your former sense of self. Your mother-in-law thinks your baby's hungry and your mother thinks you're feeding him too much. One book tells you to let your baby cry and the other book tells you to pick him up. You don't know what you believe, but you do know that the person previously known as you is clinging to a raft in a stormy sea of pastel burp cloths and bottle warmers.

What kind of mother am I? Who the hell am I and what is a "mother," anyway? How did the nine zillion other women who did this before me deal with it? I need somebody to tell it like it is, not tell me what to do.

We just wanted a book that would guide us through the choices and issues we might face without pushing an agenda, being condescending, or using scare tactics. We needed a trustworthy resource with an approach we could relate to, and without judgment. We couldn't find one. And that's how *From the Hips* was born.

This book will show you the range of possible approaches and help you find your own way of having a baby. We'll deconstruct the studies and delve into the controversies. You'll hear from pregnant women, new parents, ob-gyns, genetic counselors, lactation consultants, pediatricians, anthropologists, midwives, "old wives," and more—even the aforementioned doula (who, by the way, is a woman trained to assist and comfort new mothers during and after the birth process).

When we got pregnant, we were both living in the same city, going to the same parties; we were the same age, same shoe size, same bra size. We were friends. We bonded over the same physical dramas and difficult decisions. But we often took different approaches. A decision that left one of us completely wiped out was a breeze for the other. One of us set up the nursery months before the birth; the other didn't buy a thing till the baby was securely in the house. One of us circumcised; the other didn't. One coslept; the other had her baby in the crib right away. One of us was back in the office after a brief maternity leave; the other was home. Having babies brought us closer, but also put our differences in high relief. If two women with so much in common could have such different responses to pregnancy and parenting, the possibilities were clearly endless. We made it our mission to get input from as many new parents as possible. Hundreds of moms and dads gave their stories to this project. We do our best to avoid assumptions about our readers: We won't imply that you've got the stereotypically clueless uninvolved husband (or even that you've got a husband). Parenthood is as unique an experience as anything else, no matter how much the media tends to generalize.

Not long ago, an eight-year-old girl was watching one of us alternately hug and struggle with a squirmy toddler at a restaurant. Taking in the scene, she asked, "So, is being a mom fun? Is it, like, so great you can't believe it? Or is it so boring you can't believe it? Or is it, like, UGH! I can't stand it!" Well, as far as we can tell, it's all of those things. Sometimes in the same week, sometimes in the same day, sometimes at the same time. This book is about both sides of the story: the warm, fuzzy baby blanket and the poop that gets swept underneath. It's about the real world of new parenthood as we, and all the parents who contributed to these pages, see it. We hope it helps you on your way.

— *Rebecca and Ceridwen*

ten anti-rules
for parents-in-progress

1. everyone's an expert, but you're the authority on yourself and your baby.

Once you get pregnant, everybody seems to have something to say about what you should (or absolutely should *not*) do with yourself and your baby. But everyone's experience and perspective are different. The way you deal with pregnancy, birth, and your baby comes from who you are, where you've been, and what you believe in. So, while getting advice from friends, family, and other experts can help you along the way, keep in mind that what worked for your sister, your mother, or your best friend will not necessarily work for you . . . and vice versa. Experts—be they professionals or strangers—have ideas, but they may also have agendas. Take the advice that makes sense to you and take the rest with a grain of salt. The important thing is to be able to filter what you hear through an understanding of what matters to you and your family.

2. confidence is more important than instinct.

People often tell parents to "trust their instincts." Go with your gut and you'll be confident about your choices. But it takes confidence to trust your instincts in a world of conflicting advice! Nothing builds confidence like hard-earned experience, but in the meantime, you can help build yours by seeking supportive environments. Know yourself and what makes you feel safe and secure in who you are. Stay away from people who make you feel bad about yourself, and look for situations that make you feel stronger as a parent. Instincts are an indispensable tool, but they're worthless without the confidence it takes to put them to use.

3. strive for imperfection.

When we're pregnant, we are warned to hone our diet for ideal fetal development. We must advocate for the optimum birth and bonding experience—often fighting against the tide of hospital policy. Later, we learn tips to help our babies reach their milestones on time, or better still, early! The desire for children to succeed is as old as mothers. What's new is the mile-long list of do's and don'ts, and the mounting pressure on moms to make it all happen. An alarming number of studies focus on maternal responsibility. But no amount of fish oil, flash cards, and quality time can guarantee an A+ in motherhood. And the quest for perfection sucks parents' energy and enjoyment, leaving resentment in its wake. You may think your child will feel only the benefit of your attention, but the pressure seeps through, too. If you're trying to be a perfect parent, your child may think the same perfection is expected of him. Kids need permission to be themselves, not performers. Parents need to cut themselves some slack, maintain a sense of self, and be as wary of overparenting as they are of underparenting. We think "good enough" parenting is not just good enough, it's better.

4. parenting is out of control.

Becoming a parent inevitably means giving up some level of control. When you're pregnant, you can't control how your body responds—whether or not you feel sick, for example, or get stretch marks. And though you may be able to curtail some weight gain, we never met a pregnant woman who didn't feel "too big" by delivery time. Birth itself is the ultimate exercise in letting go. Afterward, many people are desperate to keep the baby from disturbing the peace of their lives. They worry that they'll be "chained to the couch" or "lose themselves," or become "boring parents." Having a baby will change your life whether you fight it or not. It's not that resistance is futile—it can actually be healthy. But the happiest parents we know are the ones who learn to surf the waves rather than try to conquer them.

5. there's **no such thing** as a "natural" mother.

People talk about "natural" mothering. *Natural mothers breastfeed. It's not natural to breastfeed your child beyond six months. It's natural for babies to cry. Babies only cry when we resist our natural impulse to comfort them.* For some women, it is natural to trust a doctor when it comes to their body and baby. For others, the natural way to give birth is at home with midwives and family. But one person's natural is another one's weird, or worse. We live in a culture with complex—and sometimes contradictory—rules, expectations, and ideals, and what feels natural to you depends on your point of view.

6. **shift** happens.

Babies grow, and growth means change. Sometimes this is a relief; you go to bed at the end of your rope and wake up to find that the problem has passed. Sometimes it's frustrating; just when you think you've got the hang of things, the landscape shifts and your baby enters a whole new weird/wonderful phase. Either way, it means that whatever is going on, it probably won't last forever, for better or for worse. Try not to despair when things are miserable, or get smug when things are going smoothly. Both babies and the world around them are in constant flux. If what you're doing isn't working anymore, do something else. Try not to get too attached to any one way. Keep your eyes and your mind open, and be ready to adjust your strategies accordingly. It'll help you enjoy the ride.

7. babies are **people,** not problems.

Pregnancy, birth, and, to some extent, babies, are all too often seen as problems waiting to happen. Parents can be so anxious about what to expect and what's "normal" that every hiccup becomes a potential crisis. Often, the real problem is unrealistic expectations. People expect their pregnancies and babies to develop in a certain way, and when they don't, it can be hard not to panic and try to fix what may not be broken. It's tempting to think that there is a simple, almost mathematical solution to whatever you may be facing with your baby, but raising a child is not a science. Babies are people. You can't input the same data into every one and expect the same result. Techniques may work for you as promised, or they may not. Individual people have individual needs, in infancy as well as adulthood. We don't believe in one-size-fits-all formulas for any other human relationship, so why would we expect one to work with babies?

8. frustration, resentment, anger, exhaustion, exasperation, aggravation, jealousy, nostalgia, regret, etc., don't make you a **bad** parent.

Every parent (well, almost every one) has bad feelings at one time or another. Sometimes it starts in pregnancy, when you're too big and tired to climb the stairs to your bedroom. Sometimes it starts in labor when you feel like the baby is ripping you apart. And sometimes it doesn't hit you until the baby's screaming through the fourteenth night in a row and you really, really wish you could just go out for a margarita, or read a book, or take a bath, or take a nap. Or even just sit down for five seconds without a baby in your arms or screaming in your ear. Whatever the trigger, we all have our bad days when we wish for a fleeting moment (or more) that things were a bit more like they used to be. How could we not, considering the havoc a baby wreaks on our lives? But then we look at the adorable little thing and are overcome with joy . . . rapidly followed by guilt. Well, we're here to tell you that you can love your baby and hate how your life has changed at the same time. Pretty much everyone feels this way sometimes, even if they won't admit it. Feeling mad or sad about what you're going through doesn't make you love your baby any less, and it definitely doesn't make you a bad mother or father.

9. look **forward**, not backward.

"Life as you know it is over." From the minute you're visibly pregnant, strangers on the street will stop to remind you of the radical, life-altering reality of having a baby. Certainly some aspects of your life will return to a semblance of "normal," but it's true that your old life isn't coming back. Of course, you'll miss it sometimes, but the important thing is to mourn the losses and move on to the gains. Challenge the old, depressing, and oft-repeated notion that your life "is over" by thinking toward the future. Your life isn't over, your old life as a nonparent is over—and your new life has only just begun.

10. there is **no right way.**

Remember, no matter what anyone else says, there is no across-the-board evidence that any one way of parenting is better than any other way. The best way is whatever works for you.

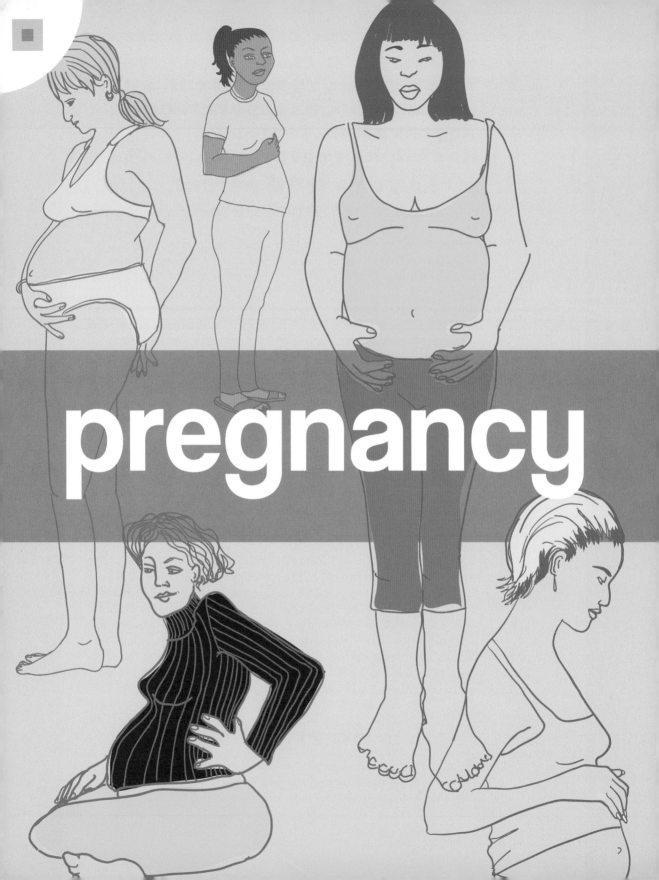

pregnancy

pregnancy, for us, was quite a trip. Our minds were opened to a whole new world of bodily functions (and dysfunctions). The monthly to weekly examinations, the parade of minor and major discomforts, the talk of germs and genes made us realize how very human, or even animal, we really are. As our bodies chugged along, our brains were busy playing catch-up, trying to absorb all that was coming in just a few short (endless) months. What would our births be like? What would our babies be like? What would our lives be like? Pregnancy gives parents plenty to worry about, if they're so inclined. New studies come out constantly, reiterating and revising the mammoth list of warnings for expectant parents to heed in the interest of optimizing their unborn children. Some take it all to heart, considering the restrictions a small price to pay for a little more confidence. Some take a more moderate approach in the interest of balance (or sanity). The two of us had very different ways of handling this anxiety. One lived pretty much by the book, the other was a little looser. Here, we'll try to accommodate both impulses: the desire for maximum information, and the freedom to make your own choices.

Pregnancy is not like a head cold that gives everyone who catches it the same basic symptoms. Different babies, different bodies, and different lives mean that pregnancy experiences are all over the map. This section will talk you through some of the changes, emotions, and options you might encounter on your way.

THE 40-WEEK CALENDAR OF PREGNANCY

Because it is not always possible to know the date of conception, pregnancies are dated from the first day of your last menstrual period (LMP). Using this calendar, pregnancy usually lasts about 40 weeks—including the 2 weeks or so before you even conceived.

FIRST TRIMESTER (WEEKS 1–13)

MOM

SOME EARLY PREGNANCY SYMPTOMS
→ See Bodily Byproducts of Pregnancy, page 45, for more on all of these.

- Missed period
- Nausea and/or vomiting
- Feeling PMSy
- Super sense of smell
- Sore boobs
- Tingly boobs
- Bigger boobs
- Fatigue
- Dizziness
- The need to pee a lot
- Heartburn
- Constipation, a lot of gas
- Skin changes
- Cravings and aversions

→ See Eating While Pregnant, page 52.

TESTS YOU MAY BE OFFERED
→ See Prenatal Screening and Testing, page 31.

- Initial prenatal blood work (first visit with your provider, or shortly thereafter), including blood type, antibody screen, hepatitis B surface antigen, STDs, cystic fibrosis screening
- Pap smear
- Urine culture
- Genetic testing, if appropriate
- Ultrasound (may happen at any point or at each visit)
- First-trimester screening: blood screening and nuchal translucency ultrasound (10–13 weeks, varies)
- CVS test (10–12 weeks, varies)

MONTH 1 0
Your baby is about the size of a grain of arborio rice (about ¼ inch long).

BABY

- Last menstrual period (LMP): 40-week pregnancy calendar begins.
- Day 1 of gestation: Sperm meets egg (conception).
- 6–12 days after conception: Fertilized egg implants in the uterus.
- Weeks 5–10: Period of greatest risk of birth defects → See Timing and Risk, page 63.
- Weeks 5–7: Heartbeat can usually be detected on ultrasound monitor.

"The 4½ week old embryo resembles a prehistoric animal more than anything else."
— Lennart Nilsson, *A Child Is Born*

SOME THINGS THAT MAY BE GOING THROUGH YOUR HEAD

→ See The Pregnant Brain, page 79, for more.

- Isolation, especially if you're not telling → See Talking About It, page 24.
- Fear of miscarriage
- Worry about what you're getting yourself into
- Worry about how your relationships might be affected
- Wonder how you'll get through 9 months of feeling like this (you probably won't have to)
- Excitement
- Ambivalence, second thoughts, anxiety . . . and guilt about not feeling just plain happy
- Disbelief, doubt that it's real

- You might look exactly the same to the outside world, or your bigger boobs and/or thicker middle might have people asking you if you're pregnant almost instantly.
- Your first visit with a healthcare provider will probably take place when you're between 5 and 10 weeks pregnant. → See Choosing a Healthcare Provider, page 27.

MONTH 2
Your baby is about the size of a fava bean (I inch long and less than ⅓ ounce).

MONTH 3
Your baby is about the size of a small deer mouse (2½ to 3 inches long and I ounce).

- Week 8: Webbed fingers and toes develop, the placenta forms and begins to function during month 2.
- Week IO: Embryo becomes fetus (all organs are developed).
- Until II–I4 weeks: Embryo/fetus has tail.

→ See The Beginning, page 24.
→ See Decisions, Decisions, page 27.
→ See The Endless No, page 62.

SECOND TRIMESTER (WEEKS 14–27)

MOM

SOME MIDPREGNANCY SYMPTOMS

→ See Bodily Byproducts of Pregnancy, page 45, for more on all of these.

- Increased energy
- Diminished nausea, vomiting
- Increased libido (for some)
- Shortness of breath
- Slowed digestion
- Heartburn
- Continued breast changes
- Abdomen achiness from stretching ligaments
- Increased vaginal discharge
- Dizziness
- Bleeding gums
- Faster pulse

TESTS YOU MAY BE OFFERED

→ See Prenatal Screening and Testing, page 31.

- Alpha-fetoprotein test (AFP) for neural tube defects if nuchal translucency was done in first trimester (15–20 weeks) or triple screen/quad screen if nuchal translucency was not done
- Amniocentesis (15-plus weeks)
- Ultrasound (at any point or at every visit)
- Targeted ultrasound/anatomy scan (18–22 weeks)
- Glucose screen for gestational diabetes (24–28 weeks)

WEEK 14 15 16 17 18 19 20

MONTH 4
Your baby is about the size of a ham-and-cheese croissant (6 to 7 inches long and 4 to 5 ounces).

BABY

- 14–17 weeks: External genitalia can be seen on ultrasound.
- 18–22 weeks: Movements become more coordinated and deliberate (although the baby has been moving reflexively since about 10 weeks).
- Sensory apparatus develops.

SOME THINGS THAT MAY BE GOING THROUGH YOUR HEAD

→ See The Pregnant Brain, page 79, for more.

- Am I still pregnant? (after you stop feeling sick but before you start feeling movement)
- More excitement about the pregnancy now that you're showing
- Irritation due to other people's advice now that you're showing
- Worry about prenatal testing
- Worry about all the other important decisions you'll have to make → See Decisions, Decisions, page 27.
- Relief if you don't feel sick anymore

- The miscarriage rate is much lower from now on.
- Your pregnancy will likely become visible to the outside world at some point during this trimester.
- The placenta takes over hormone production during weeks 14–17.
- Fetal movements can usually be felt somewhere around 20 weeks.
- Depending on availability in your area, you may need to start thinking now about any support people you would like to have around during or after your birth. → See The Birth Support Team, page 156, and Postpartum Support, page 168.

21 22 23 24 25 26 27

MONTH 5
Your baby is about the size of a bottle of shampoo (10 inches long and ½ to 1 pound).

MONTH 6
Your baby is about the size of a lobster (12 inches long and 1½ to 2 pounds).

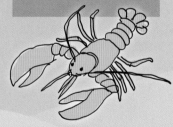

- Fetus is covered with fur called lanugo and slimy white stuff called vernix to protect the skin and aid in warmth.
- Babies born at 24 weeks have a 50 percent chance of survival.
- A 27-week-old fetus can respond to touch and light.

THIRD TRIMESTER (WEEKS 28–40)

MOM

SOME SYMPTOMS OF LATE PREGNANCY

→ See Bodily Byproducts of Pregnancy, page 45, for more on all of these.

- Back pain
- Pelvic achiness
- Insomnia
- Rib pain
- More vaginal discharge
- Digestive issues
- Sciatica
- Swollen ankles and feet
- Varicose veins
- Restless legs
- Itchy abdomen
- Belly button pops out
- More frequent peeing, leaking urine
- Braxton Hicks contractions (see page 51)
- Colostrum from the nipples (a premilk substance, see page 282)
- More fatigue
- Appetite changes

TESTS YOU MAY BE OFFERED

→ See Prenatal Screening and Testing, page 31.

- Glucose screen if you didn't get it at the end of the second trimester
- Group B strep test at 35–37 weeks
- Non-stress test to check fetal heart rate and response

SOME THINGS THAT MAY BE GOING THROUGH YOUR HEAD

→ See The Pregnant Brain, page 79.
→ See Expectations, Fantasies, and Fears, page 141.

- Ready for it to be over . . . impatient or excited
- Not ready for it to be over . . . anxious about birth and/or baby
- Feeling clumsy and unable to get around

WEEK 28 29 30 31 32 33

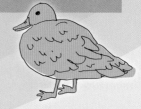

MONTH 8
Your baby is about the size of a small duck (18 to 19 inches long and 4 to 5 pounds).

MONTH 7
Your baby is about the size of a ferret (15 to 16 inches long and 2½ to 3 pounds).

34 35 36 37 38 39 40

MONTH 9
Your baby is about the size of a svelte cat (19 to 21 inches long and 6 to 9 pounds).

- Visits with your healthcare provider usually increase during the final month(s) of pregnancy.
- This is usually the time to start thinking about birth prep and/or childbirth classes.
- The average gestation in the United States is 39 weeks (figuring in scheduled C-sections and inductions).
- Only 5 percent of women give birth on their due dates.
- Babies may be born as far as 2 weeks past due date.

nesting

As the due date approaches, some women (and some men, too) feel a sudden compulsion to sort out drawers, organize closets, shop, and clean everything in sight. Though usually defined in relation to domestic chores, "nesting" may include financial or logistical planning in the home or at work. You may never feel the urge and wonder why any woman in the final throes of pregnancy would want to clean house. Some prefer to orchestrate the cleaning actions of others from a comfortable perch on the couch.

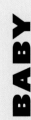

BABY

- Weight gain is a big deal this trimester (½ pound a week is the usual amount).
- Weeks 30–32: Lanugo starts to disappear.
- Growing baby has less space in the uterus, so movements are more restricted.
- Weeks 33–36: Most babies are in head-down position.

the beginning

> The Books told us to expect six months after abjuring The Pill before anything would happen—it happened the first try. So I felt "happy" and "woken up five months early."
> —anonydaddy

the test

If you are reading this, there's a good chance that you or someone you love has recently taken a pregnancy test and gotten a positive result. What goes through your head when you find out you're pregnant? Quite possibly a much wider range of emotions than you expect. Even when the news is exactly what you wanted, your response can still be surprising. Tears, shock, fear, euphoric laughter, and borderline panic attacks are all (totally normal) possibilities. For some, the plus sign or double pink line represents a definitive moment where life changes; for others it's more like a blurry beginning to a long, unpredictable transformation. → See Emotional Landscape of Pregnancy, page 79.

> I knew from the second I took a pregnancy test my life was to change completely. Although it's what I wanted, once I knew I had it, I completely freaked out.
> —anonymom

talking about it

... with partners

Your partner, if you've got one, may be hovering over the stick with you. Otherwise, you get to break the news. And there is absolutely no right or wrong way to do it. Pick up the phone, fire off a text message, stagger into the next room and scream. It's hard to predict how your feelings will mingle on this topic, or whether either of you will be able to find the right words to describe those feelings.

Both partners may feel like they should be in celebration mode, but along with the happiness, or instead of it, one or both of you may fear for your independence or feel afraid you won't be able to rise to the occasion of parenthood. Whatever the status of your relationship before, you've just taken a pretty big turn. Sharing a child represents a whole new kind of connection. It can feel both inspiring and threatening to the relationship you know and love.

can i trust the test?

By the first day of a missed period, home pregnancy tests are about 90 percent accurate. A week later they're 97 to 99 percent accurate. False positives are extremely rare. False negatives are a lot more common: You can take a pregnancy test before your period's even due, but there may not be enough of the pregnancy hormone human chorionic gonadotropin (hCG) in your urine for the test to pick it up that soon. The reason many tests suggest using first-morning urine is that hCG levels tend to be highest just after waking.

> I didn't tell my husband till around the tenth week. I had a miscarriage in the past and it just devastated him.
> —anonymom

> Part of me felt delighted to be so deeply included in the primary activity of my species. Other parts of me were extremely frightened.
> —anonydaddy

When I went to the doctor and the pregnancy was confirmed, I called my husband and he was excited. We were both really excited. Then the next day we were terrified, sitting on the couch like people in a short story—you just don't want to be those people. They don't know what to do. It was like we were on a first date. We didn't know how to talk to each other. It was totally awkward and then we were like, "Well, it's a big change," and saying stupid things like that and I am pretty sure I burst into tears.

—Ceridwen

I was away when I found out (after taking half a dozen pregnancy tests in a hotel bathroom). I immediately called my husband to tell him . . . but then my ride showed up and I was late, so I had to hang up the phone! It wasn't very romantic, to say the least, but there was no way I could have waited. I was going to be away for a whole week! Later that day I got a book about pregnancy that warned, "Be sure to tell your partner in person!" Great. Pregnant ten minutes and already I've done something wrong!

—Rebecca

I felt upset when people said, "Oh honey, you shouldn't talk about it." It made me feel like I should be ashamed if my baby didn't make it, rather than just plain devastated. And it also made me think too much about the baby not making it! Which was not a good thing since I was feeling terrible.

—anonymom

I decided to tell everyone early on—I figured if miscarriage is so common, women should be able to talk about it freely (and not have to suffer in silence).

—anonymom

. . . to everyone else

The question of who, when, and how to tell (or how to avoid telling) occupies a lot of space in the minds of newly pregnant women. It's partly superstition: counting your chickens before they're hatched. And it's partly practical: There's a high risk of miscarriage early in pregnancy, so some parents keep the news to themselves until they feel more confident.

Keeping it secret can be kind of nice, or really hard. You may be too excited to keep a lid on it. The changes of pregnancy might start to put a strain on relationships and demand explanation. (*Why are you so distant? Why didn't you come to my all-night dance party? What's with the sick-days!?*) Not telling can seal you into a kind of bubble. Feeling crummy (common in the early weeks) is isolating in itself. If you don't tell anyone about what you're going through, you can't get any support (or sympathy).

So who should you tell? If you think you would tell someone about a loss, you may want to tell them about your pregnancy so you can have their support throughout. If the idea of telling seems like it will bring you more stress than support, you can consider anonymous outlets: Some women bury themselves in books or TV shows about pregnancy. Online communities can serve the same purpose and provide a place to be (secretly) open about your pregnancy.

➜ See Breaking the News, page 96.
➜ See Emotional Landscape of Pregnancy, page 79.

things to **think** about now

- Prenatal vitamins, especially folic acid (see page 53)
- Prenatal care options (see pages 27–30)
- Dangerous foods, drugs, and behaviors in pregnancy (see The Endless No, page 62)

Right when I found
out, I took a walk . . . wanted
some time to enjoy the news
all to myself.
—anonymom

I would tell
people that I knew I
would never see again, it
was random but I guess I
just wanted to tell some
people.
—anonymom

I had gone to the
bookstore that day to try to buy a
book but I was too nervous to commit
to buying anything even though I
had two tests and a doctor's note
saying "It's definitely happening."
I felt like I had to tiptoe into the
pregnancy section of the bookstore:
It was like being a teenager sneaking
*Everything You Ever Wanted to Know
About Sex but Were Afraid to Ask* off
the shelf and reading it in the closet.
—anonymom

I didn't want to
tell my mom that I was
pregnant until I got back
the results of my amnio. . . . My
husband and I knew we would
terminate if there was a major
problem. So I didn't want to have
my mom knowing about this all
because of her religious beliefs
and personal experience. I knew
it would be hard enough to
deal with my own reaction
and emotions.
—anonymom

I enjoy my
beer and I guess not
ordering one when I
went out with friends was
as good as flashing neon
signs. I've always been a bit of
a humbug when it comes to
"the joys of parenthood," so
maybe people enjoyed seeing
me change my mind,
although they didn't rub
it in my face.
—anonymom

I have been getting
advice, which is one of the
reasons that we have only told
people who are close to us. I don't
want to hear everyone's advice on the
best blankets, cribs, towels, etc. I don't
want to hear about everyone's pregnancy
horror stories or how lucky I have it
not being sick; I just want to enjoy
how this is happening to me.
—anonymom

I don't think there's
anything wrong with lying.
The people who haven't lied at my
workplace when put on the spot have
given it away by trying to change the
subject, squirming, or ignoring the question
altogether. If anyone starts asking me before
I'm ready to tell, I plan to act offended—
"What, are you saying I'm getting fat?" That
should shut them up and embarrass them,
which, frankly, they deserve. Then
later, when I let the cat out of the
bag, I'll apologize.
—anonymom

It was
stressful for
me to go public. . . . I
was very uncertain what
it all meant and it was hard to
know how to present myself to people—
it felt dishonest to be excited and
happy when I had so many other
conflicted feelings.
—anonymom

decisions, decisions

Expectant parents can barely make it back from the first pregnancy checkup and crack a bottle of sparkling cider before the big questions start rolling in hard and fast: Will you get an amnio? What will you do with the results? Are you going to find out the sex? Will you circumcise? Go natural? Get an epidural? Return to work? Have you thought of a name?! Though these questions are often pitched as choices, some parents feel they have less say in the matter than they would like: Circumcision is expected in some cultures, the mother's income is necessary for many families, testing is widely recommended for women over age thirty-five. Plus the gravity of some of the choices can be pretty disarming: These may be the first decisions you've ever made on behalf of another person. Will this name be cause for mockery? Will the circumcision (or lack thereof) set him apart from his friends? Though the first taste of parental responsibility can feel daunting, making these decisions can also be an opportunity to discover what your "family values" might look like. You may well get input from others (in print and in conversation). But your own priorities should ideally drive your choices as much as possible; this will be *your* baby, after all!

choosing a healthcare provider

Aside from birth, pregnancy usually involves more than a dozen appointments, lots of questions, and possibly some intimate and emotional issues, so you want to find a care provider you feel comfortable with. Your doctor or midwife should make you feel confident as well as looked after; he or she also needs to be respectful of whatever ideas you have about birth. Though many first-time mothers already have an ob-gyn or family doctor, pregnancy brings up new concerns. There may have been little reason to really evaluate your physician over the course of perfunctory Pap smears or flu shots. You can always make the first appointment with a current doctor, then do some homework and thinking and switch to another doctor or midwife early on in the pregnancy if necessary. However, since providers do not always accept patients later in pregnancy, a selection is usually best made early on.

obstetrician/gynecologists

In the United States, ob-gyns are the most common healthcare providers for pregnancy and birth. They are often a part of a group practice and may work in a clinic or a hospital. An ob-gyn can care for you in pregnancy, deliver the baby, and also perform medical procedures including a C-section.

family physicians

Family physicians care for your whole family and are usually a part of a group practice. They may already know your medical history and/or can continue as the family doctor well beyond the birth. This integrated doctor-patient relationship has nice flow through various stages of life. However, family doctors don't always deliver babies or may not have delivered as many as an OB or midwife.

finding a physician

- Get a personal recommendation from someone who has given birth to a baby with the doctor.
- Consult your insurance company: A list of covered physicians in your area is often available online.
- Consult the American Medical Association (ama-assn.org) or the American College of Obstetricians and Gynecologists (acog.org).
- The Society for Maternal-Fetal Medicine (smfm.org) provides listings of specialists.
- Check consumer review websites (but realize that reviews may not be reliable).

midwives

A certified nurse-midwife is a medically trained professional who can oversee prenatal and postpartum care as well as the birth. Studies have shown that in healthy, low-risk deliveries, women are as likely to have excellent outcomes under the care of certified nurse-midwives as with doctors. They are also less likely to have gone through any interventions, such as monitoring, epidural, induction, episiotomies, and C-sections (see page 131 for more info). Midwives tend to spend more time with a laboring woman than a doctor and may also spend more time at each appointment, though this varies. Many midwives are associated with an ob-gyn in case medical intervention is necessary. Sometimes they are a part of a team of obstetric care providers. If you have any outstanding medical conditions that may affect pregnancy, she will refer you to an obstetrician or a specialist. She can also refer you to someone for prenatal testing or genetic counseling. Medicaid and most insurance plans cover certified nurse-midwife services.

There are a few classifications of midwives: The majority of midwives who deliver babies in the United States are the aforementioned certified nurse-midwives (registered nurses with training in obstetrics and gynecology). Certified midwives, who are not nurses but have been trained as midwives, are becoming more common. In some states, certified midwives and nurse-midwives are trained in the same programs. There are also direct-entry midwives, who are certified in some states, and lay midwives, who are not certified and only do home births. Local laws vary; check to see what your state requires.

finding a midwife

- Get a personal recommendation from someone who has given birth to a baby with the midwife.
- Consult progressive birth centers or birth education centers (some places have bulletin boards or online resources for local midwife practices).
- American College of Nurse-Midwives (midwife.org) offers listings of certified nurse-midwives by area.
- Go through the hospital or birth center you'd like to use. See the American Association of Birth Centers (birthcenters.org).
- The Midwives Alliance of North America website, mana.org, lists certified professional midwives (direct-entry midwives).

making the choice: things to think about

Some people are able to choose a provider without getting a lot of information up front. Chemistry and vibe might be enough for you to know who you feel comfortable working with. Many of the following issues relate to birth, which may be hard to focus on so early in pregnancy. If you want to read up on birth procedures and options to help inform your choice, check out "Birth Basics," beginning on page 120.

INSURANCE: Does the healthcare provider accept your insurance plan? Will your insurance plan cover the hospital or birth center where you plan to give birth (or the backup hospital if you plan on a home birth)? You will most likely need to talk to your healthcare provider as well as your insurance company about the specifics.

THE TEAM: Many doctors and midwives work with a team or have a backup person. Ask about other partners and meet them—ideally you'll feel okay about the whole team, any of whom may be delivering your baby. (Most people have a favorite.) Ask how the schedule works for births. If you are working with a midwife, ask about the doctors or specialists she works with in case of an emergency.

PROXIMITY: Since checkups are frequent, having someone you can get to easily will be convenient. Proximity to the hospital or birth center is also something to think about.

MEDICAL CONCERNS: If you have any outstanding or preexisting health concerns, will this person be able to give you the specific kind of care you need? In some situations a specialist will work in conjunction with a primary healthcare provider.

schools of thought

Doctors and midwives represent the two main schools of thought on pregnancy and birth practices. Doctors are associated with what is sometimes called a "techno-medical" model of care. A provider who follows this model generally considers advances in technology and medicine (such as routine ultrasounds, epidurals, and surgical interventions) as helpful to the process of pregnancy and labor. Providers who follow the midwifery model of care are more likely to see a pregnant and laboring woman not as a patient in need of medical care, but as a woman going through a normal and "natural" process. They may also see the emotional and physical aspects of labor as deeply connected. In practice, the two models often overlap. A birth with a midwife may involve medical procedures. Many doctors are great supporters of "natural" childbirth. Healthcare providers are individuals and fall at lots of different places on the spectrum.

➔ See Natural vs. Medical Childbirth: Either/Or?, page 141.

WHERE TO GIVE BIRTH: Both doctors and certified nurse-midwives deliver in hospitals (where 99 percent of births occur), but for the most part, only midwives assist labor in nonhospital settings, such as a birth center or home. (Birth centers are independent birthing facilities that may be associated with or be a part of a hospital.) If you are hoping for a home birth, you will still need to consider a backup plan (with doctor and hospital) in case of complications. Some people choose a caregiver specifically based on the quality of the hospital or birth center where they deliver. → See The Setting, page 153.

AVAILABILITY: You want someone who can answer your calls at times outside a scheduled appointment. How does the office handle questions? Is there someone else you can talk to if your doctor or midwife is not on call?

GENERAL APPROACH: What kind of information exchange feels right to you? Do you want to know every single possible outcome? Or would you prefer only the basics? Ask about the doctor's or midwife's approach to childbirth. What is his or her attitude about episiotomies (see page 130) and C-sections? Also bring up *your* ideas about pregnancy and birth, if you know what they are. How does the provider react? The caregiver should be sensitive to how you like to receive and process information, as well as your hopes and fears about pregnancy and birth.

I am thirty-eight years old and chose a midwife for several reasons—primarily because of my age and history (two early miscarriages), I felt labeled as high-risk. I appreciated the opportunity to participate more fully in my care as an informed participant, rather than a passive patient. I felt like my midwife didn't pathologize me as my former ob/gyn had. I had our daughter nine years ago with a family practitioner; she was wonderful, but this time I wanted to try something different.
—anonymom

I felt a lot of uncertainty about who we were going to work with, i.e., an OB or midwife, and ended up switching three times before finding the right fit.... Don't be afraid to dump a practitioner if it's not a comfortable fit, even though you may feel pressure from them and insurance companies not to do so. In the end you have to feel really aligned with the person/people you will be working with.
—anonymom

An obvious side of me is very comforted by the medical apparatus and the docs with their years of med school and fancy degrees, I must admit. But then again, I didn't exactly bond with my OB. Unlike with other medical things, where I go for the expertise over the bedside manner, I think I really *need* bedside manner with this stuff.
—anonymom

prenatal screening and testing

Prenatal testing is used to determine gestational age, sex, and other basic information as well as to assess potential genetic, chromosomal, and other problems. Screening tests, which include blood tests and ultrasounds, carry no risk to the fetus but provide less definitive results. Diagnostic tests, such as amniocentesis and chorionic villus sampling (CVS), are almost 100 percent accurate but carry a slight risk of miscarriage. The results of prenatal screening can be used to help expectant parents make a decision about whether to pursue diagnostic tests. Women who will be over thirty-five at the time of delivery are usually given the option of diagnostic testing. For women thirty-four or younger, amniocentesis and CVS are usually recommended only if screening or other factors indicate a higher risk. They will probably not be offered by default. If diagnostic tests are not specifically recommended, they may not be covered by insurance.

Whether the decision to undergo prenatal testing is relatively easy or gut wrenching, remember that prenatal testing is much more likely to rule out any problems than to diagnose them. Ninety-five percent of diagnostic tests come back fine.

genetic counseling

Genetic counselors are specially trained professionals with expertise in human development and genetics. They work with prenatal patients to identify their potential risks for birth defects and any chromosomal or genetic abnormalities. They can interpret sometimes complex variables (family history, genetic background, maternal age, any screening results) for parents so they can make educated decisions about prenatal testing.

resources
National Society of Genetic Counselors: nsgc.org

some factors to consider

- **What are the risks of a birth defect or serious abnormality?**
- **What are the risks of the test?**
- **Who performs the test and what is their expertise?**
- **What will you do with the information?**
- **How will the timing of the test affect your decisions?**

I had no idea making a decision about prenatal testing would be so hard. Though we really tried to "accentuate the positive," there seemed to be no getting around the fact that in order to make the decision, we would just have to sit there and weigh all these really negative outcomes against each other. Even when we found the best idea for us, it was still the best choice based on the least devastating of the potentially devastating scenarios. The negativity of that whole process was overwhelming.

—anonymom

Making decisions about prenatal testing can sometimes be stressful. There can be an alarming amount of information to process—we felt like we were back in biology class, scribbling down information about carrier genes, chromosome pairing, and cell cultures. It can be a little weird to see yourself and your partner reduced to genetic categories and statistics.

—anonymom

RELATIONSHIP OF DOWN SYNDROME INCIDENCE TO MOTHER'S AGE

This data is based on live births and does not include miscarriages, stillbirths, or terminations of Down syndrome pregnancies.

MOTHER'S AGE	INCIDENCE OF DOWN SYNDROME
Under 30	Less than 1 in 1,000
30	1 in 900
35	1 in 400
36	1 in 300
37	1 in 230
38	1 in 180
39	1 in 135
40	1 in 105
42	1 in 60
44	1 in 35
46	1 in 20
48	1 in 16
49	1 in 12

Source: Hook, E. G., and A. Lindsjo, *Down Syndrome in Live Births by Single Year Maternal Age.*

what tests can tell you (and what they can't)

About 3 percent of all babies are born with a birth defect. Many are minor; some are more serious. Birth defects that come from an abnormal number of chromosomes can be identified through diagnostic tests. The normal arrangement of chromosomes is twenty-three pairs of two (one of each chromosome from each parent). When there is a third chromosome, it's called a trisomy. Down syndrome (Trisomy 21) is the most common trisomy; 1 in 1,000 babies is born with Down syndrome. Affected children have altered facial features, mental retardation, heart defects, and other health issues. Much less common and more serious (fatal) are Trisomy 13 and Trisomy 18. The risk of most trisomies increases with age.

Other abnormalities that can be detected include:

- **Neural tube defects such as spina bifida (which can lead to various levels of paralysis) and anencephaly (a fatal condition affecting the brain and skull)**
- **Some genetic disorders, such as cystic fibrosis, Tay-Sachs, and sickle-cell disease**
- **Some types of dwarfism, hemophilia, and Fragile X (hereditary mental retardation)**

Family history can help identify risk for conditions like sickle cell anemia and cystic fibrosis. Ethnicity also plays a role: Ashkenazi Jews are screened for different disorders than people of African or Mediterranean descent, for example.

Many problems cannot be detected with prenatal testing. Though tests improve all the time, we probably won't see this changing radically in our reproductive years. What we are able to know now is light-years ahead of what our parents knew about us before we were born; and we can expect that our kids' generation will have access to even more information.

why test?

Information about fetal abnormalities can be used in a number of ways. If there is a serious or life-threatening problem for mother and/or baby, doctors can advise parents on their options, including monitoring the pregnancy more closely, preparing for a complicated birth, or terminating the pregnancy. Parents can also use the time to prepare for a baby with special needs.

risk assessment

Is 1 in 200 rare? What about 1 in 4,200? One in a million? Risk is entirely subjective. What seems very unlikely to one person can seem common to another. Partly this relates to the way a statistic is expressed: A 1-in-200 risk can sound more serious than a less-than-one-half-percent risk. A 99.5 percent chance of a good outcome sounds even better. Interpreting risk also has a lot to do with what's at stake. If there's a 1-in-200 chance of stubbing your toe when you get up from your desk, you'll probably take your chances and get up. If there's a 1-in-200 chance that getting up will give you a heart attack, you might be more likely to stay put. Assessing risk in pregnancy can be confusing. Women are told to avoid eating pâté and soft cheeses though the predicted risk of listeriosis from those foods is around 1 in 5,000,000 servings. If we are playing those kinds of odds, at what point do we accept the risk of a fetal abnormality?

Doctors usually offer diagnostic testing when the risk of a serious abnormality approaches the risks associated with the test. For a thirty-five-year-old woman, for example, there is a 1-in-400 chance a baby has Down syndrome, which is close to the risk of miscarriage from the amniocentesis or CVS test that could detect it. In all of these scenarios, it's important to remember that there really is no correct way to interpret statistics. Once emotional, logistical, philosophical factors mingle with the numbers on the page . . . a whole new set of meanings emerges.

screening tests

Screening tests are a routine aspect of prenatal care for women of all ages. Some parents may prefer to not receive any information about their babies before birth and may decline some or all prenatal screening. Though screening has gotten much more accurate, for definitive results, a diagnostic test must be performed.

ULTRASOUND: An ultrasound uses sound waves to form a picture of the developing fetus. It is often used in the first trimester to:

- **Locate the pregnancy (make sure it's in the uterus)**
- **Establish a due date**
- **Check the baby's heartbeat (this can usually be seen at about 6 weeks)**
- **Check the number of babies**
- **Check the ovaries and uterus**

Some doctors use ultrasound routinely throughout the pregnancy to make sure fetal growth is on target. Late in pregnancy these measurements may be used to make decisions about the birth. If the baby is measuring very large, an earlier birth via C-section or induction may be suggested, for example, though predictions of baby weight are not always accurate. Ultrasounds can be really fun for expectant parents, giving them a glimpse of the fetus in action. There are keepsake ultrasound businesses popping up in malls across the country, but nonmedical use of ultrasounds is controversial.

Targeted ultrasound exams during the second trimester—between 18 and 22 weeks—can reveal more information about the sex of the baby, the growth rate, the general anatomy, and possible birth defects. A targeted ultrasound (also known as an anatomy scan) can pretty accurately (95—98 percent with an experienced technician) detect or rule out serious neural tube defects. This second-trimester ultrasound may identify anatomic features more frequently seen in certain genetic conditions or chromosomal abnormalities. Known as "soft signs," these include things like bright spots in the fetal heart (known as echogenic foci), small fluid-filled cysts in the fetal brain (called choroid plexus cysts), and a single umbilical artery instead of two. Individually they are almost completely insignificant, but when several such features are noted, some physicians feel the odds are increased that the baby might have Down syndrome or another chromosomal abnormality, and offer more definitive testing through amniocentesis. Most women with these ultrasound soft signs have completely normal babies.

NUCHAL TRANSLUCENCY SCREENING: This test is also called NT ultrasound.

Screens for:	Down syndrome and other common chromosomal abnormalities (like Trisomy 18 and Turner syndrome). Recent data suggests that abnormal nuchal translucency may be a predictor of serious heart defects as well.
When:	10–13 weeks (actual windows may be narrower; check locally).
Accuracy:	About 80 percent for Down syndrome cases. When combined with blood test results, that number goes up to almost 90 percent ➜ See Combined Screening, below.
Risk:	None.
Method:	Ultrasound is used to measure the clear space on the back of the fetal neck, the "nuchal translucency." The higher that measurement, the greater the chance for Down syndrome or other serious abnormalities. Maternal age is factored in to results. Women who have a large nuchal translucency measurement should also be offered the option of a fetal echocardiogram to check the developing heart at around 18–22 weeks.

COMBINED SCREENING: This test includes a first-trimester maternal blood screening plus NT ultrasound.

Screens for:	Down syndrome, Trisomy 18, Trisomy 13
When:	10–13 weeks
Accuracy:	75–87 percent
Risk:	None.
Method:	Blood test (which measures levels of hCG and pregnancy-associated plasma protein A, known as PAPP-A) combined with nuchal translucency screen. Maternal age is also taken into account.

SECOND-TRIMESTER MATERNAL BLOOD SCREENING: This test is also called multiple marker screening test, triple screen, quad screen, and expanded alpha-fetoprotein test.

Screens for:	Down syndrome, Trisomy 18, and neural tube defects
When:	Usually 15—18 weeks
Accuracy:	Measures risk. The majority of test results showing an increased risk will be proven false by further testing or when the baby is born. In combination with first-trimester combined screening, 94 percent of Down syndrome cases can be detected. ➔ See Combined Screening, above.
Risk:	None.
Method:	Blood test. A mother's age, weight, race, and whether she has diabetes are factored in with the results from the blood test.

diagnostic tests

The two primary diagnostic tests, amniocentesis and chorionic villus sampling (CVS), are typically offered to women at an increased risk for certain birth defects, including those who:

- Will be over thirty-five at time of delivery
- Have had a previous pregnancy or child with a birth defect
- Show an increased risk of birth defects or a chromosomal abnormality from screening tests
- Have a family history that suggests an increased risk of a genetic condition that can be diagnosed prenatally (for example, sickle-cell disease)

cvs or amnio?

If you're going to do CVS or amnio, look for someone who does the procedure routinely. Amnio has been around for a long time; it's easier to find physicians who are experienced. Older data indicated that CVS was a more dangerous test. But recently studies have shown that with an experienced physician, the risk of miscarriage may actually be much lower than thought. Also, keep in mind the background risk for CVS is higher: Women are more likely to miscarry in the first trimester (whether or not CVS is involved). For many, the biggest advantage of CVS is that it is done earlier, when there is more time to consider choices or gather information. If a choice is made to terminate, doing so early on is easier physically and perhaps mentally.

> We chose the amnio because of what seemed to us a high rate of false positive and negative results for the other tests that look for the same things. I will be thirty-nine when the baby is born, so we felt we wanted to be sure that there were no genetic problems. We did have genetic counseling prior to the amnio. We felt very good about the whole experience; we liked the genetic counselor, and we had gone into the experience having discussed what we would do if there was a serious problem, so we felt well prepared for the experience.
> —anonymom

rh negative blood

If your blood type is Rh negative, you will be given a RhoGAM shot if you get any invasive testing such as CVS or amniocentesis. ➔ See Rh Negative, page 112.

AMNIOCENTESIS

Tests for: Chromosomal abnormalities, neural tube defects, and some genetic disorders

When: Anytime after 15 weeks, results about 7—14 days. A process called fluorescence in situ hybridization (FISH) can give partial results in as few as 24 hours, though it's not usually covered by insurance. (Amnios are also occasionally used in the late third trimester to assess fetal lung maturity.)

Accuracy: 99.4—100 percent

Risk: Between 1:400 and 1:1600 risk of miscarriage. The more experienced the physician, the lower the risk.

Method: A sample of amniotic fluid (containing fetal cells and therefore the baby's DNA) is removed from the amniotic sac via a long needle inserted into the uterus via the abdomen. The physician uses an ultrasound to guide the needle. The ultrasound may take a little while (sometimes up to 45 minutes), but the actual procedure takes minutes. When the needle is inserted, some women feel a prick and a little pressure or cramping while the fluid is being withdrawn. One to two percent of women experience cramping, spotting, or leakage of amniotic fluid after the procedure. Often women are advised to take time off, relax, and avoid physical stress for several hours afterward.

We did the first-trimester check for Downs and the results were so discouraging, that we ended up doing an amnio. Everything ultimately checked out okay but the stress it all generated was terrible.

—anonymom

We got some genetic counseling because my triple screen test was irregular. In the end, the data was so unreliable (dates were not exact, percentages of risks varied wildly) and we were so close to the point where we couldn't have an amnio and so emotionally attached to the idea of this baby, that we decided not to go through with an amnio. I was pretty angry about this whole process because I felt I was making a big decision based on faulty information. I wished I had never done the triple screen to begin with!! The baby was fine.

—anonymom

I was pissed that I couldn't get the results of the nuchal before deciding whether or not to do a CVS. The whole experience is really your own personal mini-hell. It is hard to channel how much anxiety I felt now that it is over, but it was really scary and I felt so alone in it all.

—anonymom

We said no to Down syndrome testing, because we came to the conclusion that either way it came out wouldn't change what we were planning.... Prior to being pregnant I thought I was going to get every test imaginable and that results would have been important to me. I don't really know what changed.

—anonymom

CHORIONIC VILLUS SAMPLING (CVS)

Tests for: Chromosomal abnormalities, some genetic disorders, but no neural tube defects (which can be detected via ultrasounds and triple screen test)

When: 10—12 weeks, results within 2—7 days

Accuracy: Greater than 99 percent. (About 1 in 100 CVS tests produces an ambiguous result called pseudomosaicism. When this happens, an amniocentesis must be done to clarify the results.)

Risk: Between 1:200 and 1:100 women miscarry after CVS. The more experienced the physician, the less risk.

Method: Using ultrasound as a guide, a doctor inserts a thin tube through the cervix and uses gentle suction to remove a tiny amount of the chorionic villi (tissue that attaches the sac to the wall of the uterus and will become the placenta). Some women feel pain during the procedure. Depending on where the placenta is (and/or other factors), a doctor may recommend a transabdominal CVS (inserting a needle through the abdominal wall)—both methods are equally safe. Testing facilities specializing in both transcervical and transabdominal CVS reduce risks, since the safest option for a particular patient will be available. One in 5 women feels some cramping after the procedure and 1 in 3 experiences spotting. Women are often asked to take it easy after the procedure, and talk to a doctor about any bleeding or cramping.

> My doctor, who is apparently "the guy" for CVS, had all the grace and finesse of a truck driver who had been up for days on crank. I've never felt such pain with a speculum before—it was as if he was trying to prepare me for labor. . . . I went in thinking it was going to be no big deal but it was so painful that my cervix contracted and they couldn't get the catheter in and he just kept telling me to relax and I kept trying to tell him it wasn't that I was anxious, I was just in pain . . . but the results were good, and I had no bleeding or leaking of anything after.
> —anonymom

finding out the baby's sex

Amnio and CVS can conclusively tell you the sex of your child through his/her chromosomes. Ultrasound can provide a somewhat less reliable read, depending on the position of the fetus and the skill of the reader. According to parenthood.com, in a survey of more than ten thousand parents, 68 percent chose to find out the sex if they could. Of those parents, 84 percent said they did so to give themselves time to reconcile feelings of disappointment if the sex was not what they had been hoping for. (In the same survey, 79 percent of parents said they had a specific gender preference.) Some women feel like finding out the sex is a kind of reward for the ordeal of invasive prenatal testing. Others find out simply because the information is available to them. With frequent ultrasounds and other tests, it can actually be more of an effort to *not* learn the sex.

PROS OF FINDING OUT

- More time to get comfortable with the idea of the gender
- More info for baby stuff: clothes, décor, etc.
- No need to come up with names for both sexes
- Makes preparing for sex-specific events after birth easier (e.g., bris)
- Can make the fetus feel more like a baby

PROS OF NOT FINDING OUT

- Gender preference may be less of an issue once you're face to face with the baby
- Allows a wider range of fantasies about who your baby might be
- Keeps you from projecting sex-specific stereotypes onto the baby before birth
- Maintains the old-school element of surprise
- Some prefer not to think of the fetus as a baby

I was a little intimidated about having a girl, I think because of my relationship with my mother.
—anonymom

I don't know how to explain but after going through labor it was just a cool "reward" to find out the sex at the end. True, we did get a lot of green and yellow clothes beforehand. But we don't really care if people who don't know us can tell whether she's a boy or girl based on what she's wearing. If they ask I'll gladly tell them!
—anonymom

I have been fine all along with not knowing but I am embarrassed to say that now that I am shopping, it is annoying me! So much stuff only comes in pink or blue, or that's all that's left in stores. But it seems too gross to find out just for shopping convenience, to me anyway.
—anonymom

I wanted to know but my husband didn't. It wouldn't have been fair if I found out because I would have slipped up somehow. It was a wonderful surprise to wait. I'm glad I did.
—anonymom

As the radiologist traveled over my belly showing pics of our developing baby she stopped on its area and I saw immediately that it was a boy. My heart just broke and I fought to hold the tears in because I really, really, really wanted a girl. I hate the way I feel because the baby is said to feel my emotions and I'd hate for him to think that he's not wanted, because he is. The real issue is that I can understand and relate to a girl so much better.
—anonymom

It amazes me that people say, Oh, I want to be surprised. It is a surprise no matter when you find out. Also, finding out early makes you feel closer to your son or daughter, it's not an it.
—anonymom

naming the baby

For a lot of people, this is the fun part. Childhood afternoons spent compiling lists of fantasy names can finally be put to productive use. But naming a baby comes with slightly more complications than naming your dolls, or pets, or imaginary boyfriends. This is a name that will be attached to a real person who will have it for life. If you have a partner, you will need to find a name you both agree on. Depending on how attached either of you is to your own ideas, and how well your tastes mesh, this can be a challenge. It can also be an opportunity to explore your aesthetics and family histories.

Some parents really don't want input from others, but it can be hard to prevent people from giving unsolicited opinions. Family members in particular can have plenty to say on the subject. If it is a tradition in your family to name babies after relatives, people may have a lot riding on your name choice, hoping you'll pick a name that honors their loved ones. But even if there's no tradition to uphold, everyone has names they love and names they hate. They may be compelled to express their opinions (in sometimes insensitive ways). If you don't want to hear about the nose-picking creep in your sister-in-law's math class who happened to have the name of your dreams, keep your mouth shut.

things to think about

- **What last name will you use?** If you and your partner have different names, you can choose one, hyphenate both, or give the baby another last name entirely.

- **Spend some time with your top name choices.** Write them down and say them aloud. Think about rhyming and sound as well as any meanings that might be inferred from the names alone or in combination.

- **Is having a popular (or less popular) name important to you?** You can find names ranked by popularity at the U.S. Social Security Administration website. Name books and sites can provide other relevant info.

resources

The Baby Name Wizard by Laura Wattenberg, babynamewizard.com

Social Security Administration Popular Baby Names: ssa.gov/OACT/babynames

choosing a pediatrician

Because your baby will need to be examined soon after birth, you'll need to pick a pediatrician before he's born—usually in the last trimester of pregnancy. If you have friends in the area who have recommendations, you can use them as a starting point. Otherwise, ask other parents, your OB/midwife, or ask your insurance company for a directory. You may want to check out the facilities and meet the doctors. It can feel a little weird to be scoping out baby doctors when you don't have a baby yet, but the doctors you talk to will most likely have seen countless nervous pre-parents and be used to any awkward questions and concerns. Finding a good pediatrician involves balancing a lot of factors. You'll want someone you feel comfortable with and confident about. You'll need an office that's accessible. You will probably have to consider whether the office takes your insurance. Pediatricians sometimes get involved in parenting issues, so you'll want to find out what the doctors' takes are on anything you feel strongly about.

The questions below can help start the discussion and give you some basic information about the practitioner and practice. Some issues may be more important to you than others.

- **How many people are in the practice? How long has each been practicing medicine?**
- **Will the same person examine the baby each visit?**
- **What hospital(s) is the practice affiliated with?**
- **What are the office hours?**
- **How can the doctor be contacted during office hours? After office hours?**
- **Is there someone else who responds to questions when the doctor is busy?**
- **Can sick children be seen in the evenings and/or on weekends?**
- **What is the waiting room like? Is there any arrangement for contagious children? Newborns?**
- **How do the doctors feel about:**
  Circumcision?
  Breastfeeding? Formula? Starting solids?
  Vaccinations?
  Cosleeping? Sleep training?
  Any other choices that are relevant to your family?

circumcision

About 60—65 percent of boy babies in America are circumcised each year. The number of noncircumcised boys has been on the rise in recent years. The narrowing of the gap has led to some controversy and made the decision to circumcise more complex than ever. This is partly because from a medical standpoint, there is no clear answer. Though the American Academy of Pediatrics (AAP) has stated that the procedure is not medically necessary, it has not taken a stand against circumcision and continues to inform parents and practitioners of circumcision's potential benefits. The good news about the official medical opinion is this: Both choices have health benefits (see "Medical Breakdown," opposite). But medical pros and cons are only part of the equation. Circumcision is a very personal choice, with nuanced considerations: Cultural backgrounds, expectations, and feelings all play a role.

Some religions demand circumcision. Different countries have different customs, too. In Europe, for example, circumcision is less common. Circumcised men tend to circumcise their sons and uncircumcised men tend not to. Parents may make the decision based on the idea that if their son doesn't look like his father or the other boys in his social milieu, there could be unpleasant emotional consequences. But if the trends continue, the locker rooms of the future will have a mix of circumcised and uncircumcised boys.

On both sides, there are passionate advocates. Unfortunately, as the debate gets heated, some harsh words can come up: "mutilation" (for circumcision) and "unclean" (for uncircumcised) are two of the biggies. Those words may help cement an opinion, but more often they are an upsetting distraction. The question is often far more complicated than the extremes suggest. Though sometimes stressful, making a decision about circumcision can be an opportunity for parents to have productive, even philosophical conversations. It can even create a useful template for future discussions about parenting.

medical breakdown

possible benefits of circumcision

- *fewer urinary tract infections:* Studies have shown an increased risk (around 1 percent) of UTI in uncircumcised boys, with the greatest risk in infants under one. Severe UTIs early in life are rare, but can lead to kidney problems later on.

- *decreased risk of STDs:* Circumcision is associated with a reduced risk of syphilis and HIV. It's also associated with a lower rate of penile human papillomavirus infection and a reduced risk of cervical cancer in female partners of men with higher numbers of lifetime partners.

- *reduced risk of penile cancer:* Research shows that uncircumcised men are three times as likely to develop penile cancer, though the overall risk for penile cancer is extremely low (9 or 10 cases in one million per year).

possible benefits of not circumcising

- *no surgery complications:* Complications occur in 1 in 200 to 1 in 500 circumcised newborns. But they are mostly very minor (mild bleeding and local infection).

- *no risk of pain:* Circumcision without analgesia has been shown to cause pain and stress. However, the American Academy of Pediatrics policy states "analgesia has been found to be safe and effective in reducing the pain associated with circumcision."

- *no potential sensitivity loss:* The exposed glans (the sensitive head of the penis) may become less sensitive, which may have an impact on sexual experience. This is highly debatable and unproven.

The question of whether a boy should "look like" his daddy runs pretty deep. To me it doesn't seem that hard to explain to a kid. The real issue seems to be less about matching outfits and more about acknowledging the father's penis as the model—the ideal. So then I thought, Will we be saving the baby from a primal wound but opening one in his father?

—anonymom

We debated it for the entire time I was pregnant. And we still think about it. When I read about a new African study showing that the risk of AIDS can be reduced if a man is circumcised, I got that familiar sinking feeling. You make a choice based on science thinking that's the rational way to go, but science just ain't that certain.

—anonymom

who performs a circumcision?

A circumcision can be done by a doctor (ob-gyn, urologist, pediatrician, family physician) or by a certified practitioner trained to perform circumcisions according to religious ritual (for Jews, this is a mohel; the ceremony is called a bris). Some midwives also perform circumcisions.

Some things to consider when researching your options:

- **What is this person's experience?**
- **Where and when will the circumcision happen?**
- **Will you be given any options about the procedure?**
- **Will analgesia be used?**
- **Do you have input into the ceremony if there is one?**

resources

cirp.org (medical information, history, statistics, and links)

circinfo.net (pro-circumcision info)

mothersagainstcirc.org (anti-circumcision info)

What was kind of cool for me about the bris was that it was the first moment for me of really realizing that I had love for this baby. I was so shell-shocked and out of it and not consciously understanding my relationship to him. Then at the moment that they took him away to do this thing that I knew was going to cause him pain, I felt, Ohmigod, I'm this kid's mother, and I need to protect him, and I felt a rush of relationship to the whole history of women before me with sons who had been hurt . . . and it was just a real feeling of tribal connection to the human race.

—anonymom

the pregnant body

Tons of different things can happen to your body during pregnancy.
They're usually influenced by one or a combination of the factors below:

- **Hormonal fluctuations**
- **More blood coursing through more relaxed veins**
- **The weight of an increasingly large uterus**
- **Growth (of placenta, baby, body, hair, etc.)**
- **Loosening of ligaments, muscles, and joints**

These factors can create any number of small or large discomforts.
Moderate exercise; small, frequent healthy meals; posture adjustments; comfortable shoes; and sleep can help take the edge off a lot of
this stuff. Ask your healthcare practitioner to help you find solutions
for any specific issues you encounter.

when to call

It's really hard to give a complete list of warning signs in pregnancy
(it's just too variable). Talk to your doctor or midwife throughout
pregnancy to find out what she thinks you should be looking out for
at each stage, and what she considers urgent. You should also call
your practitioner whenever you're worried about how you feel or have
any questions about your health or your baby's. Part of her job is to be
a resource for her patients. Here's a list of symptoms you should
never ignore:

DEFINITELY CALL YOUR PRACTITIONER IF . . .

- You're having intense one-sided abdominal pain
- You're having abdominal pain that doesn't go away
- You're having vaginal bleeding
- You're unable to keep down fluids for 24 hours
- You're very dizzy and/or fainting
- You're having pain or burning with urination
- Your vision is dim or blurry, or you're seeing double or
  have spots or sparks in front of your eyes
- You're suddenly feeling very few or no fetal movements
  (after 28 weeks)
- You've got a fever over 100 degrees
- You've got a severe, persistent headache
- You're leaking fluid from the vagina

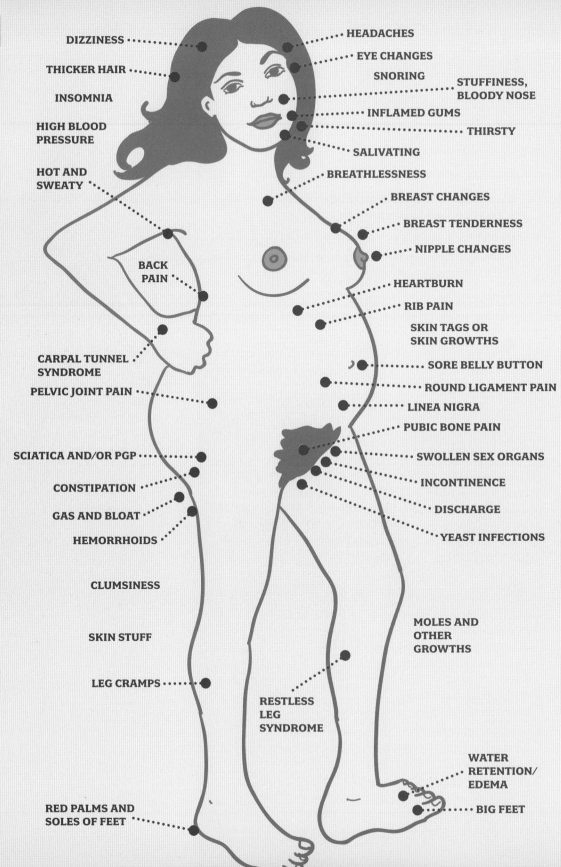

DIZZINESS

THICKER HAIR

INSOMNIA

HIGH BLOOD
PRESSURE

HOT AND
SWEATY

BACK
PAIN

CARPAL TUNNEL
SYNDROME

PELVIC JOINT PAIN

SCIATICA AND/OR PGP

CONSTIPATION

GAS AND BLOAT

HEMORRHOIDS

CLUMSINESS

SKIN STUFF

LEG CRAMPS

RED PALMS AND
SOLES OF FEET

HEADACHES

EYE CHANGES

SNORING

STUFFINESS,
BLOODY NOSE

INFLAMED GUMS

THIRSTY

SALIVATING

BREATHLESSNESS

BREAST CHANGES

BREAST TENDERNESS

NIPPLE CHANGES

HEARTBURN

RIB PAIN

SKIN TAGS OR
SKIN GROWTHS

SORE BELLY BUTTON

ROUND LIGAMENT PAIN

LINEA NIGRA

PUBIC BONE PAIN

SWOLLEN SEX ORGANS

INCONTINENCE

DISCHARGE

YEAST INFECTIONS

MOLES AND
OTHER
GROWTHS

RESTLESS
LEG
SYNDROME

WATER
RETENTION/
EDEMA

BIG FEET

44

bodily byproducts of pregnancy

As far as we know, no pregnant woman has had all of these at once!

APPETITE CHANGES:
➔ See Cravings and Aversions, page 52.

BACK PAIN: Back pain can be caused by a big belly, a shifting center of gravity, and/or relaxed joints. The pain might be in the lower back, upper back, buttocks, all over. *Exercise, side sleeping, sleeping with a pillow between the knees, good posture, flat shoes, chairs with back support, stretching, and heat may help. Avoid, if possible, twisting, overreaching, and carrying heavy things on one side. Ask your doctor about medication if pain is a big problem.*

BIG FEET: Loose ligaments and joints as well as fluid retention can cause feet to flatten and widen, and even move up a size. They may or may not shrink afterward. *Wear comfortable, bigger shoes. Support hose, elevating feet, or orthotic inserts can help.*

BREAST CHANGES: Big boobs, sore boobs, visible veins, dark nipples. *A supportive and comfortable bra can help, even during sleep (avoid underwires).* ➔ See Body Image, page 55.

BREATHLESSNESS: Hormones can speed up breathing rate, while the uterus can press on the lungs and diaphragm. *Breathing gets easier when the baby drops. Stand tall, breathe deep. Talk to your doctor or midwife if worried.*

BROKEN BLOOD VESSELS, SPIDER VEINS: ➔ See page 57.

CARPAL TUNNEL SYNDROME: Swelling in the wrists can put pressure on nerves and cause some pain or numbness in fingers. *Ease up on repetitive motions with hands, lift things with your whole hand, and type with wrists straight and hands lower than elbows. Avoid sleeping on your hands. Try wearing a brace or get physical therapy.*

CLUMSINESS: Balance can be thrown off by changing weight and shape. Loose ligaments may also contribute. *Try to cut yourself some slack if your self-image rests on being graceful; move slowly and carefully.*

CONSTIPATION: Sluggish bowel, cramped intestines, and iron supplements may be to blame. *Eat fiber. Drink fluids. Exercise or try a stool softener (not laxatives, though).*

DISCHARGE (VAGINAL): Due to general increase in mucus manufacturing. Should be odorless, colorless.

DIZZINESS: Dizziness may come from increased circulation and decreased pressure in blood vessels. *Eat frequent small meals, get up slowly, lie on side, not back; get fresh air or put head between knees. Call your doctor or midwife if you faint or if dizziness is accompanied by other problems such as swelling.*

EYE CHANGES: Fluid retention can temporarily affect vision. Estrogen might also make eyes dry and sensitive and/or vision blurred. *Wear contacts less or update lens prescription if necessary.*

GAS AND BLOAT: Due to hormones, water retention, slowed-down bowel. *Eat slowly. Forgo gassy foods: beans, cabbage, cauliflower, etc.*

GLOW: ➔ See Skin and Hair Stuff, page 57.

HEADACHES: Headaches can be caused by a few things: hormones, caffeine withdrawal, congestion, tension, exhaustion . . . etc. *Fresh air, low lights, rest, hot or cold compresses, caffeine, and frequent meals (to avoid blood sugar drop) can help. Tylenol can be used sometimes (talk to your doctor about frequency and see "The Endless No," page 62, for more on meds while pregnant). Persistent headache with blurred vision may be related to preeclampsia; call* *your doctor or midwife.* ➔ See Preeclampsia, Pregnancy-Induced Hypertension (PIH), or Toxemia, page 109.

HEARTBURN: Slower digestion and relaxed muscles in the throat can lead to upward swill of stomach acid. *Spicy, greasy, acidic food (especially before bed) may exacerbate. Talk to your doctor or midwife about calcium-containing antacid. Eat small meals and/or crackers (to neutralize stomach). Elevate head at night.*

HEMORRHOIDS: Varicose veins in or around the anus are called hemorrhoids. ➔ See page 179 for info and treatment.

HIGH BLOOD PRESSURE: Often, blood pressure goes down; sometimes, it goes up. *Since high blood pressure is associated with preeclampsia, doctors monitor for it.* ➔ See High Blood Pressure, page 107, and Preeclampsia, Pregnancy-Induced Hypertension (PIH), or Toxemia, page 109.

HOT AND SWEATY: Metabolism is up; so is body temperature. *Cool down as best you can.*

INCONTINENCE: The uterus can put pressure on the bladder, making it hard to keep from peeing all the time (or by accident). *Frequent peeing (and Kegels) may help.* ➔ See Kegels, page 58.

INFLAMED GUMS: Hormones can make gums swell and bleed easily. Plaque is also more likely to stick during pregnancy. *Brush and floss frequently. Go to the dentist regularly.*

INSOMNIA: Can come from change in hormones, physical discomfort, stress, or all. *Exercise, light dinners, fresh air, warm milk, warm bath, a small snack before bed, pillows between legs, and a body pillow can all help.* ➔ See page 50.

ITCHY SKIN: Itchy (and sometimes red or dry) skin is common in pregnancy and can be a result of skin stretching, hormones, dry skin, or preexisting skin conditions. About 1 percent of women develop an itchy rash on the abdomen late in pregnancy. *Moisturize, wear loose natural fibers, avoid overheating, try not to scratch too much. Talk to your doctor about any rashes.*

LEG CRAMPS: Sharp temporary pain in the calf. These mostly happen at night and may be the result of a decrease in circulation, dehydration, or low levels of potassium, magnesium, or calcium. *Massage leg, stretch, drink more water, eat foods high in above minerals. Bananas are sometimes recommended.*

LINEA NIGRA: ➔ See page 57.

MOLES AND OTHER GROWTHS: ➔ See page 174.

NIPPLE CHANGES: Nipples and areolas get darker and larger. Bumps around the nipple may appear more prominent. *Nipples go back to normal (or normalish) after pregnancy.*

PELVIC JOINT PAIN: The loosening of pelvic joints and ligaments can put excess pressure on the pelvic area, and causes pain in the hips and groin (usually in the second trimester and onward). *An obstetric physiotherapist can recommend pain management ideas. Avoid breaststroke when swimming, climb stairs one step at time, rest lots. Tell OB/midwife; it can affect aspects of delivery (like epidural use).*

PUBIC BONE PAIN: When the pelvic ring separates or opens, it can put pressure on the surrounding areas, causing sharp pains in pubic bone area. *If severe, doctor can refer physical therapist.*

RED PALMS AND SOLES OF FEET: Might happen from increased blood flow. *It's temporary.*

RESTLESS LEG SYNDROME: Leg(s) can feel uppity and tingling, and keep you (and anyone else in your bed) awake at night. *Try changes in sleeping position, mobility. Avoid caffeine at night. Try eating foods high in calcium, potassium, and magnesium. Meditation and massage can help.*

RIB PAIN: Uterus presses against ribs. Kicking can make it worse. *Gets better when baby drops. Try moving around to see if baby will shift position.*

ROUND LIGAMENT PAIN: A brief, sharp pain around

lower abs from the stretching of the tissue that supports the uterus. Usually peaks between 18 and 24 weeks, then fades. *Avoid sudden movement (like getting up or turning too quickly). Your doctor or midwife can recommend stretches. Rest.*

SALIVATING: During the first half of pregnancy, there may be lots of saliva, and a bitter and/or swollen tongue. This might be the result of not swallowing due to nausea. *Try fruit, small snacks, gum, lemon candy, mints, rinsing mouth.*

SCIATICA AND/OR PGP: Pressure on the sciatic nerve can cause pain to shoot down the legs, pins and needles, or numbness. It may be Pelvic Girdle Pain (PGP) if the pain is on one side, jumps from side to side, and/or is in hip area. *Good posture, flat shoes, side-lying (with pillow support), and acupuncture may help. Avoid too much sitting or lifting. Talk to a doctor or midwife physiotherapist about support belt/exercises.*

SKIN STUFF: ➜ See page 57.

SKIN TAGS OR SKIN GROWTHS: Moles may get bigger during pregnancy. Sometimes little skin growths appear—like little "tags" of skin. *Skin tags may go away by themselves, or they can be surgically removed. Check any mole changes with a dermatologist.*

SNORING: Snoring can come from the swelling of nasal passages and extra congestion. *Try sleeping on your side. Snoring has been associated with high blood pressure. If you are snoring loudly, frequently, or losing sleep, tell your doctor.*

SORE BELLY BUTTON: Navel area may feel tender or sore from expanding waistline. It usually peaks at around 20 weeks, then goes away. *Massage or use hot or cold compresses. Call your doctor if red or persistent.*

STUFFINESS, BLOODY NOSE: All veins, including the little ones in the nose, are affected by increased circulation. *Humidifier, fluids, elevated head, vitamin C, and gentle nose blowing can help.*

SWOLLEN SEX ORGANS: This can happen from water retention, enhanced mucous membranes, hormones . . . ➜ See Pregnant Sex, page 92.

THICKER HAIR: ➜ See page 57.

THIRST: A pregnant woman often needs extra fluids to help maintain increased blood supply and amniotic fluid production. *Drink plenty of water.*

URINARY TRACT INFECTIONS: Increased pressure on bladder and changes in the urinary tract make UTIs common during pregnancy. Symptoms include painful and/or frequent urination. *Antibiotics are the usual treatment. Call your healthcare provider.*

WATER RETENTION/ EDEMA: This is very common in feet, ankles, hands, and fingers. Estrogen can cause water retention, and the pressure on veins can slow the drainage of fluid. *Drink lots. Elevate legs. Try support stockings. Avoid tight clothing and standing for too long.* ➜ Sudden swelling is associated with preeclampsia; see page 109.

YEAST INFECTIONS: The vagina can be more accommodating to yeast due to an estrogen boost. *Talk to your doctor about medical treatment. Wear cotton underwear (and/or none at night); wipe front to back. Avoid tight pants and unnecessary "feminine" products and perfumes.*

super smelling

Increased sense of smell in early pregnancy is caused by a rise in the hormone estradiol (an estrogen). This hormone creates a hypersensitivity to smell and, occasionally, distorted or phantom smells. There's a theory that these super smelling abilities are a way to keep pregnant women away from dangerous food or chemical toxins during the early, vulnerable stage of embryonic development. The fact that some things that smell bad to pregnant women aren't particularly healthy (coffee, alcohol, smoke) is sometimes used to illustrate this. It's not clear whether the connection is that direct, as all kinds of strong smells can be repugnant to pregnant women, toxic or not. Sensitivity to smell is also related to morning sickness—in a 2000 study at Stanford University, women cited strong odors as a frequent nausea trigger. Any pregnant woman who's ever retched at the smell of frying onions (or for that matter, her husband) will find this association rather obvious. → See Scent of a Human, page 93.

"morning" sickness

Over half of pregnant women feel sick at some point in their first trimester, sometimes in the mornings, but often throughout the day. Those queasy/pukey feelings are officially known as Nausea and Vomiting of Pregnancy, or NVP for short. The absolute cause of the condition is not known, but it is thought to relate to hormone levels (which is why morning sickness is sometimes said to correlate to a lower level of miscarriage). Sensitivity to smells also plays a role. Sick feelings usually kick in at around 4—6 weeks. Most women find they're feeling better by the early second trimester, but a few have to contend with nausea for their entire pregnancies. The feelings can range from a mild upset stomach to a more severe (and rare) version, called hyperemesis gravidarum (HG). Some medications exist to help manage nausea during pregnancy, so if it's a real problem for you, you can ask your healthcare provider. → See Sick, Tired, and Miserable, page 84.

My husband's smells last night were making me crazy—I had to crack a window in a *blizzard*. I don't know what it was, something very sweet and all too human—gnarly. I think I need to get some flowers in here—some nonsickly sweet-smelling flowers.
—anonymom

I suffered through it and found relief by avoiding bad smells, eating frequently, and trusting my instinct. It also helped immensely once my husband started making his morning coffee in the garage :)
—anonymom

Once my "morning" sickness set in, it never left. Not for a second. It was like having food poisoning, but the nausea never lifted. I tried every medication and every natural remedy. I would throw up while wearing those stupid Sea-Bands. The doctors did not take me seriously until I'd already lost too much weight.
—anonymom

I have two modes, nausea/empty stomach or tired and full.
—anonymom

things that can help

- Keeping small amounts of food in your stomach at all times
- Not forcing yourself to eat foods that are unappealing
- Smelling, sucking, or chewing on mint- or lemon-flavored things
- Drinking fluids between meals instead of with meals
- Sea-Bands (acupressure bracelets)
- Ginger (tea, crystallized, or supplements; ask your provider first)
- Vitamin B_6 (ask provider)
- Acupressure and acupuncture (ditto)

fatigue: the view from the couch

Pregnant women often feel more tired than usual, especially very early and very late in pregnancy. In the beginning, you're producing a lot of progesterone, which can make you feel sleepy and physically depressed. Meanwhile, your body is working much, much harder than usual to produce extra blood volume and build the placenta. Many women find they can't get through the day without a nap, or pass out as soon as they get home from work. Feeling sick can also make you tired, or just make you want to lie on the couch and wallow. Iron deficiency can contribute to fatigue, as well. Late in pregnancy, many women are simply too tired to move much, because the increased weight and pressure make it such a mammoth effort.

things that can help

- Naps, naps, naps
- Hydration (but not much before bed or you'll be waking up to pee all night)
- Moderate exercise
- Prenatal vitamins
- Iron-rich foods (or iron supplements if your provider suggests them; see "Anemia," page 104)

> It definitely helps to eat a little bit all day. Whenever my stomach starts to get empty, I know I'm in trouble. And the books all say after you hit the twelve-week mark it'll go away. Yeah, right! For me it was more like fifteen weeks, but I still puked periodically through my third trimester.
> —anonymom

> I was so tired I could hardly stand up in the middle of the day. Waves of sleepiness like crappy, nausea-inducing sleeping pills mixed with jetlag and a hangover. Truly not a good state for decision making, socializing, eating, moving, or doing anything at all but count the days until trimester two.
> —anonymom

massage during pregnancy

Massage is fine in pregnancy as long as there are no complications and the massage therapist has been trained in prenatal work. Prenatal massage can reduce stress and discomforts. Some therapists prefer to wait until after the first trimester to begin doing body work on pregnant women. If you want to get a massage early in your pregnancy, it may be helpful to ask your doctor or midwife if she can write you a note okaying the work. A prenatal massage may feel different from massages you had before you got pregnant; the therapist may work less deeply, or just work on different parts of your body. Prenatal therapists are trained to avoid certain strokes and areas that might stimulate labor (if you're overdue, you can ask your therapist whether those techniques might be appropriate for you). Prenatal massage may be covered by insurance.

sleep and pregnancy

In the National Sleep Foundation's 1998 Women and Sleep poll, 78 percent of women said that they had more disturbed sleep while pregnant. Sleep problems in pregnancy can happen for both physical and emotional reasons. Any of the discomforts of pregnancy (from hormonal changes to leg cramps to anxiety) can keep you awake when they happen at night. Pregnant women understandably lament their sleep situation, wondering "When will my sleep be back to normal?" The physical issues that kept you awake are likely to improve after you recover from birth. But there may be (lots of) other things keeping you awake afterward!

Here are some of the common reasons pregnant women have trouble sleeping, and some things that might help:

COMFORT ISSUES First it's sore breasts, then it's an increasingly cumbersome belly. You'll probably need to experiment with different sleeping positions throughout pregnancy. By the last trimester, sleeping on the side is usually recommended. The left side, particularly, because it increases blood flow to the fetus. But in most cases it's not necessary to stay on the left side all night. A mountain of pillows and padding will make it easier (or at least possible) to find a relatively comfortable position. Lying flat on the back in the second half of pregnancy (some say after 16 weeks) can put pressure on the vena cava, a major blood vessel, and cut off some of the fetus's oxygen flow. Elevating one hip with a pillow can prevent this.

HAVING TO PEE Pregnant women often find themselves waking up a lot to pee at night, especially in the first and last trimesters. To decrease night pee runs, don't drink a lot before bed.

DREAMS Strange, unusually vivid, and even disturbing dreams are common in pregnancy. Sometimes these dreams are about pregnancy or parenthood. Sometimes they're about totally unrelated or even seemingly antithetical stuff; reunions with exes and dramatic encounters with strangers are common themes. Hormones may help intensify pregnant dreams, but the transformation is plenty of fodder in itself.

➜ See Pregnancy and Anxiety, page 84.
➜ See Bodily Byproducts of Pregnancy, page 45.

> Okay, get this—last night I dreamed I had sex with Michelangelo's *David*—though the situation between his legs was a bit more "functional" than the real one! Ha.
> —anonymom

> During pregnancy and in my first year as a new mom, I have had more anxiety dreams/nightmares than I can count. I have never been one to worry or be anxious; I have always been very laid back, but I woke up in a cold sweat due to nightmares four out of seven nights.
> —anonymom

> I had a lot of orgasmic dreams while pregnant (probably because I wasn't having any sex at all during that time).
> —anonymom

> I've had beautiful labor dreams, but my baby in some of my dreams has been really cold and has unfeeling eyes, which I have taken as a reminder that it takes babies a while to respond emotionally and I have to prepare myself for a baby who won't be able to smile or love me right away.
> —anonymom

kicking and hic-ing: fetal movements

Women usually feel the baby move at around 20 weeks, sometimes sooner, sometimes later. The first movements can be very faint (often described as a fluttering, and may be mistaken for gas). Later in pregnancy, the movements get much more pronounced. Babies may move more after the mother has eaten, due to an increase in blood sugar—though every baby has its own particular rhythms or patterns. Moms can also feel a baby's hiccups, which are common and may start midway through pregnancy. Some moms report feeling shudders or twitches, too. Sometimes doctors recommend tracking movements starting at around 28 weeks— at least four to six movements or kicks an hour is considered a good sign. You can talk to your doctor about fetal movements and what to look out for.

colds and congestion

Pregnant women can be congested from swollen membranes in their nasal passages, so they often feel as if they have a cold even when they don't (or the symptoms of a cold may be enhanced). A respiratory infection can also feel worse when your lungs are squished by a growing baby. And lowered immunity makes it easier to catch whatever is going around, so women pretty commonly get colds while they're pregnant. Elevating the head with pillows can help relieve congestion. Colds can also be treated with hot liquids, humidifiers, or menthol rubs. Some cold medication is considered safe during pregnancy, especially after the first trimester—ask your doctor.

fever/flu

Since pregnancy alters a mother's immune system, she may be at slightly higher risk of complications from the flu (like pneumonia). In 2004, the U.S. Advisory Committee on Immunization Practices (ACIP) recommended that pregnant women receive a flu shot (if they are pregnant during flu season). Other ways to prevent infection: Clean hands often and try not to touch your mouth, nose, and eyes. Avoid contact with sick people if you can. If you do get sick, try to get as much rest and fluids as possible. Fevers are associated with a higher risk of birth defects, so many doctors recommend taking Tylenol to reduce them, especially in early pregnancy. If you develop a fever, check with your doctor to see if she recommends you take anything or come in for a visit.

braxton hicks contractions

Many women experience sporadic, irregular contractions during pregnancy. Often described as Braxton Hicks contractions, they may be strong or intense but they do not represent the beginning of labor. The uterine muscle

the beast within

Crushing exhaustion, violent vomiting, and urgent cravings can make pregnant women feel like they are at the mercy of a mighty parasitic entity . . . not a cute little baby. Zealous kicks can inspire comparisons to fetal Bruce Lees on a belly-busting rampage. Or, more mildly, the Rockettes. Whatever your favored analogy, the mother is quite literally where the baby lives and what the baby eats. Some scientists have proposed that pregnancy is actually a battle for resources between the mother's body and the fetus's. The idea is for the baby's body to get what it needs and for the mother to keep her own body from being overly depleted. This tug-of-war scenario may not be so cuddly, but it seems that nurturing, even on a cellular level, involves give-and-take on both sides.

is flexing, but the cervix is not dilating. It can feel like a tightening that sweeps over the belly and then subsides, or more like a cramp. Some consider Braxton Hicks contractions "false labor"; others prefer to think of them as a warmup, or rehearsal, for labor. They help with uterine muscle tone and increase blood flow to the placenta. You may feel them as early as the second trimester (or sooner in subsequent pregnancies). Often they are intense only later in the pregnancy. Some women never really notice them. They are often stronger when lying down or resting and tend to go away when moving around. A warm bath, lots of fluids, some deep breaths, and/or changing position can usually ease any discomfort.

eating while pregnant

We live in a culture obsessed with food and dieting, so it should come as no surprise that the question of what to ingest while expecting is a matter of major focus (and heated debate). Add to that the complex personal relationship many women have with food, and you've got a recipe for anxious eating.

A lot is said about aiming for perfect nutrition during pregnancy. But it's not always realistic to expect yourself to eat half a dozen servings of organic leafy greens every day. Plus, the psychological impact of this pressure can be rather unhealthy. Your baby will benefit from your eating the healthiest possible foods, but will probably manage fine on whatever you eat—within reason. Everyday food risks are amplified in pregnancy, because your immune system is compromised and your fetus is vulnerable. Deciding what to eat can sometimes feel like a juggling act between getting the nutrients you both need and avoiding the foods that gross you out or might make you sick. Some people would rather follow a diet that keeps them from having to make too many choices. But diets can feel oppressive and really aren't necessary if you have an idea of basic nutrition and food safety during pregnancy.
→ For "forbidden foods," see The Endless No, page 62.

cravings and aversions

Pregnancy is often associated with an intense, insatiable desire for bizarre foods—or combinations of foods, e.g., the famous cliché of pickles and ice cream. And cravings are often equaled or bested by powerful food aversions, especially during the first trimester. Morning sickness can also be directly tied to food cravings—frequently, women find that their nausea can only be quelled by eating very specific foods. Herein lies the root of the familiar image of an expectant father on the supermarket checkout line at midnight. Even when nausea is not involved, desires for certain foods during pregnancy can feel much more urgent than at other times. A craving may be a message from your body about what it needs, and this communication often occurs at high volume (more like a shriek than a casual suggestion). Sometimes these messages get lost in translation or filtered through an emotional fog: a craving for a margarita may actually be a craving for salt . . . or for the uncomplicated life you had before you got pregnant.

"the pregnancy diet"

There are lots of tailored diets for pregnant women, but the bottom line is pretty simple: Eat a balance of food groups, try to avoid processed foods and bad fats, stay hydrated, and be aware of freshness and vitamin content. There may be a list of banned foods a mile long but there is no list of foods you *have* to eat. → See The Endless No, page 62.

Around 300 extra calories a day are usually suggested for appropriate weight gain. This is a guide and not a mandate; you may need more or less depending on your weight or how much you usually eat. If you're worried about your ability to consume all necessary nutrients (due to aversions, banned foods, morning sickness), talk to your doctor or midwife.

attitudes about eating

There can be something life affirming about eating while pregnant and feeling like the food you consume is actually the building blocks of your baby. Some people see pregnancy as a rare opportunity to eat what they want without worrying about it. This may even be the first time some women can remember when they didn't regard every meal as a potential threat to their svelte figures. They can finally indulge, bolstered by chants of "You're eating for two!"

Others find pregnancy a time of increased obsession about eating. Rather than feeling liberated from their food and body-image anxieties, they obsess about their inevitable weight gain and try to control it aggressively, "make every calorie count," and eat only the most nutrient-rich foods to efficiently nourish their growing babies. The highly structured diets found in many pregnancy books tend to enhance this anxiety. Finding a middle ground between being conscious of what you eat and obsessing over the nutrition/fat ratio of every item you put in your mouth may take a little effort, but is probably worth it for your pregnant psyche.

eating disorders

Whether it's due to concern for the baby's health or a newfound relationship to the pregnant body, moms who have battled eating disorders often notice a real improvement in body image through the process of

folic acid in early pregnancy

The chances of neural tube defects are reduced significantly by 400–800 micrograms of folic acid per day in vitamins or enriched foods. The neural tube (which grows to form the central nervous system) closes 5–6 weeks after conception, so it's most important in very early pregnancy. Folic acid supplements are sometimes recommended even before conception for this reason. Folic acid can also be found in foods, but some studies have shown supplements to be more effective.

weight gain

Weight gain depends on many factors: prepregnancy weight, height, age, ethnicity, body type, fitness level, mobility, degree to which cravings and aversions rule your appetite, changes to diet, how many babies you're carrying, and metabolism. Weight gain is important for fetal growth. If you're underweight, you need to gain more weight. If you're overweight, less. You can ask your doctor about what kind of weight gain she sees as appropriate. → See Boobs, Bellies, Butts, and Other Areas of Expansion, page 55, and Multiples, page 107.

resources

National Association of Anorexia Nervosa and Associated Disorders: ANAD.org or hotline, 847-831-3438

Eating Disorder Referral and Information Center: Edreferral.com or 800-843-7274

having a baby. Some of these women even experience a permanent change of attitude toward food and their bodies. Others find that eating disorder symptoms creep back in once the baby is born. Eating disorders such as anorexia, binge eating, and bulimia may persist through pregnancy. Even if the symptoms are not as severe, anorexic or bulimic women can feel tremendous amounts of guilt and anxiety. The shame associated with these illnesses can prevent women from talking to their doctors. But open communication is crucial: Active eating disorders during pregnancy can lead to a range of significant health and developmental problems for the baby. They can also lead to serious health issues for the mother. Your ob-gyn needs to be aware of the disorder so that she can offer dietary guidance as well as monitor or prevent any health problems. Emotional support is just as important. Bad body image is very tangled up with low self-esteem in general, and eating disorders are also associated with postpartum depression. Making an anonymous call to a hotline can be a good first step in seeking treatment (group and/or individual support). Even those who feel "cured" of an eating disorder during pregnancy may benefit from support sooner rather than later.

obesity and pregnancy

Since one-third of adult women in the United States are obese, obesity and pregnancy is a serious concern. According to the American College of Obstetricians and Gynecologists, obesity increases the risk of a whole range of problems for mother and baby. Lowering weight prior to the pregnancy can reduce a lot of these risks. Once pregnant, good nutrition and exercise can help ensure a healthy pregnancy. Trying to lose weight while pregnant is not recommended. Instead, most doctors recommend that obese women control their weight gain, aiming to gain only 15 pounds during pregnancy.

Sometimes doctors feel uncomfortable addressing obesity with their patients, and vice versa. Other doctors obsess on weight in a negative, unproductive way. But since this is a health issue, it's really important that a dialogue be established. If you are concerned about your weight, make sure to discuss the following with your ob-gyn: all potential complications, a nutritional program, whether to meet with an anesthesiologist before delivery, and the option of screening for gestational diabetes in both the first trimester and later on if the first test was negative.

resources

Big, Beautiful, and Pregnant: Expert Advice and Comforting Wisdom for the Expecting Plus-Size Woman by Cornelia van der Ziel and Jacqueline Tourville

Your Plus-Size Pregnancy by Brette McWhorter Sember and Dr. Bruce D. Rodgers

body image

There's a huge amount of anxiety about what having a baby will do to your appearance. Will you get fat? Saggy? Flabby? Or "bounce back"? Will your body make you proud? Miserable? Both? Pregnancy can make you feel like your body is totally out of control, but this feeling can also, oddly enough, provide some body image relief. A pregnant mother may discover a new confidence in her creative body. Many women go through body-image fluctuations the whole way through, feeling powerless sometimes and powerful at others. There are so many influences at work: hormonal changes that can affect energy and emotions, negative associations with weight gain, new abilities and disabilities, and built-up expectations.

boobs, bellies, butts, and other areas of expansion

Bigger boobs are one of the first signs of pregnancy. For the less well endowed, this can be a thrill, giving formerly flat-chested women the chance to throw around some serious cleavage. For those who came to pregnancy already bearing bazongas to reckon with, pregnancy can have the opposite effect, sending the expectant mother hurtling into a world of G cups and double-wide bra straps. You may have heard this before, but it's worth reiterating: It's this boob inflation, not breastfeeding, that causes any postbaby sagging.

It has been said that pregnant women do not begin "showing" until around 4 or 5 months, on average, the first time around. This defines showing as the point at which you begin to look undeniably pregnant instead of possibly just fat. Many women do experience a "thickening" around the middle very early in pregnancy. This can make it difficult to wear tight clothes comfortably, even during those first weeks.

If your belly is considerably larger or smaller than people seem to think is "normal" for that time period, you'll probably hear about it from various busybodies. But in reality, the range is huge! If there is a real size concern, you will hear about it from your healthcare practitioner.

Why do women gain weight in places nowhere near the baby? Partly, it's genes; some women are programmed to carry their babies like basketballs in the front, and others put a layer of fat over their whole bodies. Heredity, metabolism, energy levels, sickness, food aversions, cravings

under the microscope

Pregnancy is not a sickness, but pregnant women are patients: examined, assessed, measured, weighed, prodded, and generally seen as bodies first and people second. We have doctors sticking things into us (sometimes in front of our partners). We have hour-long discussions with strangers about the details of our genes, and see countless vials of our blood and pee. All this medical monitoring can affect how we feel about our bodies and ourselves. The attention on your body may make you feel taken care of or special. But if you're already anxious about your health, doctors, or hospitals, pregnancy can heighten that anxiety pretty quickly. Women with high-risk pregnancies, chronic illnesses, or disabilities may have to work extra-hard to convince themselves that pregnancy is a normal part of the human experience and not a life-threatening disease. Pregnancy can also be hard on the hypochondriac, since it provides myriad new possibilities for assessing and diagnosing "symptoms," not to mention a whole new person on whom to imagine their impact. Some people feel that the viewing of pregnancy in a medical context undermines women's confidence, especially when it comes to birth.
→ See Natural vs. Medical Childbirth: Either/Or?, page 141.

> I wore tight-fitting, body-hugging outfits because I loved my belly and I thought I looked fantastic! I was proud of how I looked and wanted to show it off, I guess.
> —anonymom

. . . it's really hard to control the way your body decides to swell. Diet and exercise can make an impact, but won't change *the way* your body puts on baby weight. Water weight gain and swelling can lend more puffiness. (Pregnant bodies actually store water *between* fat cells, causing an overall appearance of weight gain.)

I felt good and loved that my never-flat stomach could now be free! No more holding it in.
—anonymom

Being a full-figure gal, I didn't really start to show until my seventh month. I now have the full harder belly look going on with the duck waddle in my step.
—anonymom

For a while I was feeling like I actually looked sexier while pregnant—maybe because I thought my bigger belly was making everything else look so skinny . . . but now that I am in the third trimester, I'm fixated on how fat my thighs look compared to prepregnant. . . . I wonder if they will ever return to their formerly svelte selves???
—anonymom

Everyone kept saying "You won't need maternity clothes until the fifth month" but that was totally not true for me. I had someone ask me if I was pregnant in the second month! Granted I was not my thinnest at the time, but I was also really bloated and thick in the middle from the pregnancy starting very, very early.
—anonymom

The puffy ankles were pretty tough to handle. They happened to me at about month eight. Also, the point at which you gain weight but not in your stomach . . . that gave me a feeling of helplessness because there isn't a thing you can do about it.
—anonymom

The belly—I loved everything about it, and it makes people—strangers, even—feel enthralled with you. I never felt so gorgeous in my life, even though I had lost my petite size-six body to an extra sixty—that's right, sixty!—pounds.
—anonymom

In a certain way, it's very fascinating to discover the changes—like your own little science experiment.
—anonymom

I didn't really show or need maternity clothes until right around the middle of the sixth month. And I never did get really huge the way some people do. People kept telling me how small I looked until it began to bug me, as though implying I wasn't eating properly or taking care of the baby. By the end, though, I *felt* huge—all swollen and waddling.
—anonymom

I am into my thirteenth week and it would be pretty hard for anyone to guess I was pregnant. My body looks different to me but I guess it's still subtle. In some ways this means it still doesn't feel real and when I do show, perhaps it will be all the more shocking?
—anonymom

skin and hair stuff

That "glow" people are always talking about is not just a reflection of overwhelming joy. Because pregnant bodies produce more blood, skin can seem brighter and pinker. Blood volume and water retention can plump things out a little (sometimes minimizing wrinkles). Hormones can cause an increase in oil production, which lends a sheen that can look gorgeous or grimy, depending. But hormones affect the skin in many different ways. Pregnant women may have better, clearer skin than ever before. Or break out with pimples. Acne medication is not safe during pregnancy, but you can talk to your OB or dermatologist about topical treatments.

Stretch marks are a common side effect of pregnancy (more than half of women get them). These marks, the result of skin stretching too much or too quickly, can show up as early as the second trimester or not until after the baby has been born. Pregnant women around the world slather themselves with slime in efforts to prevent the dreaded marks, which can range from white to red to deep purple. But when it comes to stretch marks, it seems that if you're going to get them, you're going to get them, regardless. How much weight you gain and how fast as well as whether you're genetically predisposed all factor in to whether or not you'll be in the mark-free minority. The bad news is that stretch marks are permanent; the good news is that they fade after the baby's born. They may or may not be visible, and creams and/or laser treatments may or may not reduce them.

Some women get spider veins (clusters of blood vessels) or varicose veins. Heredity makes you more susceptible to these issues. To minimize varicose veins, keep circulation going, put your feet up, try not to sit for very long stretches, and avoid cinching tights or socks. Spider veins and varicose veins often fade or recede after the baby is born.

Nipples and areolas get darker during pregnancy. Many women develop "linea nigra," a darkish line of pigment leading from their pubic bone up to the navel. Some pregnant women experience skin color changes around their eyes, nose, and cheeks known as chloasma, or the mask of pregnancy. Sun exposure may trigger pigment changes or make them more visible. Darker-skinned women are more likely to notice these changes.

Increased oil production can help make hair look shiny . . . or greasy. Many women have thicker hair during pregnancy, caused by changes in the natural cycle of hair growth and loss. Hairs fall out much less frequently, resulting in more hair on the head overall. Things reverse after the baby's born, when a lot of the hair that was retained during pregnancy falls out at once.

exercise

The basic principles of exercise apply to pregnant women as they do to all people: Regular and moderate doses can boost energy, flexibility, strength, cardiovascular fitness, circulation, and mood. Working out can be good for your posture and digestion as well as help prevent aches and pains. Activity is generally considered fine throughout pregnancy as long as there isn't much risk of slamming into anything, falling, or being hit (horseback riding and skiing, for example, are not recommended). But it's a good idea to discuss any exercise you plan to do with your doctor or midwife, especially if you have a high-risk pregnancy or any complications. → See High-Risk Pregnancy, page 103.

Some things to think about:

- You are pumping a lot more blood than before (50 percent more by the thirtieth week) so your heart rate tends to be faster, and blood pressure lower. It's also easier to get out of breath when pregnant. Some say that if you cannot carry on a conversation while exercising, your body is probably working too hard.

- Overheating is not recommended in pregnancy, so keep this in mind when contemplating cardio, Bikram yoga, saunas, etc. → See Hot Stuff, page 78.

- There may be specific moves or positions to revise or eliminate—teachers or trainers can help you.

- If you worked out a lot before you got pregnant, you may be able to do more than is typically recommended for pregnant women. Everyone's threshold is different.

THE PELVIC FLOOR: The pelvic floor is like a hammock slung from front to back with muscles crossing over and interlacing around the urethra, vagina, and anus. These muscles are at work during orgasm, excretory activities, and birth. They are sensitive and elastic, unless they have been stretched and weakened from a particularly intense labor (or from a number of labors or over time). A slack pelvic floor can lead to incontinence and urinary tract infections as well as pelvic organ prolapse—a rare but potentially scary situation that occurs when the muscles can no longer support the organs, causing them to fall into or out of the vagina. This area can be strengthened by doing Kegel exercises.

> Squats help lower back pain go away. Putting your back up against a wall and squatting down. It's really the only thing that helped me.
> —anonymom

kegels

Kegels are exercises designed to strengthen the pelvic floor muscles. Kegels can be done by contracting and releasing the muscles around your vagina in sets of ten or so. You can also try the "elevator technique," tightening the muscles progressively as if your pelvic floor were an elevator going up to the first, second, third, and fourth floors, and gradually releasing as you lower the "elevator" down. Ideally Kegels should be done a number of times a day during pregnancy and postpartum.

your body, everyone else's business

At no other time in your life would it be okay for someone to come up to you and say, "You're huge!" But this could happen to you every day when you're pregnant. It is never pleasant to be asked if you're carrying twins when you're not. It's even more unpleasant, after the humiliated, mumbling "No . . ." to be asked, "Are you sure?" And if you're most definitely *not* huge, you may hear that you're too skinny. Or not eating right. When your size isn't inspiration enough for commentary, your shape may be. There is a widespread (and totally unsubstantiated) belief that the way you carry your pregnancy sends secret messages about the sex of your baby or how your birth will pan out. In fact, the way you carry your pregnancy sends not-so-secret messages about how your body is built.

Pregnant bodies are, it seems, public property to evaluate and judge, and even to touch without asking. Unfortunately, there isn't much you can do to prevent people from saying annoying things. And in our experience, witty comebacks are a lot easier to come up with once you've seethed in silence for ten minutes and are well out of earshot. Unsolicited pregnancy commentary can serve a purpose: It provides warmup for the onslaught of unsolicited advice and opinion you'll get once the baby's born. If you learn to tune it out while pregnant, you'll be better prepared later.

I think I've always felt that as a woman, my body was somehow public property. But then, when I got pregnant, I couldn't believe how those comments went from covert to overt; who would say anything about your boobs to your face if you weren't pregnant?
—anonymom

If one more person asks me if I'm having twins, I'm going to scream, "No, I'm just fat, OK???"
—anonymom

I can't tell you how many people would talk to me about the shape of my belly, the position of my belly—half the time I would be fine with it, but there were times I would just come home and curl up in a ball and cry "*I don't want it anymore.*" It was like when someone notices your boobs when you're not thinking about your boobs and it throws you off.
—anonymom

Most people are lovely and kind. Some, however, do not realize how insensitive their comments might be . . . . There are those who feel the need to tell me it looks like I'm carrying twins (when in fact it's only one little boy). One girl even went so far as to say "No, I know you've got to have twins in there. You'll see I'm right when they're born!!" What???? Wow. What can I possibly even say to that?
—anonymom

I just think that it's odd that once you become pregnant, you're all of a sudden on a meat hook for people to just go ahead and say anything they darn well please. I wouldn't walk up to someone in the street and say, "Hey, you've got a big pouch there or a giant double chin!"
—anonymom

I came through a recent pregnancy without gaining much weight (a combination of being freakishly tall and losing my appetite completely), and found myself fielding a range of odd reactions, from predictable envy to a surprising amount of anger. I started to feel as if I was betraying some historical prerogative. The most common thing I heard: "If I were you, I'd look at pregnancy as permission to eat and get really fat." This stuck with me; what an interesting comment on women and denial.
—anonymom

getting bigger in a small-minded world

For a long time, pregnancy was somewhat isolated—and insulated—from the usual obscene pressure we place on women to attain physical perfection. Maternity clothes made a point of concealing rather than revealing a woman's shape. The pregnant uniform was some sort of secular burka comprised of muumuus and tent dresses, decorated with adorable ribbons (or businesslike ruffles if you were wearing the professional version). We've come a long way, baby. Sort of. The first nail in the old-school coffin may have been Demi Moore appearing naked and pregnant on the cover of *Vanity Fair* in 1991. She was pregnant yet sexy. Everyone was outraged! And then inspired. Slowly, pregnancy fashion started getting cooler. Then it started getting more and more revealing. Now pregnant women are finally allowed to be hot, sexy, gorgeous women . . . who happen to be pregnant. Clothes are tight instead of tents. Bellies are bared. We're all for the celebration of the pregnant shape, but the sexification of pregnancy has come with a price: Women are not just "allowed" to be hot while they're carrying a kid, they are expected to be. And since our culture's idea of hot is about as broad as a tightrope, this means that pregnant women are now subject to the same exact scrutiny as nonpregnant ones.

This "hot mama" mania has been fueled by a huge celebrity breeding frenzy. Every magazine seems to feature a spread lauding some superstar for her remarkable ability to keep her cravings under control. It's a little sad that the minute pregnancy was emancipated from its frumpy, sexless status, it immediately became another stage on which women could feel judged about how they look, or how they fail to live up to an ideal. You have some choice in the matter: Turn away from the celebrity sightings (this can mean lots of turning, but it is possible) and turn toward real body sightings to see just how different pregnant women's bodies can be.

documenting your pregnancy

Women with artistic inclinations (and even those without them) may have the urge to creatively capture their pregnancies. There are lots of ways to do this: journals, photographs, paintings, scrapbooks, songs. Then there's the classic plaster-of-paris belly cast, which gives a three-dimensional impression. These documentations can help make an ephemeral time seem more real, or help you remember what it was like later on.

Getting things down on paper (or film, or whatever) can also help you express and capture feelings that might not be easily communicated otherwise. Pregnancy art doesn't need to be considered in terms of an audience—though it certainly can be—it may just be a way of helping you process this incredible time for yourself.

fashion: dressing your pregnant self

The explosion of the maternity fashion industry has made pregnant dressing a lot less challenging. It's now pretty much possible to at least extend some of your style sensibility to your pregnant self. If looking fashionable while pregnant is important to you, there are no shortage of options for trendy, classic, boho, chic, rocker, athletic, sexy, or country-western maternity wear (if you're willing to pay the price in dollars and/or shopping time).

Some moms have a strong desire to stay hip and stylish while pregnant. Losing a fashion edge can bring up anxieties about "letting themselves go" and succumbing to the baby or even losing their identity. Other people couldn't care less about how they look, or can't stand spending money (whether they have it or not) on clothes they'll wear for only a few months, or even weeks at certain stages. They may want the cheapest wardrobe possible, or make do on what they can scrounge from friends or reinvent from nonmaternity clothes. Either way, pregnancy, as endless as it seems when you're staring at a closet full of undesirable options, is a brief phase in your fashion career. Your sartorial strategy for these months will not make or break the rest of your stylish life.

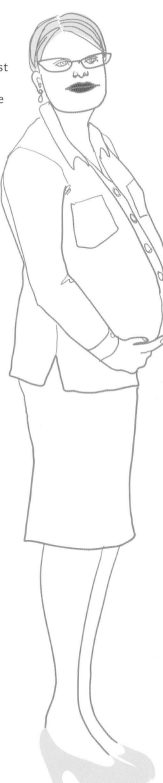

common fashion concerns of pregnancy

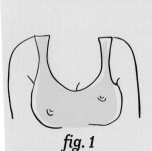

fig. 1

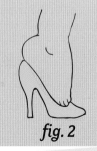

fig. 2

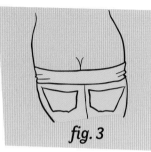

fig. 3

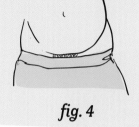

fig. 4

the endless no

A knowing eye can pick out a pregnant person, not by what she looks like, but by what she does. Or more specifically by what she *doesn't* do: what she turns down at a party, or how she refuses to set foot in the freshly painted lobby. Having a baby in the modern world can be one long tiptoe through the no-no's. More and more of the things we eat, drink, absorb, and inhale have become suspicious. Things are considered guilty until proven innocent. And since testing on pregnant women is rare (and risky), things are not often proven innocent.

Today's hypercautiousness is a backlash against yesterday's ignorance, when people thought the placenta was impervious and no harmful substances could pass through. It's taken a lot of tragedies for people to accept that this is not even close to the case. Now that we know, it's like we've opened Pandora's box. It seems like everything everywhere is a potential risk. Danger lurks at the dinner table, in the litter box, even in the air we breathe if we're in the wrong place at the wrong time. If you take the warnings at face value, it can be hard to walk down the street without feeling like you're dodging dangers with every step. Filtering the information can start to feel almost as problematic as filtering the toxins—but ignorance is only blissful if everything turns out fine. We need to find a way to balance caution with confidence. This may mean taking the warnings with a grain of salt. Or it may mean diving headfirst into the data and radically changing your life to lessen every suspected risk. Most of us probably settle somewhere between running for the hills and burying our heads in the sand.

All these prohibitions do carry an important message, though: As much as we want to protect our babies, ultimately, total protection is an impossibility. While our babies grow inside us, we all do the best we can and bet on the overwhelmingly good odds that they'll be okay. Just as we will be, after they're born.

This chapter is a pretty in-depth listing of everything that's considered questionable during pregnancy, why, and what you can do to try to lessen the risk if you're so inclined. If you don't care to delve into the details, you can check out the food chart below, skim the headings, or skip the chapter entirely and find out from your care provider what she really sees as crucial.

> Being sober among lushes is never as fun. —anonymom

> All I wanted for nine-ten months was beer and sushi. It was a constant battle. I ate a lot of avocado and chocolate chip cookies. I felt like they were my substitutes. —anonymom

resources

The Panic-Free Pregnancy by Michael S. Broder
The Complete Organic Pregnancy by Deirdre Dolan and Alexandra Zissu

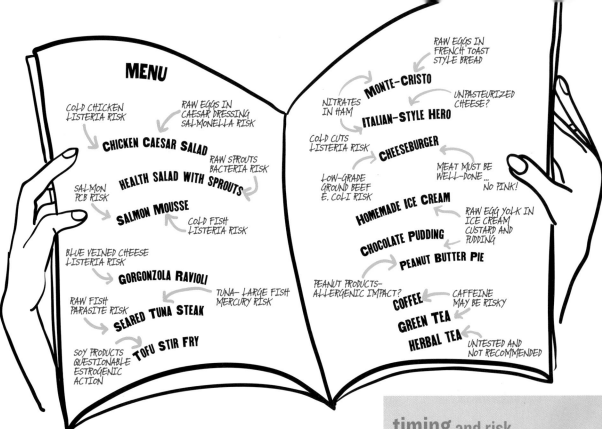

MENU

COLD CHICKEN
LISTERIA RISK

RAW EGGS IN
CAESAR DRESSING
SALMONELLA RISK

CHICKEN CAESAR SALAD

RAW SPROUTS
BACTERIA RISK

HEALTH SALAD WITH SPROUTS

SALMON
PCB RISK

SALMON MOUSSE

COLD FISH
LISTERIA RISK

BLUE VEINED CHEESE
LISTERIA RISK

GORGONZOLA RAVIOLI

RAW FISH
PARASITE RISK

TUNA– LARGE FISH
MERCURY RISK

SEARED TUNA STEAK

TOFU STIR FRY

SOY PRODUCTS
QUESTIONABLE
ESTROGENIC
ACTION

RAW EGGS IN
FRENCH TOAST
STYLE BREAD

MONTE-CRISTO

NITRATES
IN HAM

UNPASTEURIZED
CHEESE?

ITALIAN-STYLE HERO

COLD CUTS
LISTERIA RISK

CHEESEBURGER

MEAT MUST BE
WELL-DONE …
NO PINK!

LOW-GRADE
GROUND BEEF
E. COLI RISK

HOMEMADE ICE CREAM

RAW EGG YOLK IN
ICE CREAM
CUSTARD AND
PUDDING

CHOCOLATE PUDDING

PEANUT BUTTER PIE

PEANUT PRODUCTS–
ALLERGENIC IMPACT?

COFFEE

CAFFEINE
MAY BE RISKY

GREEN TEA

HERBAL TEA

UNTESTED AND
NOT RECOMMENDED

forbidden foods

Did you think food was *good* for you? Sucker. We're not talking your run-of-the-mill trans fats here. That ten-dollar organic sandwich you're holding is a breeding ground for bacteria. Salad bar? An orgy of organisms. Between the mercury, the PCBs, and the risk of parasites, you may as well forget about fish. So much for those omega-3s. Meat could have *E. coli* or other germs if it's not cooked through. But don't let it burn! That's carcinogenic. And check for nitrates, too; those can't be good for your baby. Considering vegetarianism? Don't forget that magazine article you read about the dangers of soy!

How the hell is a pregnant woman supposed to eat? Ultimately, it's about risk assessment. We can't know for sure what's going to make us sick and what isn't. What we know is what's more likely to be harmful, though just *how much* more likely may be a little harder to figure out. The following pages cover the major factors in the world of pregnancy food safety.

timing and risk

During the very early weeks (before a missed period) the embryo has not yet implanted in the uterus. So exposure to a drug or another teratogenic (fetus-damaging) substance at this time may prevent implantation and cause a miscarriage, but it will not cause birth defects. Some call this the all-or-nothing phase, and it's why women are often told not to worry about any drinks they had before they knew they were pregnant—provided they found out right away. The weeks immediately following the missed period are the ones in which the embryo is most vulnerable to major birth defects. After 8 weeks of development (that's 10 weeks of pregnancy on the 40-week calendar) the risk of major defects decreases, but the risk for neurological, brain, and growth issues goes up.

63

FOODS CONSIDERED RISKY DURING PREGNANCY

There are varying opinions on these guidelines; speak to your healthcare provider to find out what he or she recommends. More details on risk factors are given throughout this chapter.

FOOD	POTENTIAL RISK
DAIRY	
Unpasteurized dairy products: raw milk, soft cheeses like Brie, bleu cheese, queso fresco (unless they're made with pasteurized milk)	Listeriosis → See page 65.
EGGS	
Undercooked eggs and foods that contain them	Salmonella bacteria
MEATS	
Cold cuts, deli meats, hot dogs, leftovers (unless heated to steaming hot)	Listeriosis
Liver	High levels of vitamin A, which may be harmful to a fetus
Raw or rare meat	Toxoplasmosis, other bacteria → See page 66.
Refrigerated pâté and meat spreads	Listeriosis
FISH	
Farmed salmon, some local freshwater fish	PCBs → See page 73.
Raw/undercooked fish, especially shellfish	Parasites, bacteria → See The Story wih Sushi, page 65.
Refrigerated smoked fish (unless hot)	Listeriosis
Swordfish, shark, king mackerel, tilefish, other large fish	High mercury content → See fish chart, page 74.
FRUITS AND VEGETABLES	
Peanuts and peanut products (with family history of food allergy)	Possibly increased chance of allergy in allergy-prone children (more research is needed)
Raw sprouts	Bacteria
Unpasteurized fruits/vegetable juice	Bacteria → See page 65.
Unwashed raw fruits and vegetables	Toxoplasmosis, bacteria
BEVERAGES	
Alcohol	Fetal Alcohol Spectrum Disorder → See page 68.
Caffeine	Lots of caffeine associated with miscarriage → See page 67.
Herbal teas	Unknown effects on pregnancy → See page 70.

FOOD-BORNE ILLNESS: Because pregnancy affects the immune system, pregnant women are more vulnerable to illness from contaminated food (and illness can be harder to treat because medication may be unsafe). However, most forms of food poisoning do not pose a direct risk to the fetus, with the exceptions of listeriosis and toxoplasmosis, which can be very dangerous, even fatal, to a fetus in development.

GENERAL FOOD SAFETY PRECAUTIONS:

- *Raw foods are more likely to be contaminated than cooked ones.* Wash all raw fruits and vegetables carefully. Pre-washed packaged salads are at especially high risk for contamination. Do not use, or rewash them thoroughly before eating.

- *Cooking foods further reduces the chance of bacterial infection.* Meats should be cooked through for the lowest risk.

- *Store meats away from other foods in the fridge.* Keep kitchen and fridge surfaces clean, especially after they have come into contact with raw meats.

- *Keep your refrigerator below 40 degrees F to reduce bacterial growth.*

- *Reheat refrigerated foods thoroughly; use them promptly.*

- *Always wash hands before and after handling foods.*

LISTERIOSIS: Listeriosis is caused by the bacteria *Listeria monocytogenes*. According to the CDC, there are about 2,500 cases of listeriosis in the United States each year. Pregnant women account for about a third of these cases. The risk of listeriosis is very small (it affects about .02 percent of U.S. pregnancies, or 1 in 5,000). *Listeria* risk is highest in pâtés, unpasteurized cheeses, deli meats, and smoked fish, but it can be present in any raw food, even on the skins of vegetables and fruits. The disease can cross the placenta, causing miscarriage, stillbirths, or health problems for the baby after birth. Infected babies have a high mortality rate. It can also be fatal for the mother. So healthcare providers suggest that pregnant women take prevention guidelines seriously, even though cases are rare. Listeriosis has an incubation period of from a few days to eight weeks. Symptoms in pregnant women can resemble the flu, but there may be no symptoms. A blood test can confirm the disease, which is treated by antibiotics. Early treatment lessens the chance that the fetus will be infected.

resources

Centers for Disease Control and Prevention/Foodborne Illness Line (24-hour recorded information): 888-232-3228 or cdc.gov/foodsafety

U.S. Food and Drug Administration Center for Food Safety & Applied Nutrition: 888-SAFEFOOD or cfsan.fda.gov

the story with sushi

Sushi is one of pregnancy's most famous prohibitions. But is it really a serious risk? Here's the deal: Raw fish can be inhabited, very occasionally, by parasites. The risk is higher for home-prepared sushi and with certain kinds of fish (freshwater, in particular). Because sushi is a raw food, it also can harbor bacteria. This risk is higher with prepackaged sushi than freshly made sushi. Parasites don't present a direct threat to a fetus, but they can compromise a pregnant woman's health, and if left untreated could theoretically interfere with the fetus's nutrition. Some people think these consequences are too great even if the chances are minimal. Others feel that eating sushi in a reputable establishment with high-quality fish is not a major risk. Those who do choose to eat sushi should be aware of the mercury content. Many popular sushi fish are at the high end of the mercury scale.

→ See chart, page 74, for details on the best and worst sushi fish regarding mercury consumption.
→ See Mercury, page 73.

to minimize risk

- Avoid pâté, unpasteurized cheese, deli meats, and smoked fish.
- Wash raw foods thoroughly before eating.
- See the food chart on page 64 for foods to avoid.

TOXOPLASMOSIS: Toxoplasmosis is a parasitic infection. The best-known source of infection is cat feces, but you can also get it from eating under-cooked infected meat, raw eggs and milk, and from contact with infected soil, which may contaminate fruits and vegetables. Toxoplasmosis can cross the placenta and cause severe problems in a newborn. It's rare—only .01—.02 percent (or 1—2 per 1,000) babies born in the United States each year are infected. The risk of serious damage is greater early in a pregnancy. Toxo-plasmosis often has no symptoms, but it can cause fever, fatigue, sore throat, and/or swollen glands. The infection can be treated with antibiotics, which can help prevent or reduce impact on the fetus. If you've had toxoplas-mosis before, you may be immune. A blood test can confirm whether or not you're likely to be susceptible.

to minimize risk

- Wash all fruits and vegetables.
- Cook all meats past the pink point.
- Avoid contact with cat feces (especially important with outdoor cats).
- Wash hands after gardening and/or wear gloves.
- Wash hands after contact with high-risk foods.
- See the food chart on page 64 for foods to avoid.

THE SOY CONTROVERSY: Soy has been touted as a miracle food and even a cancer cure. But soy products have raised some concern lately, largely because they contain phytoestrogens, which are suspected of lowering tes-tosterone and potentially affecting development of the fetal reproductive organs. This is a relatively new (or new-to-the-public) theory, so it's not clear how it will shake down when there has been more research. For now (at the point of this writing, anyway) soy is not considered a particular concern in pregnancy.

to minimize risk

- Vary your diet.
- Don't eat huge quantities of soy while this question remains unanswered.

NITRATES AND NITRITES: Nitrates and nitrites are found in water and foods, largely in processed meat products. Nitrates in food products are not considered a particular problem for pregnant women (though since they are carcinogenic, they are not the healthiest food choice). But nitrates in well water can be dangerous.

to minimize risk

■ **If you use well water, get your water tested for nitrates, which can be reduced by filters.**

CAFFEINE: There's a general agreement that caffeine should be limited during pregnancy, but a lot less agreement about what the limits should be. In 1980, as a result of a study that linked caffeine with birth defects in rats, pregnant women were discouraged from drinking caffeinated beverages. This rat study was later questioned considering the rats were given doses equivalent to more than fifty cups of coffee per day. Women who drink a lot of caffeine (which is defined as five, six, seven, or more cups of coffee per day, depending on the study) have a higher risk of miscarriage, birth defects, or stillbirth. Recent studies suggest similar effects at lower doses, so it's often recommended that pregnant women drink as little caffeine as possible. Some say a cup of coffee a day (or equivalent) is fine; others are more cautious. Caffeine content varies (a cup of coffee can range from 65 to 300 milligrams of caffeine depending on strength and size; caffeinated soda is usually 20—80 milligrams).

Green tea may be risky for another reason. The tea's cancer-fighting ingredients can interfere with folic acid absorption. Drinking large quantities of green tea during early pregnancy may increase the risk of neural tube defects.

to minimize risk

■ **Limit or avoid caffeine.**

ARTIFICIAL SWEETENERS: Artificial sweeteners are considered safe in moderation during pregnancy, with the exception of saccharin (and cyclamate, which is banned in the United States). Stevia, a natural sugar substitute, is not approved for use as a food additive and therefore not recommended for pregnant women. Many herbalists claim that stevia is completely safe, and that the controversy stems from the challenge the sweet herb poses to the artificial sweetener business.

to minimize risk

■ **Use artificial sweeteners in moderation or avoid.**

ALCOHOL: It is known that in high and/or frequent doses, alcohol is very dangerous to the health of a growing fetus. Fetal Alcohol Spectrum Disorder can cause major developmental and emotional problems, facial disfiguration, slow learning, and other really, really bad stuff for your baby. Because no safe level of alcohol consumption has been medically proven, most doctors prescribe zero alcohol during pregnancy. This recommendation is echoed throughout the world, although some have a more relaxed take on very moderate drinking during pregnancy.

At this point there is no real way to measure the exact risk of an occasional glass of wine affecting the fetus. Some think even a sip is irresponsible while others think the prohibition on alcohol is extremist. The fact that many of our mothers drank during pregnancy is often used as an example. We now know that different women's bodies process alcohol in different ways, which makes it even more difficult to set a safe threshold.

In the end, all parenting behavior, both pre- and postnatal, is a matter of choice. If you do choose to drink a little during pregnancy (especially if you do it in public), be prepared for judgmental responses from others.

to minimize risk

- **Avoid alcohol during pregnancy.**

sympathetic abstinence

If you can't drink, does that mean your partner can't drink, either? Some couples take a "We're in this together" approach—the nonpregnant party cuts out or cuts down on alcohol and other forbidden fruits to avoid tempting the mother-to-be (or else, nauseating her with his barfy booze breath, or embarrassing himself in a lone drunken stupor). Others are less chivalrous and more pragmatic: "What's the point of not drinking? *I'm* not pregnant." Some pregnant women feel like it's unfair to drag a loved one into a world of unnecessary denial. They may feel guilty, not pleased, to see their partner abstaining—or prefer that a partner pull their weight in other ways. Whatever you decide, having the support of your partner can make it a lot easier to give up ingredients that were formerly part of your culinary lifestyle. You may need your partner's cooperation, for example, to keep certain foods out of the refrigerator if you find them hard to resist. And patience during your seven-minute interview with a waiter about the safety of various menu items is always appreciated.

→ See Adjusting to Life with a Vessel, page 80.

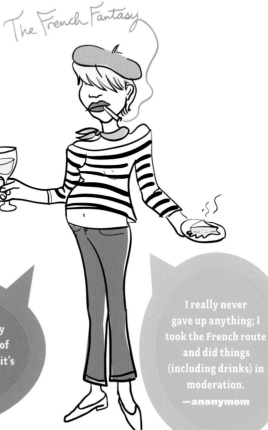

The French Fantasy

> I lived in London while I was in my first trimester and my doctor recommended two glasses of wine a day (yes, not a week!!—Hey, it's okay America!!!).
> —anonymom

> I really never gave up anything; I took the French route and did things (including drinks) in moderation.
> —anonymom

DRUGS AND MEDICATIONS: Under normal circumstances in the modern world, pills are one of the first lines of defense against any ache or pain we may come up against. But we're told to avoid drug use during pregnancy if at all possible. What are the risks of drug use during pregnancy? What's okay and what isn't?

There are varying opinions on the safety of medication use by pregnant women, and the opinion most definitely varies with each medication. The question is really about weighing the risk of the drug against the risk of the illness. When a mother has a life-threatening condition, the stakes can help clarify the choice. But when it's a matter of her comfort, things get a little more confusing.

In general, the first trimester is considered the time of greatest vulnerability to drugs (with exceptions—some drugs, aspirin, for example, are most problematic in the last trimester). A few drugs must absolutely be avoided during pregnancy. The acne drug Accutane, for example, has been strongly associated with birth defects and must not be taken by women who are or may become pregnant.

Drug use during pregnancy is something that should always be discussed with your healthcare provider. Although many over-the-counter medications are considered safe during pregnancy, some are not. Your doctor or midwife will have access to information about individual drugs and can give you a recommendation about how to treat whatever might be causing you trouble. Self-medicating when you're pregnant is a risky proposition. → See Emotional Landscape of Pregnancy, page 79, for antidepressant information.

fda pregnancy-drug categories

The FDA classifies drugs according to how much is known about their safety during pregnancy. These classifications help healthcare providers make decisions about which medications to recommend:

A Adequate, well-controlled studies in pregnant women have not shown an increased risk of fetal abnormalities to the fetus in any trimester of pregnancy. Very few medications are in this category.

B Animal studies have revealed no evidence of harm to the fetus; however, there are no adequate and well-controlled studies in pregnant women.

OR

Animal studies have shown an adverse effect, but adequate and well-controlled studies in pregnant women have failed to demonstrate a risk to the fetus in any trimester.

C Animal studies have shown an adverse effect and there are no adequate and well-controlled studies in pregnant women.

OR

No animal studies have been conducted and there are no adequate and well-controlled studies in pregnant women.

D Adequate, well-controlled or observational studies in pregnant women have demonstrated a risk to the fetus.

However, the benefits of therapy may outweigh the potential risk. For example, the drug may be acceptable if needed in a life-threatening situation or serious disease for which safer drugs cannot be used or are ineffective.

X Adequate, well-controlled or observational studies in animals or pregnant women have demonstrated positive evidence of fetal abnormalities or risks.

RECREATIONAL DRUGS: Recreational drug use is totally discouraged during pregnancy. Many drugs have known negative effects, ranging from higher risk of miscarriage to birth defects to addiction in the newborn. Others, marijuana in particular, are less conclusively harmful (according to information available at this point) but have been associated with some neurological or behavioral problems. Since drugs are sometimes taken in combination, figuring out what causes what is complicated. The general recommendation is to avoid drugs altogether during pregnancy, and if you can't, to seek help.

SMOKING: Smoking is harmful during pregnancy. There's a lot of information about how smoking negatively affects babies, partly because there are so many people who subject themselves to the experiment. Despite warnings, many pregnant women still smoke. A 2002 count put the number at somewhere above 10 percent. Smoking during pregnancy is associated with increased risk of miscarriage, stillbirth, premature delivery, and Sudden Infant Death Syndrome. The risk goes up most with maternal smoking but a lot of secondhand smoke increases risk as well. There are also questions about the long-term effect of smoking on babies.

to minimize risk

- **Quit smoking as soon as you know you are pregnant.**
- **If you can't quit, cut down as much as you possibly can and discuss options with your healthcare provider.**
- **Avoid regular exposure to secondhand smoke.**

resources

National drug help hotline: 800-662-4357

Substance Abuse and Mental Health Services Administration (including facility locator): dasis3.samhsa.gov

Information on smoking-cessation practices for pregnant and postpartum women: pregnets.org

HERBS: Many doctors suggest avoiding herbs during pregnancy altogether, largely because their effects are even less studied than those of pharmaceutical medications. When there are recommendations, they are often contradictory. Some say chamomile tea is safe—even recommended for its calming and anti-inflammatory properties. Others say chamomile should be used cautiously or completely avoided because it can cause uterine contractions. Why so much confusion? Well, herbs are a lot less regulated than pharmaceuticals. This means it's harder to get an authoritative answer on what's safe. It also means that concentrations can vary tremendously. So while most people would agree that a cup of commercially processed chamomile tea is not a problem, a massage with concentrated chamomile oil might be more questionable.

Culinary herbs are fine to consume in normal amounts. Infusions made from food products such as citrus peel, ginger, cinnamon, mint, lemongrass, blackberries, rose hips, etc., are considered safe to drink in weak blends and in moderation. Many say supermarket-style herbal teas are also fine to drink. You can check with your doctor or midwife to get her opinion. If you're really interested in going the herbal route during pregnancy, it's important to consult with an educated herbalist (not just the clerk at the health food store) and keep your health practitioner in the loop. There are lots of herbs contraindicated during pregnancy for very good reasons.

RASPBERRY LEAF TEA: Raspberry leaf tea is often recommended during pregnancy for its supposed benefits in labor and childbirth. Studies of this positive effect are inconclusive, though many women believe the tea has helped them have shorter and easier births. At any rate there is some question about whether the tea is safe in the early part of pregnancy or if it may stimulate the uterus at a time when stimulation would not be beneficial. Those who are at high risk for miscarriage or preterm labor especially should avoid the tea until they are full term.

to minimize risk

- Avoid medicinal herbs during pregnancy, or consult an herbalist before using any.

resources

Herbs for a Healthy Pregnancy: From Conception to Childbirth by Penelope Ody
Wise Woman Herbal for the Childbearing Year by Susun S. Weed

I used to be a pretty heavy herbal tea drinker. My kitchen shelves were overflowing with bags of mint with rose petals, cans of spice infusions, and boxes of detox blend. I found out I was pregnant while I was away from home, sick with a cold, and eager for comfort. I knew I couldn't take anything, but surely some herbal tea couldn't hurt? I wanted to be sure, so we made a special trip to the health food store to try to research and stock up on the healthiest, safest options for my new situation. I flipped through a few books and found many of my favorite teas were off the okay list. Who knew mint and chamomile were uterine stimulants? I kept seeing recommendations for raspberry leaf tea. Back in my hotel room, I snuggled into the chintz armchair with a steaming hot cup and my new pregnancy guidebook, drinking in the aroma of my new extracareful existence. Three soothing minutes later, I turned the page to find a bold box: "Do NOT drink Raspberry Leaf Tea in the first trimester! May Cause Miscarriage!" How soothing.
—Rebecca

licorice

A recent study showed that pregnant women who consumed two and a half packages of true black licorice a week were twice as likely to experience premature labor as women who ate none. Licorice can increase prostaglandins, which are hormone-like substances that can encourage labor. Most popular licorice-flavored candies (like the kind you'd get in a supermarket or at the movies) do not contain actual licorice.

fear of a toxic planet: an activist aside

If you think environmental protection is about tree-hugging and the looming global-warming threat, we've got some disturbing news. Human beings are in fact a *part* of the environment. We are being polluted along with our planet. Nothing is a clearer, or scarier, indication of this than the fact that a newborn baby has already come into contact with hundreds of toxic chemicals by the time it is born. A study of ten babies born in 2004 at two independent laboratories found an average of two hundred different chemicals in the newborns' cord blood:

Of the 287 chemicals we detected in umbilical cord blood, we know that 180 cause cancer in humans or animals, 217 are toxic to the brain and nervous system, and 208 cause birth defects or abnormal development in animal tests. The dangers of pre- or post-natal exposure to this complex mixture of carcinogens, developmental toxins and neurotoxins have never been studied.

—Environmental Working Group, *BodyBurden: The Pollution in Newborns*

We're not saying this to freak you out about the safety of your baby. Lots and lots of healthy babies are born, year after year, after much more significant exposure to toxic chemicals than is likely in day-to-day life. Touching your dog's flea collar is not cause for panic. Neither is getting an occasional lungful of tailpipe from a passing bus. In all likelihood, the place where you live and the water you drink and the air you breathe are just fine.

But do we really want to just give up and let things be? Fights rage on in the government about the sanctity of life from the moment of conception. If the fetus is so sacred, shouldn't someone be regulating the chemicals that are believed to do fetal harm? When it comes to the individual, there's plenty of regulation. Don't eat this, don't drink that. We're told to avoid even a sip of alcohol in pregnancy: No safe threshold has been established. Safe fetal thresholds haven't been established for any of the other toxins in the world around us, either. But those, we don't have a choice about. Protecting our environment is the same as protecting our children. If we don't do it, who will?

resources

Having Faith: An Ecologist's Journey to Motherhood by Sandra Steingraber

Collaborative on Health and the Environment: healthandenvironment.org

Environmental Working Group: ewg.org

Natural Resources Defense Council: nrdc.org

The Sierra Club: sierraclub.org

taking charge of toxins

Many of the toxins a mother has been exposed to are stored in her body, sometimes for months, sometimes for years, sometimes forever. It's not always possible to prevent those toxins from being passed on to the fetus. But there are some things you can control. Here's what you need to know to minimize exposure.

LEAD: Lead exposure during pregnancy can increase risk of miscarriage, low birthweight, and developmental delays in the baby. Lead can be found in drinking water (from lead pipes), in the soil and air (from industrial waste), and in leftover lead paint. Lead paint was used in most U.S. buildings before it was banned in 1978.

minimizing exposure

- Avoid contact with chipping or peeling paint.

- Do not strip or sand paint during your pregnancy. If there is stripping or sanding going on, leave the house until all the dust is removed.

- Let the tap run for a few minutes before collecting drinking water from old pipes. A water filter also helps.

- You can also avoid eating or drinking from crystal glassware and lead-glazed ceramics, though it's unclear how much of a risk these materials might pose.

MERCURY: Mercury is a neurotoxin that is amplified when it gets ingested by marine life. The major risk for mercury exposure in pregnant women is eating contaminated fish. The higher a fish is on the food chain, the greater the concentration of mercury. The lists that follow, from the Natural Resources Defense Council, detail which fish (and sushi fish) are highest and lowest risk for mercury exposure and offer dietary recommendations for pregnant and nursing mothers. See the next page for details.

minimizing exposure

- Highest mercury fish: Avoid.

- High mercury fish: Eat a maximum of three (6-ounce) servings monthly.

- Lower mercury fish: Eat a maximum of six (6-ounce) servings monthly.

- Lowest mercury fish: Can be eaten more frequently.

PCBs: Polychlorinated biphenyls (PCBs) are industrial chemicals. They are thought to be carcinogenic. Some studies have shown that PCBs may have an impact on fetal brain development when ingested in large quantities during pregnancy. Banned in 1976, PCBs have had a persistent effect on the environment and can still be found in high concentrations in fatty fish.

minimizing exposure

- Avoid eating game-caught fish from local lakes and streams, which are often contaminated with PCBs. Or check your local resources to confirm safety.

- Farmed salmon has high levels of PCBs, both due to feeding practices and high fat content. Wild salmon is significantly lower in PCBs.

GUIDE TO MERCURY IN FISH

HIGHEST MERCURY
Grouper
Marlin
Orange roughy
Tilefish
Swordfish
Shark
Mackerel (king)

HIGH MERCURY
Bass (saltwater)
Croaker
Halibut
Tuna (canned, white albacore)
Tuna (fresh bluefin, ahi)
Sea trout
Bluefish
Lobster (American/Maine)

LOWER MERCURY
Carp
Mahimahi
Crab (Dungeness)
Snapper
Crab (blue)
Crab (snow)
Monkfish
Perch (freshwater)
Skate
Cod
Tuna (canned, chunk light)
Tuna (fresh Pacific albacore)

LOWEST MERCURY
Anchovies
Butterfish
Calamari (squid)
Caviar (farmed)
Crab (king)

Pollock
Catfish
Whitefish
Perch (ocean)
Scallops
Flounder
Haddock
Hake
Herring
Lobster(spiny/rock)
Shad
Sole
Crawfish/crayfish
Salmon
Shrimp
Clams
Tilapia
Oysters
Sardines
Sturgeon (farmed)
Trout (freshwater)

© Natural Resources Defense Council. See nrdc.org for more information, including which fish to avoid for environmental impact.

GUIDE TO MERCURY IN SUSHI

HIGHEST MERCURY
Kajiki (swordfish)
Saba (mackerel)

HIGH MERCURY
Ahi (yellowfin tuna)
Buri (adult yellowtail)
Hamachi (young yellowtail)
Inada (very young yellowtail)
Kanpachi (very young yellowtail)
Katsuo (bonito)
Maguro (bigeye, bluefin, or yellowfin tuna)
Makjiki (blue marlin)
Masu (trout)
Meji (young bigeye, bluefin, or yellowfin tuna)
Shiro (albacore tuna)
Toro (bigeye, bluefin, or yellowfin tuna)

LOWER MERCURY
Kani (crab)
Seigo (young sea bass)
Suzuki (sea bass)

LOWEST MERCURY
Aji (horse mackerel)
Akagai (ark shell)
Anago (conger eel)
Aoyagi (round clam)
Awabi (abalone)
Ayu (sweetfish)
Ebi (shrimp)
Hamaguri (clam)
Hamo (pike conger; sea eel)
Hatahata (sandfish)
Himo (ark shell)
Hokkigai (surf clam)
Hotategai (scallop)
Ika (squid)
Ikura (salmon roe)

Kaibashira (shellfish)
Kaiware (daikon-radish sprouts)
Karei (flatfish)
Kohada (gizzard shad)
Masago (smelt egg)
Mirugai (surf clam)
Nori-tama (egg)
Sake (salmon)
Sawara (Spanish mackerel)
Sayori (halfbeak)
Shako (mantis shrimp)
Tai (sea bream)
Tairagai (razor-shell clam)
Tako (octopus)
Tamago (egg)
Tobiko (flying fish egg)
Torigai (cockle)
Tsubugai (shellfish)
Unagi (freshwater eel)
Uni (sea urchin roe)

PESTICIDES AND HERBICIDES: Studies have shown that first-trimester exposure to pesticides and herbicides from nearby industrial spraying was associated with a higher rate of birth defects. Extended (1-month) exposure to pesticides and insecticides in the home or work environment during early pregnancy was associated with a much higher rate of stillbirths. No evidence shows that using insect repellent with DEET increases the chance of birth defects or problems in pregnancy, but some suggest limiting its use.

minimizing exposure

- Avoid pesticides whenever possible, including home and garden use.
- If pesticide application is necessary, remove yourself from the area, ventilate, and take care to protect food and food-prep areas from pesticide residue.
- Pregnant women who live in agricultural areas where pesticides are used should consider relocating for weeks 3—8 (gestation), when the fetus is most vulnerable.
- Apply insect repellent to long sleeves and long pants rather than skin.
- Eat organic when possible, or choose low-pesticide produce.

NONSTICK AND STAIN-RESISTANT PRODUCTS: Perfluorooctanoic acid (PFOA) is a chemical found in items such as nonstick pans, stain-resistant coatings, and microwave popcorn bags, to name a few. PFOA has become somewhat controversial and is being investigated as a possible carcinogen, though no link has yet been shown. The EPA has reached an agreement with major manufacturers of PFOA products to phase out the chemical by 2015. PFOA can be found in the vast majority of newborns' cord blood.

minimizing exposure

- Teflon pans should be used on low temperatures and not heated empty.
- Microwaving food in glass or ceramic is safer than cardboard or plastic.

pesticides **on produce**

Studies that link pesticides/herbicides to birth defects refer to acute exposure, not residual chemicals on foods. There is very little data on whether pesticides on foods have health risks for the general public or pregnant women. The government assures us that eating food treated with pesticides is safe, but some are skeptical. Organic produce has no pesticides by definition; some produce is not organic but is pesticide-free. Peeling fruits and vegetables as well as washing can help reduce the pesticides, though some will probably remain.

Some foods are more likely to be contaminated than others. These are the most and least pesticide-heavy conventionally grown produce (after washing). For more details, see foodnews.org.

TWELVE MOST CONTAMINATED	TWELVE LEAST CONTAMINATED
• Apples	• Asparagus
• Bell peppers	• Avocados
• Celery	• Bananas
• Cherries	• Broccoli
• Imported grapes	• Cauliflower
• Nectarines	• Corn (sweet)
• Peaches	• Kiwi
• Pears	• Mangos
• Potatoes	• Onions
• Red raspberries	• Papaya
• Spinach	• Peas (sweet)
• Strawberries	• Pineapples

PAINT AND SOLVENTS: Painting during pregnancy is generally discouraged, but it's not clear whether there is any real risk in using latex paints for limited time and with adequate protection. Oil-based or lacquer paints contain organic solvents that are hazardous in pregnancy. Pregnant artists should also be aware that many art paints contain lead and other potentially dangerous materials. Dry-cleaning solvents are also toxic.

minimizing exposure

- If you do decide to paint, ventilate and wear protective clothing to minimize skin contact.
- Avoid bringing paint-stained clothes into your living environment or washing them with your laundry.
- Avoid oil-based paint, turpentine, and other solvents, particularly during the first trimester. Avoid using powdered pigments during pregnancy.
- Avoid dry-cleaning chemicals.

resources

The Artist's Complete Health and Safety Guide by Monona Rossol
Arts, Crafts & Theater Safety, 212-777-0062, or
ACTSNYC@cs.com or artscraftstheatersafety.org

beauty products and treatments

There are chemicals in almost everything we put on our bodies, from hair spray to toenail polish. Many of us take for granted that these products are tested and safe, but testing of cosmetic products is actually quite limited. Cosmetics do not have to undergo government testing before reaching the shelf. According to the Environmental Working Group, "research shows that the industry itself has safety assessed just 11 percent of the 10,500 chemical ingredients used in personal care products." If ingredients have not been tested much at all, they certainly haven't been tested on pregnant women! Whether any of these substances pose a risk during pregnancy is unknown. In general, most people (including doctors) seem to see hair-, skin-, and body-care products (shampoos, moisturizers, lotions, etc.) and other things that are applied topically as fairly safe during pregnancy. But there are some ingredients that are questioned by consumer safety organizations and others.

The chemicals listed below are found in a huge quantity of the products we use on a daily basis, so it seems unlikely that normal use during pregnancy presents any major health threat. If you discover any of them in your favorite products, don't feel compelled to discontinue their use. Much of this research is still preliminary and it's not at all clear that there is any risk. If you prefer, you could look for another product (try health food stores) to limit your exposure.

PHTHALATES: Phthalates are used for lots of purposes in cosmetics—as emollients, plasticizers, and to help products penetrate the skin. They're found primarily in perfumes, hair sprays, deodorants, perfumes, and nail polishes. Studies have linked phthalates to birth defects in animals, which has raised questions about the safety of these ingredients. Some cosmetic companies have taken note of this worry and are phasing out phthalates from their products, particularly nail polishes.

label awareness *Dibutyl phthalate, DBP, diethyl phthalate, dibutyl ester, phthalic acid, and dimethyl phthalate*

PARABENS: Parabens are antimicrobial preservatives, and can be found in an estimated 75—90 percent of cosmetics and body products. A 2004 study from the *Journal of Applied Toxicology* questioned the safety of parabens because they were found to mimic the female hormone estrogen and suspected of contributing to cancer, specifically breast tumors. Other studies have questioned the impact of parabens on the fetal development of reproductive organs.

label awareness *Butyl-, ethyl-, methyl-, propyl-paraben*

METHYISOTHIAZOLINONE (MIT): This antibacterial/antifungal ingredient is found in shampoos and lotions. MIT has been under some question since 2004 study results from the University of Pittsburgh showed that the chemical harmed developing nerve cells in rats. It is unclear whether the risk extends to humans or whether normal exposure presents any risk.

label awareness *Methyisothiazolinone, MIT*

HAIR DYEING, BLEACHING, STRAIGHTENING, PERMING: Despite popular belief, there is no real indication that moderate use of hair treatments is unsafe in pregnancy. The familiar image of a pregnant woman with roots halfway down her head was inspired by a twenty-year-old study that found a slight increase in miscarriages among hair-care professionals who did a large number of chemical treatments weekly. More recent studies (1990s) did not show the same association. Although data do not show any risk of chemical hair treatments at any point in pregnancy, there are some even less risky options for the extracautious.

to minimize risk

- **Wait until the first trimester is over to chemically treat your hair.**

- **Choose a process that does not require leaving chemicals on the scalp for an extended time.**

- **Use dye with a minimum of chemical ingredients, such as vegetable dye.**

resources

A Consumer's Dictionary of Cosmetic Ingredients: Complete Information About the Harmful and Desirable Ingredients in Cosmetics and Cosmeceuticals by Ruth Winter

The Safe Shopper's Bible: A Consumer's Guide to Nontoxic Household Products by David Steinman and Samuel S. Epstein

Household Products Database: householdproducts.nlm.nih.gov

HOT STUFF (SAUNAS, HOT TUBS, STEAM ROOMS, HOT BATHS, ELECTRIC BLANKETS, SUN): Because abnormally high body temperatures have been associated with a higher risk of birth defects, pregnant women are told to avoid getting overheated. If you do go into the heat, limiting your exposure can limit your risk (10 minutes maximum is recommended). Electric blanket use has been associated with a possible increase in the first-trimester miscarriage rate.

to minimize risk

- Avoid or limit time in hot tubs, saunas, or steam rooms.
- Avoid electric blankets.
- Don't let yourself get excessively hot in the sun or during exercise.
- Keep bath temperatures below 100 degrees F.

TANNING: Aside from potentially raising body temperature, tanning is sometimes discouraged during pregnancy because the skin is more sensitive. In general, moderate tanning is not considered especially dangerous. Tanning beds should be avoided during the first trimester because of a possible link between UV rays and folic acid deficiency. Self-tanners are sometimes suggested as an alternative, but some suggest avoiding them or waiting until after the first trimester because, like most cosmetics, it's unclear whether the active ingredients penetrate the skin.

treatments that may have to wait

Cosmetic procedures such as Botox and other injectables as well as some chemical peels are often discouraged during pregnancy. Spa wraps, which can raise the body temperature, may also be unsafe.

resources

The Complete Guide to Everyday Risks in Pregnancy and Breastfeeding by Gideon Koren

March of Dimes Pregnancy and Newborn Health Education Center: marchofdimes.com/pnhec

Motherisk: motherisk.org

Organization of Teratology Information Specialists: otispregnancy.org

the pregnant brain

emotional landscape of pregnancy

One of the big challenges of pregnancy is adjusting to adjusting. The way you feel about yourself and your situation will very likely go through as many changes as your physique. One day you'll be reveling in your special status. The next, reviling life in pregnant limbo. The emotions are endless.

Some feelings you might have over the course of your pregnancy (or over the course of an afternoon):

> I feel proud to be pregnant … very happy and content.
> —anonymom

Anxious Crazy Excited Regretful Overwhelmed Guilty
Frustrated Lazy Alone Fulfilled Calm Meta- Giddy Angry
Content Important Sad Confused Connected Attached Happy

> I *loved* being pregnant, I felt very connected to the life inside of me and felt privileged to have the ability to carry a child.
> —anonymom

> I am amazed. What an incredible thing we can do!
> —anonymom

> Frantic one minute. Calm another.
> —anonymom

> I am depressed that I don't have more energy to get simple things done (e.g., wash my hair, fill the dishwasher, make dinner for my family).
> —anonymom

> I'm worried I'm going to crash after the birth.
> —anonymom

> I was totally surprised about the doubts that surfaced regarding whether I actually want to be a parent or not.
> —anonymom

> I'm happy but finding it hard to express with all the queasy-making progesterone flowing.
> —anonymom

> I'm excited for labor and birth. I'm excited to meet this little person who's growing in my body. I'm excited to share all of this with my partner. I'm excited to see him as a father. I'm excited about seeing someone who looks like the two of us. I'm excited to watch this kid grow up and become him- or herself. A lot of being pregnant is really just feeling ill and uncomfortable. But when I think about how I feel about being pregnant, the crappy stuff fades into the background.
> —anonymom

relationships in pregnancy

Pregnancy doesn't just swell your body and rewire your brain; it can also alter your relationships. One study found that women described their relationships in pregnancy as more changing than stable throughout. Sometimes the changes are predictable, like when you have friends or family members who are freaked out by the idea of you starting your own family. But your pregnancy may summon deeper, more surprising feelings in the people around you. These feelings often have more to do with what's going on in their lives than your pregnancy. Many of the relationship issues that happen in pregnancy are preludes to parenting ones. The "Becoming a Parent" part of this book discusses relationships with friends, family, and partners. → See It Takes a Village (But Maybe Not the One You're Living In), page 218.

adjusting to life with a vessel

Being a partner to a pregnant woman can be a lot of work. Pregnancy may make her less available, less predictable, and more needy. Besides being focused on her new role and changing body, she may also be anxious or annoyed about all the things she is supposed to avoid and feel resentful if her partner doesn't get how hard that can be: "How could you let those people light up while I was asleep on the couch?" "What were you thinking, giving me a half-cooked hamburger?" Though the queasiness and exhaustion can be a huge drag, those discomforts do serve a purpose; they constantly remind a woman that she's pregnant. A partner has no such internal reminders, and can thus take a lot longer to get the gist of things. Spouses and partners may want to get involved right from the get-go, but pregnancy and birth are undeniably the pregnant woman's domain. While they're often welcome, and even expected, at certain key prenatal checkups (like for the first heartbeat or a detailed ultrasound), partners can sometimes feel literally pushed aside as the ob/gyn directs her attention to the mother.

Though less obvious, changes that partners experience can be powerful. Some expectant fathers experience what's known as sympathetic pregnancy or, more fancily, couvade syndrome. A father may gain weight, feel nauseated, or experience other pregnancy symptoms. There's a lot of speculation about what causes couvade; one theory is that the extra pounds represent some kind of deep longing on the part of the man to carry some of the weight and feel engaged in the process. But the partner often finds himself carrying burdens beyond the body: finances, home safety, job security, savings, benefits, insurance, shopping for and assembling nursery furniture, etc.

It can be difficult to express frustration to a woman who's already preoccupied with her own frustrations. Your own complaints may seem selfish in the face of all her hard work. But if you ignore your feelings, you may end up acting intolerant of or even hostile toward your partner during the pregnancy. Sometimes finding another outlet can give you a place to vent without guilt. Other recent or expecting partners to pregnant women may be able to relate. Books and websites can also be good sources of support, info, and tension-dispelling laughs. → See The Good Daddy: Provider Anxiety, page 202.

I know that my partner missed me, missed playing chess and drinking with me into the wee hours of the morning. We both missed having sex.
—anonymom

I remember when she first got pregnant and was tired and sick all the time and I just couldn't believe it was that bad—since I wasn't experiencing anything I just kept thinking "Sheesh, she is so lazy and helpless. So she's a little tired, so what, I'm tired all the time and I still get up and go to work, why can't she?" I guess I didn't realize at all how bad it actually was. And since she wasn't showing at the time, it was hard to really "get" that she was pregnant. I also was a little angry that I had to quit smoking even though she was the one who was pregnant. Now that I've quit, I'm happy I did, but at the time I didn't understand why I had to do things differently if I wasn't the one who was pregnant.
—anonydaddy

I feel the support of my husband, but sometimes I think he underestimates the effects of pregnancy on women. I guess one truly needs a first-hand experience to understand what it's like. I still do most of the cooking, cleaning, and all of the food shopping.
—anonymom

I was anxious that I would never be able to provide for this child properly. That I would never be able to enjoy a life I'd only recently begun enjoying. That the quality of my work would suffer. That I'd miss my friends. That I'd never see a movie again. That I wouldn't have time to read. That my marriage would shift from a sexy partnership to a twenty-four-hour child-rearing service. That no matter how deep and lovely the bond I formed with my child, eventually it would somehow, someday, "go bad." That I wouldn't be able to avoid the weirdness between parents and children that nobody avoids. All of these anxieties, to some extent or another, have been borne out. Wonderful things have happened, too. It all balances out. Or appears to enough that I can tell myself it's all balancing out.
—anonydaddy

As a childless couple we have had the freedom to do whatever we wanted, in terms of lifestyle choices/habits. Now we have to consider and plan for how our current and future choices will affect our child. This requires more communication and negotiating, which has strengthened us as a couple.
—anonymom

Because the pregnancy came so suddenly, my wife had to quit a half-dozen bad habits at once, and didn't have energy for the good ones. No smoking, no booze, no antidepressants; less gym and socializing with friends at fashionably late hours. I had no worries that my wife wouldn't change overnight for the good of the kid. It was that so much change so fast might expose a weakness in our relationship, an incompatibility that we hadn't realized or addressed over months of trying to conceive. In (sexually deprived) moments of anxiety, I thought she'd changed from my wife to its mother, and she wouldn't change back again.
—anonydaddy

From the moment you find out you are pregnant, your life is irreversibly changed, altered. Men get nine months of oblivious bonus time before reality sets in. I am sure once the baby comes, things change.
—anonymom

resources

Be Prepared: A Practical Handbook for New Dads by Gary Greenberg and Jeannie Hayden

The Birth Partner: Everything You Need to Know to Help a Woman Through Childbirth by Penny Simkin

Confessions of the Other Mother: Non-Biological Lesbian Mothers Tell All edited by Harlyn Aizley

The Expectant Father: Facts, Tips and Advice for Dads-to-Be by Armin A. Brott

The Father's Almanac: From Pregnancy to Preschool, Baby Care to Behavior, the Complete and Indispensable Book of Practical Advice and Ideas for Every Man Discovering the Fun and Challenge of Fatherhood by S. Adams Sullivan

Pregnant Man: How Nature Makes Fathers Out of Men by Gordon Churchwell

New dad blog: daddytypes.com

pregnancy and depression

Until quite recently, depression was considered unlikely during pregnancy. Even women who had been depressed beforehand were expected to be temporarily "cured" by hormonal changes. But recent studies have shown what many have already learned from experience: Lots of women do indeed become depressed in pregnancy (sometimes even if they're on antidepressant medication). The *Journal of Women's Health* found that depression affected 1 in 5 of the 3,472 pregnant women they polled. Depression in pregnancy can be a continuation of depression before pregnancy or it can be triggered by changes in brain chemistry or life struggles while pregnant. A study from the National Institute of Mental Health asked 201 pregnant women who were being treated for depression to choose whether or not to continue their medication, then studied the results. Of the women who stopped taking drugs, 68 percent became depressed during pregnancy, as did 26 percent of those who stayed on their meds. Although many cases are minor, it is important that depression be diagnosed and treated in pregnancy as in any other time of life. Untreated depression may lead to self-destructive behavior such as smoking, drinking, and poor prenatal care, all of which can have potential long-term negative impacts on a baby. Studies have also shown that depressed women have higher risks of certain complications and preterm births.

Signs of depression (usually continuing for 2 weeks or more) include:

- **Persistent sadness**
- **Difficulty concentrating**
- **Sleeping too little or too much**
- **Loss of interest in activities that you usually enjoy**
- **Recurring thoughts of death, suicide, or hopelessness**
- **Anxiety**
- **Feelings of guilt or worthlessness**
- **Change in eating habits**

> There are so many assumptions made by the world about pregnancy, that the mom loves it, that it is a beautiful experience, that pregnancy = joy for every woman.
> **—anonymom**

TREATING DEPRESSION DURING PREGNANCY: Women who are depressed can be treated with talk therapy or support groups. Light therapy can be helpful for some people. The use of medications for depression in pregnancy is a complex issue. Many of the drugs used for depression have not been thoroughly tested on pregnant women, and some are already associated with problems. Still, since depression involves serious risks for the mother and baby, it is not always advisable for women to stop taking medication during pregnancy. Women who have any of the above symptoms or become pregnant while on antidepressant medication should discuss their options with a healthcare provider, ideally with both an OB/midwife and a psychiatrist or psychopharmacologist.

resources

Beyond the Blues: A Guide to Understanding and Treating Prenatal and Postpartum Depression by Shoshana S. Bennett and Pec Indman

Pregnancy Blues: What Every Woman Needs to Know About Depression During Pregnancy by Shaila Kulkarni Misri, M.D.

sick, tired, and miserable

Feeling sick and exhausted for weeks on end can take an emotional toll. Some definitions of morning sickness even include depression and anxiety as symptoms. Intense fatigue is a symptom of depression, too. Not being able to easily do the things you are used to being able to do (like getting from the couch to the bed) can make anyone feel less than optimistic. And the timing doesn't help; it's like you've just started off on a marathon and someone whacks you in the shins. Being on bed rest can be similarly depressing. ➔ See Treating Depression During Pregnancy, page 83, and Bed Rest, page 111.

> One of the hardest things for me right now is that there's just the idea of the baby, and the reality of feeling crappy. It's so hard to imagine what the balance will be like and sometimes hard to even remember what I'm going through all this aggravation for. Hopefully when the baby is born, it won't be so lopsided, all about what I'm losing and nothing tangible in its place.
> —anonymom

> I know when this beautiful baby comes out, I will fall in love so deeply and totally; however, now is a different story. I feel like no one prepared me for how crappy I would feel—Sick and Tired—all the time. I know I only have another month or so of this feeling, but how does that knowledge help me get stuff done now???? What if I never want to eat my favorite foods again? Will I ever want sex again????... I don't understand women who seek this out all the time.... I doubt I'll have another one and go through this again.... I know it's temporary, but the feelings are still there.
> —anonymom

pregnancy and anxiety

CONNECTION AND DISCONNECTION: You may feel attached to your baby from the moment you find out you have conceived. Or you may find it hard to connect to something so abstract, a "baby" you know only as a dot on a screen, a disembodied noise they tell you is a heartbeat, or even just two lines on a stick. You may grow increasingly attached as time goes on, gradually or in stages, as milestones of pregnancy are passed and you feel more secure. Some people feel only a vague sense of connection until they feel the baby move, or even until it's born and beyond. ➔ See Bonding Pressure, page 198.

FEAR OF LOSS AND THE UNKNOWN: A lot of pregnancy anxiety is driven by the fear of loss—either loss of the baby altogether or loss of "the baby of your dreams." A lot of women are very attuned to the fear of loss during pregnancy and may feel it as a constant or intermittent stream of anxiety. Worries may also be centered around high-risk times. There are endless things to worry about, before you have the baby and after. There's prenatal testing to wait for. Then fear of something happening during the birth. Then SIDS. Having a child is by definition a risky proposition, because where there's love, there's something to lose.
➔ See **Birth**, page 118.
➔ See The Existential Vulnerability of the Human Condition, page 199.

> I have experienced a tremendous amount of anxiety throughout this pregnancy.... I was given a less than 5 percent chance of conceiving and am considered a high-risk pregnancy, so I fear losing the baby.
> —anonymom

PREGNANT PROGNOSTICATION: Women who have had miscarriages sometimes speak of having had a sense that "something wasn't right." It's true that in some cases there are clues that the pregnancy might not continue. And it may also be true that people can have an emotional connection (or lack thereof) that correlates, at least in hindsight. But it's also true in a lot of cases that anxiety or a sense of disconnection or foreboding does not equal a problem with the pregnancy. And sadly, many pregnancies that felt perfectly okay have ended in miscarriage.

It's only natural to want some kind of control over the uncontrollable reality of pregnancy. Trust in a sixth sense or gut feeling can be a really attractive (and valuable) concept, but it can also be a little dangerous. There is a lot of inherent anxiety in pregnancy for many women, and to think that this anxiety is a warning sign could be crippling. Having a bad thought does not mean something bad is happening. Even when the subject is more benign, as when people ask a mother whether she has an idea about the gender of the baby she's carrying, this pregnancy prognostication can have weird undertones. If she's wrong, is she lacking some maternal instinct? It can be reassuring to think that if something were amiss, we'd get some kind of sign. Sometimes we do, sometimes we don't.

A STRESSFUL SITUATION: Pregnancy is stressful for so many reasons. Exhaustion. Physical discomforts. Worry about everyone's health. And life itself can be pretty stressful, too, for reasons it's not always possible to control. But pregnant women are often asked to avoid stress, since research has suggested that high stress levels can pass on to a fetus, contribute to pregnancy complications, and maybe even potentially affect brain development and performance later in life. Yet a 2006 study found that children born to women who faced moderate stress in mid to late pregnancy were actually more advanced in several areas at age two. Stress is often unavoidable. It's a part of everyone's life to some degree. So while it's definitely a good idea to try to minimize stress however you can, it's definitely a bad idea to stress out about being stressed out.

→ See Massage During Pregnancy, page 49.

As each day passes I become more convinced that I might not be carrying the spawn of the devil—something that I felt sure of for about five nightmarish weeks. . . . Nobody told me that besides being insanely ill, bedridden, and on a strict carb diet, that I might also feel totally ambivalent and depressed. It's probably a good thing too, or else I would have had these tubes tied at puberty . . . and I'm only partly kidding. It's only been in the past week that I've started to feel somewhat human again and I've even actually begun to integrate vegetables and other nonwhite foods into my diet (whoopee) along with a little beer (thank God).

—anonymom

I am constantly worried that there is something wrong with my baby. I don't know why, but for some reason the feelings of worry and anxiety are so much stronger than the feelings of excitement. I am worried the baby will have a disease or a neurological problem or a physical problem or some other things that none of the tests can detect. It's not that I don't trust the tests, I just know there are so many things they can't pick up. I also know there is nothing I can do about it until he's born and that all this worry is bad for him, but I just can't seem to do anything about it.

—anonymom

[I had a] constant worry that I would miscarry. I remember walking around with all my muscles clenched trying to hold it in. I would be sure that any small leakage of fluid was blood and was forever ducking behind bushes to be sure that I wasn't bleeding (not actual bushes . . . but you know).

—anonymom

I could never really get it when TV moms "lost their baby" after an accident, etc. It seemed so weird to be attached to something you've never seen or touched. Now that I am pregnant, though . . . I feel like I've already invested so much time, energy, love, thought into this little critter and I just weep and weep when I think that it could all be taken away. Miscarriage is a cruel tragedy. I wish I believed in God because I would be praying nonstop. Actually, maybe I will anyway.

—anonymom

I recall my first baby shopping experience as if it were yesterday. It definitely took away from some private special feeling of *my* baby (my life) and replaced it with a pretty ghastly image of *the baby,* crammed into some injection-molded car seat structure, padded and propped before heinous toys, surrounded by belittling pastels.

—ceridwen

PRENATAL CLAUSTROPHOBIA: Babies, babies everywhere. Who knew there were so many babies out there in the world, on the street, in the mall . . . in utero and out? And it's not just the adorable guys themselves, it's the extensive accoutrements: strollers, carriers, cribs, car seats, bathtubs, etc. Both of us left our first pregnant visit to a baby superstore dazed and hyperventilating. Though it may have manifested itself as a fear of suffocating under masses of puffy pastel bumpers, the real fear was that we would be eradicated by the massive tidal wave of parenthood. For a lot of people this anxiety is wrapped up with a fear of losing individuality, since the world of babies seems to already have its sensibility defined. It is, of course, possible to carve out your own aesthetic and philosophical approach to parenthood, but many people feel like they have to work extrahard to do it. → See Baby Stuff: What to Buy, page 99.

dr. internet and the dangers of self-diagnosis

When a pregnant woman gets anxious about something related to her health or her baby's, she has a few options. She can page through a book and see what the author has to say. She can call her doctor, and probably wait a while to get a response. Or she can get online and instantly peruse any of the thousands of pages of articles and studies available. The world of Internet medical research can be a mixed bag for anyone, but for pregnant women, the situation can get really crazy. Say you've got a headache. You figure you'll plug in "headaches+pregnancy" just to make sure everything's okay. Ten minutes later, you've diagnosed yourself with preeclampsia and are pretty sure that both you and your baby's lives are in danger.

A headache may indeed be a sign of something serious, but the chances are, it isn't. At any rate, it's close to impossible for you to accurately diagnose yourself based on what you read on the Internet.

Internet medical information can be sketchy and difficult to decipher. It's really hard to tell what's coming from a reliable source, and whether the author has an agenda you don't know about. Doctors are trained to evaluate research and to see things in context. When you are up at 2 A.M. manically cross-referencing acog.com with marchofdimes.org with a blog post recounting the tragic story of someone's cousin, you're not even seeing straight, much less seeing things in context. And though you may eventually come across some information that soothes you enough to allow you to shut down the computer and go back to bed, on the way to that information, you may have come across a few sites that made you think you might be about to drop dead. There's a good chance that those worrisome possibilities will be the ones that come back to haunt you in the middle of the night.

what if i'm a bad parent?

There are infinite versions of bad-parenting anxiety. Some worry they are not patient enough, or rich enough, or level-headed enough, or too selfish, too ambitious, too anxious. Others fear they will crumble with the difficult decision-making or fail to set a good example. Sometimes fears are inspired by memories from childhood. Will I be overbearing or put too much pressure on my kid? Will I make him a neurotic mess? How will I succeed where my parents failed, or manage to succeed like they did? In addition to inner voices, there are all those voices in the world: When a friend says "I can't imagine you as a mother!" it may be purely a reflection of this person's limited imagination. But it can feel like a confirmation of your own deep-seated fears. Even comments like "You'll make a great mom!" can make an expectant mother cringe with anxiety *("What if I'm not?" "What does that even mean?" "I better live up to this!!")*.

Sometimes pregnancy itself can seem like a preliminary test of your parenting skills: The exhaustion of the first trimester might be a foreshadowing of postpartum sleep deprivation. If you handle it with grace the first time, you pass the test. But what if you don't? Does that mean you'll suck at being a mother? Or that you just really don't like being tired? Probably the latter. Fears of being a bad parent may loom large during pregnancy, but they are a very normal part of adjusting to your new role and working out what you want for your child. There are many aspects of pregnancy that do prepare women for parenthood—one of the biggest ones might just be learning to filter out "bad parent" pressure.

→ See It's Just a Fantasy, page 89.
→ See Beyond Good and Evil, page 201.

> It sucks how most of the things you read about being pregnant don't really acknowledge that you might feel this way. Sometimes it makes me feel like I'm being a bad mother before I'm even a mother.
> —anonymom

children of abuse

People who have been abused often desperately want to protect their children from going through the kind of pain they did, but breaking the cycle isn't always easy. Some parents who endured abuse do go on to abuse their children. Most do not. The risk increases for very young parents, drug users, and those living with violent partners. Mental illness and depression also make abuse more likely. If you are a child abuse victim and haven't already explored your feelings about your abuser in some kind of therapy, it's a crucial step to take now that you're a parent. Even if you feel you've come to terms with your experience, having a child may bring up new issues. Support and counseling can make a huge difference in helping you parent in a positive way.

resources
Breaking the Cycle of Abuse: How to Move Beyond Your Past to Create an Abuse-Free Future by Beverly Engel

Spare the Rod: Breaking the Cycle of Child Abuse by Phil E. Quinn

Support and resources for adults raised with unhealthy control: controllingparents.com

Prevent Child Abuse America: preventchildabuse.org

> I don't feel like myself. . . . I feel like a part of me has died.
> —anonymom

> My biggest fear is that I will change so much that I won't be "me"—of course I know I'll always be me, but I'm just so scared that after the baby is born I won't be able to (or want to) do the things that I think are totally who I am.
> —anonymom

> I had a bad night last night—a small breakdown about my body not being able to do things I need it to do—the baby was wriggling all night: hiccups, kicking my bladder. I just wanted to *escape*, which led me to try and "take control" with all my perky To Do lists, which made me feel like I'm no longer a spontaneous girl (all I do now is "keep it together" so I can be strong for this transition) and so I started to cry.
> —anonymom

> I have been trying so hard to keep a happy face on all the time. I had a yoga teacher refuse to allow me to take a class and I thought, Great, another fun thing I used to do, my life is over. I burst into tears on the sidewalk (yay hormones!). Everyone keeps saying congratulations and I keep thinking holy shit.
> —anonymom

> People were kind to me, wanted to talk to me, men held open doors for me, and I just felt special, like I was the only woman in the world who'd ever been pregnant.
> —anonymom

> Honestly, the attention is wonderful. Feeling special, feeling like you're doing this amazing thing, and having other people recognize that and reach out to help take care of you.
> —anonymom

pregnant identity

The identity shift that comes with pregnancy can be subtle or obvious. You may feel like a different person the minute you confirm that there is another person growing inside you. Or you may not have any sense of essential change until you are face to face with your baby. It might not sink in for weeks, months, or even years afterward. How much you change and how it feels to you are entirely personal. Here are some of the common identity issues parents-in-progress may encounter.

→ See **Becoming a Parent**, page 174, for more on identity and parenthood.

you are special

A pregnant woman is both powerful and vulnerable. She's in her own special category, somewhere between a bomb trailing a sparking fuse and a velvet box holding a precious, fragile prize. She's got the whole world in her uterus. Or the future, anyway. This magical, venerable position can really inspire people to pull out the kid gloves. A pregnant woman may find herself treated/subject to chivalry like never before. This can make a person feel valuable. Or it can make her feel weak and handicapped. It can also vary a lot depending on your mood or who's doing the gentle handling. Even those who don't enjoy this feeling during pregnancy can find themselves missing it a little when it's gone.

so this is what i'm here for!

Pregnancy can be a time when everything seems to click into place, when you suddenly feel like you've got a really good reason for being on the planet. Things that seemed stressful and irritating can fall by the wayside compared to the importance of what's brewing in your belly. It can be much easier to feel focused and energized with your eye on such a monumental prize. Having a baby inside you can also be a reminder that you're a living being, actually *growing* for the first time in your adult life, part of the life cycle of the natural world.

life in the transit lounge

Have you ever made a stopover overseas, en route to a foreign country? If so, you may be familiar with the "passengers in transit" phenomenon. For those who haven't had the pleasure, the transit lounge is effectively a holding pen for travelers to hang out in until they get on the plane to their final destination. No customs, no payphones. Nothing to do, except wait. The transit lounge isn't even technically in a country; it's just in an airport. Having done a fair amount of traveling ourselves, we were reminded of this limbo-land when we got pregnant. Pregnancy is a nine- to ten-month waiting room. When you're pregnant for the first time, you're not yet a mother, but you're not *not* a mother, either. You can't do what you used to do before you were pregnant, which separates you from your childless friends. But you don't know yourself as a parent, either, so you can't yet relate to what your parent friends are going through. This in-between feeling can make it hard to connect with people on either side. But for some women, being "nowhere in particular" can feel like a pleasant, if odd, break between the old life and the one to come.

it's just a fantasy

Pregnancy is a time of intense focus on the *idea* of babies and parenthood, but for first-time parents, the reality is still a step away. At this point, basically, it's all in your head (and your midsection). Which can translate to lots of curiosity, excitement, anxiety, or impatience. Seasoned parents sometimes joke that no one has a less realistic view of parenthood than a pregnant couple who are still free to imagine that they will "get it right," having not yet been thrown into the

> I think it was hard for me during my pregnancy to picture what life would be like with a baby—the best I can describe it was that it was like being a senior in high school, about to leave for college. I knew that it would be a transformation, but was unsure whether I could hack it—although I had friends who had been there (to parenthood) and loved it.
> —anonymom

> I keep trying to think about strategies for how I will be able to keep doing what I want to do after the baby comes. But then when I really think about it, it's impossible to know what I will want to do in that situation because I've never been in it before. I know it's pointless to spend energy worrying but it's hard.
> —anonymom

> Being pregnant is like walking over a plank-and-cable bridge. Behind me, on one bank, is the tribe of women who are not mothers. They drink wine, stay up late, skip meals, change lovers, study Sanskrit, and write grant proposals for a five-year study of tropical cloud forests. In front of me, on the other bank, is the tribe of mothers. They arrive at meetings late, leave parties early, are badly in need of haircuts, know way too much about the care and feeding of guinea pigs, and have to hang up now.
> —Sandra Steingraber, *Having Faith*

> I still see my friends for movies/dinners/walks. And that's lovely. But I miss having a few glasses of wine, frankly. I miss feeling young and spontaneous and irrational and *fun*. I know, I know, it's worth the sacrifice. And I know I will get used to it and continue to find more creative ways to entertain myself. It doesn't help that I seem to be surrounded by people who are either very single or are parents with many kids (and therefore I never see them!).
>
> —anonymom

> I missed drinking, but more than that I didn't know what to do with myself! Since I was twenty, my social life involved cocktail hour and restaurants and cooking and there was no way I was cooking!! Yucko. At first I hid out, but then I learned to go out without drinking (or eating sushi, cheese, etc., etc.).
>
> —anonymom

> It was a surreal time. Not drinking was very strange. I never thought of myself as a big drinker, or of my friends as big drinkers, but *God!* we did nothing, went nowhere without it being drink centered. This was very strange. I would feel bored and boring by the end of most evenings.
>
> —anonymom

ring. But then again, optimistic fantasies can help expectant parents get through the pregnancy, the waiting, and the tension, not to mention the birth.

➜ For more about anxieties regarding your baby and yourself as a parent, see Pregnancy and Anxiety, page 84.

it's hard to party when you're the host (organism)

Hitting the party circuit when pregnant can be a tricky proposition. It's not just skipping out on the alcohol that can make it so hard; it's the hours on your feet, in a quite possibly smoky room . . . enduring conversations about things you might not be interested in talking about (i.e., not pregnancy or babies). Once you remove the cheese platter, smoked salmon roll-ups, and open bar from a cocktail party, you're basically left with a room full of blabbing people and a long line for the bathroom. If happy hours or wine-drenched dinner parties played a big role in your pre-pregnant life, you'll definitely have some adjusting to do. For some this means getting really good at talking to (and trying not to judge) friends who are at various levels of inebriation. For others it means bagging the party scene altogether. Many women find the early days the most exasperating—with all your changes on the inside and the pregnancy quite possibly a secret, it can be hard to keep finding excuses for bailing on your social life. Once your belly starts getting cumbersome, people might be more forgiving when you duck out of a bachelorette party early or make only a passing appearance at the company Christmas booze-up.

domestic violence **during** pregnancy

Every year, more than 300,000 pregnant women are victims of domestic violence. Abuse is more common than gestational diabetes or preeclampsia. But while all women are screened for these complications if they're getting good prenatal care, few doctors routinely screen for abuse. Abuse during pregnancy can directly injure the fetus, as well as increase the risk of complications and the chances that a mother will engage in other risky behaviors, such as drinking and smoking. If you or someone you know is experiencing domestic violence during pregnancy, tell your doctor, or contact one of the organizations below so you can get help.

resources

American Institute on Domestic Violence: aidv-usa.com/Resources.htm

National Domestic Violence Hotline: ndvh.org

I remember crying in the middle of Fifth Avenue after seeing *Lost in Translation* because that life of random and whimsical meetings and exotic (if desolate) hotel rooms was gone to me. Perhaps it was my age, but the pregnancy seemed to be stealing some part of my youth. At times the responsibilities of parenthood made me feel good: the suspended adolescence thing had been going on for too many years (decades). But the sadness of losing a life where spontaneity could rule the day was crushing. It was like I had to detach myself from a life of detachment.

—Ceridwen

"mommy brain"

Many women feel like their brains turn to mush over the course of their pregnancies, making them more forgetful, distracted, or spaced out. This phenomenon is sometimes called mommy brain. But scientific research has not shown any impact on mental acuity during pregnancy. One study found that when pregnant women were tested against non-pregnant ones, the two groups performed equally well. The pregnant women, however, perceived themselves as having impaired memory and attention. Though it's possible that the study didn't pick up on subtle changes, it's also possible that the myth of "mommy brain" stupefying women through history really is just a myth. Katherine Ellison's 2005 book, *The Mommy Brain: How Motherhood Makes Us Smarter,* discusses how pregnancy and new motherhood actually improve intelligence.

I went to parties when I was pregnant and engaged in the usual chitchat. "Hi, I'm so-and-so. Nice to meet you. So, what do you do?" I'd tell them, "I'm a writer and an artist." And they'd look at me like I was insane. Eventually it would become clear that they weren't asking "What do you do?" but "When are you due?" The ubiquitous urban banter staple had been replaced. This happened over and over again. I missed it almost every time. I know it was just stupid small talk, but it was hard not to project: Suddenly, everything was irrelevant compared to when my baby was being born.

—Rebecca

resources

PREGNANCY MEMOIRS

Every pregnancy is different. Reading personal accounts can remind you how true this is. And maybe give you some perspective on your own.

Increase by Lia Purpura

Knocked Up: Confessions of a Hip Mother-to-be by Rebecca Eckler

Love Works Like This: Moving from One Kind of Life to Another by Lauren Slater

Misconceptions: Truth, Lies, and the Unexpected on the Journey to Motherhood by Naomi Wolf

Navel-Gazing: The Days and Nights of a Mother in the Making by Jennifer Matesa

Pregnancy Stories: Real Women Share the Joys, Fears, Thrills, and Anxieties of Pregnancy from Conception to Birth by Cecelia A. Cancellaro

Waiting for Birdy: A Year of Frantic Tedium, Neurotic Angst, and the Wild Magic of Growing a Family by Catherine Newman

SUPPORT AND GUIDANCE

Magical Beginnings, Enchanted Lives: A Holistic Guide to Pregnancy and Childbirth by Deepak Chopra, M.D., David Simon, M.D., and Vicki Abrams, C.C.E., I.B.C.L.C.

The Pregnant Woman's Comfort Book: A Self-Nurturing Guide to Your Emotional Well-Being During Pregnancy and Early Motherhood by Jennifer Louden

The Spirit of Pregnancy: An Interactive Anthology for Your Journey to Motherhood by Bonni Goldberg

→ See Birth resources, page 142.
→ See Emotional Resource Rescue, page 204.

I feel like the closer I get to having the baby, the more I start freaking out about the reality of it. I get really worried about logistical stuff—like from now on I will never be able to just blow off laundry or some crap I hate doing, because it just won't be an option. On the other hand I think on some subconscious level, that was one of the motivations for having a kid in the first place: no more excuses!

—anonymom

pregnant sex

Sex while pregnant: You might love it. You might hate it. Or hate it and then love it, and then hate it. You may love it but feel that something is missing. Or hate it but feel driven to have it. You may want to do it all the time. You may never ever want to do it until someone tells you that sex can help induce an overdue labor and then do it out of desperation. You may want to do it, but find no willing partner. Or your partner may be really into it while you're really repulsed.

Plenty of women who expected to be happy, liberated sex goddesses through pregnancy then find themselves entirely numb for the better half of it. Lots of dads who had previously considered pregnancy entirely not hot are surprised to discover how unbelievably exciting their partner's swelling bodies can be. Though you may hear that sex is totally fine while pregnant, there is no telling whether you will *feel* totally fine about having it. Sex drive ebbs and flows, and for most women, the pregnancy period is on the ebby side. Confidence that the flow will return will keep anxiety from exacerbating the situation.

Here are a few of the more common sexual feelings a pregnancy can spark (or snuff out). . . .

intimacy and isolation

When you're feeling like you've transformed from a person into a person factory, it's hard to concentrate on romance. Your body may feel foreign. You may be so wrapped up in what's going on inside you (consciously or not) that you can't possibly summon the energy for a hug, much less full-on sex. The process of growing a baby inside you can seem intimate enough to preclude any other intimate connection. Meanwhile, your partner may be feeling alienated, too. While you're consumed with your own physiological drama, your partner's probably hanging out on the lonely outskirts, wondering whether he'll ever be allowed back in.

three's a crowd

Some couples end up feeling like they've got company during pregnant sex. But the image of the fetus being present or poked during sex is largely a matter of imagination. Sex will not harm or agitate a growing fetus. All evidence shows that the pleasure a mom feels during sex is fine for the baby. Nonetheless, for some people a distracting three-way vibe persists. Some parents even find it more comfortable to have sex with a sleeping infant nearby than they do with a growing fetus in the womb.

loving it

The idea that what's growing inside is a product of love (and sex) can make pregnancy a romantic time for one or both partners. Partners might lust for a pregnant woman's swollen boobs, her "ripe" and

I always thought I'd be the kind of person to get into the sexy-momma thing when pregnant and doing it all the time, *but* no such luck. Everything feels so different down there (like there's already something in there, so why add anything else?) and also, zero sex drive. Zero, zero, zero even when I try to do it myself, it ain't happening.
—anonymom

I would personally be happy to do it a lot more now; he just is not into me. All my friends say they were feeling so off sex but their husbands were up for it as much as ever, if not more! I guess I am just lucky.
—anonymom

voluptuous body. With birth control no longer an issue, spontaneous or truly recreational sex can be a new thrill. Pregnant women might feel extrasensitive or supercharged with hormonal urges. Hormones can cause increased blood flow to the genitals, which can intensify sex. We've also heard from many women who describe a kind of itch for sex that often has very little to do with love, romance, passion, or even their partner. Pregnant women may have vivid sexual (even orgasmic) dreams. Since hormones change over the course of pregnancy, these kinds of urges may be stronger at varying times. We've talked to couples who enjoyed heaps of lusty sex throughout trimester two, but then got turned off later in the game. We've also heard from women who gleefully masturbated through the final sluggish few weeks of the ninth month. An urge for sex can strike at any time, in a huge variety of ways . . . or not at all.

scent of a human

A pregnant woman's hypercharged sense of smell is not necessarily a bonus in the sack. A lot of women are shocked to discover, at some point early on in the pregnancy, that their partners quite simply reek. This may be obvious when there's garlic or smoke or Scotch involved, but just the basic smell of another living creature can be enough to turn a pregnant woman's stomach. Partner stench can be intolerable during the first trimester, and may or may not linger throughout all three. Powders, potions, and obsessive dental hygiene may or may not improve the situation. Luckily for the human race, a woman's sense of smell returns to relatively normal levels after the baby is born.

blech

Many people feel just plain turned off by pregnant sex. Part of this may have to do with the shape of the woman's body falling outside the ideal. Part of it may have to do with associations with motherhood as the antithesis of sexuality. ➜ See Where's the Mystique?, page 212.

No matter what kind of *ideas* you may have about pregnant sex, sometimes the feeling just isn't there. This can be a huge disappointment or no biggie, depending on your expectations. When one partner finds pregnancy to be a huge turn-on (or at least not a problem) and the other is just not feeling it, there can be some confusion about what to do, and whom to please. There's also the issue that in our culture, pregnant women are often thought of as "patients." We have as much in common with sick people as sexual ones, and sickness is not very erotic. ➜ See Under the Microscope, page 55.

I loved my body early in the pregnancy. I wanted to have sex all the time.
—anonymom

So many girlfriends were like, "Wait for the second trimester! That's the horny part." Not for me. My poor man has been handling it well, but it's like nothing is connected right. I have no desire, no drive, and no way to warm things up. I was looking forward to the sexy trimester . . . now I'm getting stressed I won't want it even after the birth (crazy unnecessary stress at this point).
—anonymom

I think I only had sex with my husband four times during my entire pregnancy! I don't know what was worse, his b.o. or his breath.
—anonymom

Somehow my only desire for sex came at night . . . in my dreams, often with ex-boyfriends or strangers.
—anonymom

pressure to be hot (from inside and out)

An active sex life can be a rebellion against the stereotype of the nonsexual mother: My sexuality *will not* be taken down by motherhood! It may be the urge to keep your partner happy. Or other parts of your prebaby self intact. Of course, the desire to remain hot and sexy throughout pregnancy may or may not coincide with your hormones, emotions, or the way your partner feels.

last-chance pressure

Along with the ubiquitous "Your life is over!" warnings you'll probably be hearing from the second you announce your pregnancy, you may begin to get pressure to maximize your couple time ASAP. After all, this is your last chance . . . to go to dinner, see movies, sleep, have sex. Not very relaxing or romantic, and quite possibly not all that realistic either. The imminent arrival of the baby can make this a passionate time, fleeting and that much more intense. Some people do well under pressure. But for a lot of people, pressure creates anxiety and kills any hope of getting in the mood. Even if you can get past the forced intimacy, it's hard to live the remains of your prebaby life when you're no longer living your prebaby life. Baby talk may end up a big topic at that all-important candlelit dinner.

Try to separate your desires from what you feel pressured to do, and try not to feel overly freaked out by threats of looming life transformation. Yes, things will be changing radically very soon, but they've already started to change. You need to respect where you are, not just cling to the coattails of your former existence. If spending romantic time together under pressure makes you feel more stressed out, it's not really serving the purpose of savoring the last morsels of freedom. Getting a nudge isn't always a bad thing, but sex is always better when you want to do it than when you feel like you should.

love your body (or at least accept it)

In an attempt to enjoy your pregnant body, you can do yoga, swim, have massages, read books about how great and cool your pregnant body is, walk around naked, cover yourself in special oils and tonics, wear sexy silky clothes, and just generally treat your body like the temple that it is. Of course, you may not have the time or money for any of this stuff, or you may try any variety of these things and still feel horrible, unsexy, huge, and barely energetic enough to flip through a copy of *Fit Pregnancy*. Sometimes the pressure to feel positive about your body all the time can backfire. The glowing goddess trip may not be the one you're on, but whatever you can do to push your self-image away from the "hate" side of the spectrum can have a positive impact on your sex life. Solo sex takes self-love to a whole new level. Whether it's a consequence of overwhelming appreciation, frustration, or boredom, masturbating can be a great thing to do when you're pregnant. Making yourself feel good can actually improve how you feel about your body and your self.

> I have a lot of sex dreams but then when it comes down to getting down to business, it's usually hopeless for me. Sometimes I feel like I'm missing out on my last big opportunity to have sex before I am constantly interrupted by baby stuff. But somehow that's not really much of an aphrodisiac, either.
> —anonymom

> I always knew there would be logistical issues (for example, being huge) but I didn't really predict that there would be huge lapses of time when I would forget that feeling good was even an option! It's like my body is otherwise engaged and can't function in two ways at once or something.
> —anonymom

> I am so into how I look pregnant. I've got that glow, I'm super curvy/round and soft looking. I love my cleavage. It helps having a man who is so into what my body looks and feels like.
> —anonymom

> I definitely did not feel sexy while pregnant!
> —anonymom

> I decided that pregnancy should be a time for me to indulge. So I get massages every other week, I sleep a lot, I rent movies, read books, and don't go out much, I have the occasional glass of wine, I eat chocolate, I eat meat and dairy (I was vegan before I got pregnant), I sleep in, I call in sick to work, I masturbate a lot, I take long baths, I spend a little more money on beauty products, I get my legs waxed, I let my partner cook dinner and I eat it in bed.
> —anonymom

> My partner and I have definitely discovered a new closeness through being pregnant. We're still crazy in love with each other and silly (and probably annoying) like brand-new couples often are, and being pregnant has brought out a whole new dimension of love in our relationship.
> —anonymom

sex safety

Sex is almost always okay during pregnancy. If you are at risk for preterm labor, or are in another specific high-risk category, your healthcare provider may tell you that sex is not a good idea. Semen contains prostaglandins and orgasm releases oxytocin; both can cause contractions. In a normal pregnancy, sex will not trigger premature labor. Sex is also an issue for women whose placenta covers the cervical opening, because it can cause bleeding. If your healthcare provider has not told you to abstain from sex, it's safe to assume you've got a green light. There is no sexual act that is not safe during pregnancy, with one exception: Forcibly blowing air directly into a pregnant woman's vagina can in rare cases cause an embolism, a life-threatening situation. Aside from that, the only safety issues are the ones that come up whether you're pregnant or not—protecting yourself from sexually transmitted diseases.

Mild cramping and spotting after sex and/or orgasm are common in pregnancy.

getting creative

Pregnant sex has practical considerations. You probably won't want to do a whole lot of kissing if you're grossed out by your partner's breath. As your belly grows, you might find your position options get increasingly limited. Your sex life may benefit from a little creativity and flexibility, which can mean getting into contortions, or trying out stuff that didn't seem appealing (or necessary) before. It might mean changing the definition of "having sex." Vibrators and other sex toys are also generally considered safe during pregnancy. Oral sex can circumvent "poking the baby" anxiety. There are also hands and other body parts to consider. You might be doing it a lot more if you include doing it . . . differently.

95

the pregnant life

working through pregnancy

There is generally no reason a healthy pregnant woman needs to stop working, unless her work involves specific safety hazards. Heavy manual labor has been associated with a higher risk of complications including premature birth, hypertension, and preeclampsia. Working with chemicals is also potentially risky during pregnancy. If there is any question about the safety of your working environment, get as much information as you can about your work materials and situation and bring them to your OB/midwife for consideration. You can also see the resources below for more information on occupational safety. Being at risk for preterm labor and certain other factors can also affect your ability to work during pregnancy; your healthcare provider can help you figure out whether you need to make changes.

What happens if your provider suggests you change your duties or workload but your boss doesn't go for it? Unfortunately, there's not much recourse for pregnant women in the workplace. Your company's responsibility is limited. They're under no legal obligation to give you a less-risky job, permanently or temporarily. And they have no responsibility if your pregnancy becomes complicated after strenuous physical labor. If your job provides disability insurance, you may be able to get that. But if not, you may have to make a tough decision: Either stick with the work against your doctor's recommendation, take time off, using sick days or part of your maternity leave, or quit.

➔ See The Balancing Act, page 226.

breaking the news

Telling your boss about your pregnancy is a complicated prospect. No matter how good your relationship is, your boss will need to consider how your situation will impact your job and hers. If your work has been affected by your pregnancy (or will be), you'll need to talk about that. But the big question is usually what will happen after the baby's born. If you are committed to your work and know that you plan to return, reassuring your boss may help quell any anxiety. But if you think there is a good chance that you might not come

> I definitely wanted to hide it from people I worked with for as long as I could . . . not because I thought my job would be in jeopardy but because I felt like it was a personal thing that they shouldn't be privy to. After all, you have to have sex to be pregnant and I don't really like sharing that type of thing with work colleagues!
> —anonymom

resources

National Institute for Occupational Safety and Health: cdc.gov/niosh

Occupational Safety and Health Administration: osha.gov

> I told pretty much everyone right away. I planned to wait to tell work until my eight-week ultrasound, but it kinda seemed odd that I was napping in my car every day, and running to the bathroom to hurl, so one Friday, I just posted it on the board at work (after advising my boss) so that was done!
> —anonymom

back after your maternity leave, you'll have to decide how to handle the situation. The benefit of being honest with your boss (besides just being honest) is that you'll give her more time to find a replacement, and that you'll have the opportunity to train that person to make the transition smoother. If you treat your company respectfully, you may get better recommendations later if you decide to go back to work at some point, or they may even hire you back. The downside of telling her you're leaving in advance is that you don't get the benefit of your maternity leave. Though leave is unpaid, some moms choose to take it anyway if they're not 100 percent sure whether they want to work after their babies arrive. → See Maternity and Paternity Leave, page 236.

dealing with coworkers

If you're not lucky enough to have the kind of job where you actually can crawl under your desk and nap when you have a free moment, you'll have to struggle through any pregnancy discomforts while simultaneously managing to at least appear productive. If you're not ready to tell your coworkers early on, you may need to come up with some excuses for your behavior. It may be hard to keep people from suspecting pregnancy, especially if you're vomiting, not just feeling queasy or wiped out.

The people you work with can have a variety of responses to your pregnancy, pleasant and unpleasant, helpful and irritating. There may be an urge to set you apart from other employees, as if you're in a different category now. This may feel sweet or chivalrous ("Let me help you with that door") or a little insulting ("I'll handle this . . . you've got other things to worry about now"). Competition can also be an issue, especially if there is any question about you resuming your role after the baby is born.

> Men that I work with definitely act like I am "the pregnant girl" or "the mommy" almost as though they are more aware that I am not a male now.
> —anonymom

> I am mostly put off by people at work who think I am some kind of invalid now and can't do anything for myself. They wring their hands and say, "Oh, you shouldn't be lifting that, or you shouldn't have to do this, or you shouldn't be around that room freshener," etc.
> —anonymom

your rights: professional protection

Since 1978, working pregnant women have been protected by the Pregnancy Discrimination Act. Here are some of the major points:

- Employers cannot refuse to hire a pregnant woman because of her pregnancy unless she is unable to do her job.
- A pregnant woman cannot be refused employment because of prejudices against pregnant workers from within the company or among its clients or customers.
- Pregnancy-related medical conditions must be treated on the same basis as other medical conditions in the workplace.
- Benefits must be equally available for pregnancy- and nonpregnancy-related concerns.
- Employers are required to hold a job for pregnant women on leave for the same amount of time as an employee on sick/disability leave.

For more information on the Pregnancy Discrimination Act (as well as where to turn if you feel you are experiencing discrimination due to your pregnancy) see the U.S. Equal Employment Opportunity Commission website at eeoc.gov.

→ For Maternity and Paternity Leave, see page 236.

keeping comfortable at work

ON YOUR FEET: Standing exacerbates varicose veins and swelling in the lower body. Support hose can help both conditions. Shifting your weight regularly and taking frequent rests can also help take the pressure off.

AT A DESK: See if you can get a chair with decent back support. It also helps to be able to adjust the chair as your body grows. Or bring in some pillows for added support and comfort. Elevating your feet with a footrest (or whatever you can find) can also help keep your back comfortable, and may help keep swelling in your feet down later in pregnancy. Try to get up and stretch when you can.

AT THE COMPUTER: Use of a desktop or laptop computer is considered safe during pregnancy. However, pregnant women are more prone to carpal tunnel syndrome, which affects the wrists, hands, or fingers and can make holding a newborn difficult. If you spend a lot of time at the computer, it's a good idea to be proactive about ergonomics before the problem starts.

→ See Carpal Tunnel Syndrome, page 45.

getting around

If your pregnancy is going relatively smoothly, there shouldn't be many restrictions on your travel (local or long distance) for most of your pregnancy. Comfort is a factor, though. If you're feeling sick, travel may be more difficult. Later in pregnancy, sitting still for long periods can be increasingly uncomfortable. Sometimes people (e.g., flight attendants, other passengers) can be really helpful, making your trip as easy as possible. But you may find that people are less accommodating to a pregnant women than you'd like. To avoid having patients go into labor too far from home, many doctors don't recommend long trips within the last month of pregnancy. Some airlines restrict travel for women after a certain point in pregnancy (usually 36 weeks). A note from your care provider can sometimes circumvent this if travel is necessary.

Whatever travel method you choose, there are safety precautions to consider; some of these are pregnancy-specific and others apply across the board.

traveling safely

IN CARS: Always wear your seat belt. Do not turn off air bags. The risk of being injured or trapped by a seat belt or air bag is very, very small; the risk of being injured by not having those things in place is higher.

IN TRAINS OR BUSES: Hold on to railings or seats if you must move around while the train or bus is in motion.

IN PLANES: To reduce the (very small) risk of blood clotting, do calf exercises while seated and move around at least once an hour. Compression stockings can also help. Nonpressurized cabins (as in small aircraft) are questionable during pregnancy due to low oxygen conditions at high altitudes.

AT YOUR DESTINATION: If you're going somewhere unfamiliar, you may want to research hospitals in the area, or get a recommendation for a local OB/midwife through a friend or your country's embassy. Local private doctors may or may not be willing to help patients from out of town; it can feel reassuring to have a number regardless.

baby stuff: what to buy

There are varying opinions about what new parents really, *really* need to buy for a new baby. Some people feel sufficiently equipped only once the house and nursery have been kitted out with the very latest in baby gizmo-tronics. Others feel annoyed, overwhelmed, or even offended by the idea that they need to go on a shopping bender just because a baby is coming into their lives. Many people we've talked to felt some combination of excitement ("We just brought home the crib!") and anxiety ("I had a massive emotional breakdown trying to buy a crib").

The baby-stuff industry is huge and thrives on convincing every parent that x-million gadgets, blankets, warmers, bottles, educational toys, stimulating toys, soothing toys, teething toys . . . are not just useful but essential. The fact is what you really, *really* need is a place for baby to sleep, diapers and clothes, and some food. The food might be you. The bed might be yours (if you cosleep). Taking into account those very elemental concerns, here's a list of what most parents consider to be . . .

"essential" needs

CAR SEAT: required (by law) for bringing home baby from the hospital in most cases. ➔ See Car Travel, page 359.

STROLLER AND/OR BABY CARRIER: ➔ See Getting Out and About, page 354.

SLEEP SETUP: crib, bassinet, cradle and/or cosleeper, etc. ➔ See Sleep, page 332.

DIAPERS: Lots of disposables (a baby can go through as many as fifty-plus a week) or two to three dozen cloth diapers (and some diaper covers). Cloth diapers can also be used for burps, spills, and wiping up. ➔ See Diapers: Cloth vs. Disposable, page 263.

RECEIVING BLANKETS, BURP CLOTHS: These cotton baby blankets/cloths are useful for swaddling, covering furniture, your lap, shoulder, etc. Get at least a few; if you give birth at a hospital, you'll likely be able to take some home with you.

CLOTHES: Depends on the season, but generally about six to eight soft cotton newborn nightgowns or one-piece sleepers (front opening is easiest for changing), soft cotton hats, and some layers. You do not need shoes at this stage. When purchasing fancy baby clothes, remember that babies grow . . . *fast*.

FEEDING EQUIPMENT: ➔ See Feeding Your Baby, page 274, for info on pumps, nipples, and bottle choices.

BABY-CLEANING GEAR: A bathtub or insert, fragrance-free baby soap, diaper rash cream, baby wipes (some prefer unscented or water and cloths for newborns), a couple of baby towels (optional), alcohol and cotton Q-tips for cord care, and, if necessary, petroleum jelly for circumcision care. ➔ See Bathing, page 257, and Genitals, page 265.

BABY MEDICAL SUPPLY KIT: These typically include a thermometer, infant Tylenol, nail clippers, and nasal aspirator. Baby first-aid kits are often sold in one packet at drugstores.

FOR THE MOTHER: If you give birth in a hospital, some of these may be provided.

- Sanitary napkins (thin and thick)
- Squirt bottle (for gentle cleaning)
- Stool softeners
- Tucks or other medicated soothing wipes
- Motrin
- Breast pads
- Breastfeeding nipple cream and/or soothing nipple pads

➔ See Healing, page 176.

and some other stuff you may want to consider

DIAPER DISPOSAL: If you are using disposable diapers, you can use a regular trash can with a lid and/or purchase some plastic bags to seal the smelly discards, or you can buy a special diaper disposal unit that usually comes with its own liners. These tend to keep the smell to a minimum though liners need to be continually replenished.

BABY MONITOR: Depending on the arrangement of space in your home, and how deeply you sleep, you may want to have one of these to alert you to goings-on in the nursery. Some love the type with a motion detector that goes under the crib mattress (it beeps if there is a pause in the baby's movement/breathing). Others find it too stressful since it can go off randomly and give you a heart attack in the middle of the night.

CHANGING TABLE: You will be changing your baby a lot. For years. An official changing table isn't required (any desk or baby mat on a stable surface can do just fine, but consider how easy it is for you to access it over and over and over again). It is very helpful to have a regular spot set up for changing routines.

GENTLE DETERGENT: Since new babies can have sensitive skin, people often suggest using detergent that's either specially designed for babies or that's free of dyes, perfumes, and harsh chemicals. (Some think this is less important than others.) It's often recommended that new clothes, burp cloths, and blankets are washed before they're used, because fabrics may be treated with chemicals that can be irritating.

ROCKER, GLIDER, NURSING CHAIR, AND/OR FOOTSTOOL: These can help you find a comfortable position for feedings, though they are often quite pricey (except for the footstool). If you're not partial to rocking, you can use any chair or couch (or bed) for feedings.

NURSING PILLOW: Specially designed pillows can help you raise a young baby to the breast, making it easier to get a good latch. Some provide back support for the mom as well.

DIAPER BAG: You can use any big bag or tote for baby gear, though these days there are endless diaper bag options, often with various perks, like straps that fit right on a stroller, a changing mat that folds out, pockets for easy access, etc.

BOUNCY SEAT/VIBRATING SEAT/SWING: These products try to simultaneously address the baby's love of motion and the parents' need to put down the baby somewhere. Some babies can chill out in a bouncy seat all day long; others scream the minute they touch one. Trying various options out at friends' houses or in a cooperative store may give you some inkling of whether your baby will take to a specific style or movement.

FEEDING CHAIR: Once your baby starts eating solid foods, you'll need somewhere for him to sit. Many parents feed babies in bouncy seats or car seats early on, but eventually upgrade to a feeding-specific seat. There are two basic seating options in the world of baby feeding . . . high chairs and booster seats.

We joined the booster camp by necessity (must conserve every square inch of space in our NYC apartment). I coveted groovy Euro high chairs that I couldn't import or fit in my home. But now I'd recommend a booster seat to anyone, and here's why. Using a booster helped our kid understand from day one (or day 185, which was around when he started eating solids) that eating was a family affair. He was at the table with us from the get-go, start to finish. Yes, it's true that we had to cover our fine, hand-crafted walnut table with a far less fine piece of fluorescent pink vinyl. But now I get lots of compliments on my creative solution to kid splatter. And while I can't say with any authority that his seating had anything to do with it, our kid, so far, has been eating up a storm with a minimum of food-based home decoration. (Of course, every night may be the night he grinds his soup into the couch.) For us, meals are a social event, and I think sitting together reinforces that priority.

—**Rebecca**

We were given a really swank Scandinavian high chair as a gift and were pretty thrilled since we never had any designer furniture before. This thing is like a piece of art. Funny that it should also be the most abused piece of furniture in the house. We love to pull the chair up to our dining table and eat with our baby, but we also like to plant the chair in the middle of the kitchen, give him a tray full of finger food, and let him go nuts while we do dishes and/or cook our own meal. Since some booster seats do come with their own trays, and some folks have kitchen tables, the high chair is not necessary for this kind of multitasking meal scene. In fact, there's nothing a high chair can do that a good booster can't. And boosters can travel. Our high chair does, however, transform into an older kid chair and then an adult chair, so we will have this "piece" in our lives forever!

—**Ceridwen**

brand bullying

We live in a consumer culture. The necessities may be few, but the options are countless. The proliferation of baby-bling and miracle inventions is apparent on the pages of every parenting magazine. Depending on your point of view, this can be inspiring or outrageous. Some people are really into the latest thing and are willing (and able) to pay the price. Ergonomics may mean nothing to you, but pushing around that expensive piece of radical industrial design may be the highlight of a gearhead parent's day in the park. Others oppose costly baby stuff on grounds of conspicuous consumption. Different strokes (and strollers) for different folks: Everyone has their own bank accounts, values, and priorities to consider.

Research can help you figure out how to make your own choices, although some people feel overwhelmed by ratings, reviews, features, and factors. If you ask a bunch of friends (especially those who are in a roughly similar financial situation as you) what they liked and disliked in baby gear, you'll probably get some really good and very specific advice. They may even give you some stuff they're done with. Buying secondhand is a great way to save money, but some things are best bought new, like mattresses, car seats, breast pumps, and baby-feeding gear.

→ For information about strollers, car seats, and baby carriers, see Getting Out and About, page 354.

baby showers

A baby shower can be a practical way to get parents stocked up on baby gear (and save them some money). Still, baby showers are not for everyone. Some don't believe in buying gear for an unborn baby, whether for religious or superstitious reasons. Some just find showers a little freaky. Most essentials can be selected (online or on hold at actual stores) and purchased after the baby is born. It may be hard to make complex consumer decisions in the hectic newborn period, so bigger purchases can be mulled over and debated prebirth. Gift registries can cut down on returns.

resources

Baby Bargains by Denise and Alan Fields
Consumer Reports Best Baby Products:
consumerreports.org

when things get complicated

Here we cover a few of the more common and/or serious complications of pregnancy. Some of them are no big deal; others are a bit more serious. This list is intended as a brief overview—*not* as a medical guide. Some resources for more detailed medical info are listed below, but your best resource is your healthcare provider. Good prenatal care is designed to help detect risks and prevent or treat problems quickly. Many preexisting medical conditions can affect (or be affected by) pregnancy—always talk to your doctor or midwife about any concerns and all medical history.

high-risk pregnancy

A pregnancy is classified as high-risk when a healthcare provider determines that there is a greater-than-usual chance of problems that could endanger the mother and/or baby. A high-risk diagnosis can be the result of one specific problem or a combination of factors that the doctor sees as predisposing a woman to complications. High-risk pregnancy means different things to different people; or more specifically, to different doctors. Because age increases the risk of some complications, pregnant women over a certain age are sometimes considered high-risk by default. Thirty-five is the classic cutoff, but some doctors do not consider women over thirty-five to be high-risk unless there are other concerns. Multiple pregnancies are generally considered high-risk, as are pregnancies of women with certain preexisting health conditions, such as diabetes. Developing a pregnancy complication such as preeclampsia or gestational diabetes will also move a pregnancy into a high-risk category. If your pregnancy is considered high-risk, you may have to change providers or see a high-risk doctor as well as your regular provider.

High-risk pregnancies can require lifestyle changes; sex and/or exercise may, for example, be discouraged. Bed rest may be recommended for some conditions. High-risk pregnancies require more doctor visits and tests and generally necessitate hospital births. They can be stressful both physically and emotionally; support from the people around you and from other women who have been through similarly difficult pregnancies can really help.

resources

The High-Risk Pregnancy Sourcebook by Denise M. Chism
When Pregnancy Isn't Perfect: A Layperson's Guide to Complications in Pregnancy by Laurie A. Rich
National High Risk Pregnancy Support Network: sidelines.org

resources

Mayo Clinic Guide to a Healthy Pregnancy (dry, medical, very comprehensive)

1000 Questions About Your Pregnancy: Everything Every Expecting Woman Needs to Know by Jeffrey Thurston, M.D., F.A.C.O.G. (an old-school OB tackling nearly every medical concern in great detail)

The Whole Pregnancy Handbook: An Obstetrician's Guide to Integrating Conventional and Alternative Medicine Before, During, and After Pregnancy by Dr. Joel Evans and Robin Aronson (the subtitle says it all)

Resources for specific conditions are listed throughout this chapter.

complications

anemia

Anemia in pregnancy is common and treatable. Pregnant women are routinely tested. Unless it is severe, anemia is unlikely to harm the baby—though it has been linked with preterm labor and low birth weight. It can also make you feel really tired. The usual cause of anemia is iron deficiency. Iron supplements and/or an iron-rich diet can prevent or treat anemia. Iron supplements may cause constipation or nausea; you can try different vitamin brands, lots of water with meals, and extra fiber in your diet. Foods containing vitamin C can also increase iron-absorption. Iron-rich foods include:

- **Red meats, shellfish, poultry (dark meat)**
- **Fortified breakfast cereals and oatmeal**
- **Leafy greens, baked potato (in skin)**
- **Cooked beans**
- **Raisins, dates, prunes, figs, apricots**

asthma

The effect of pregnancy on preexisting asthma varies from person to person. Studies have indicated that about a third of asthmatic women experience no change, a third improve, and a third get worse. If asthma is well treated and under good control, there is no greater risk of complications during pregnancy and birth than there is for nonasthmatic women. Uncontrolled asthma can be dangerous. According to the Lung Association, asthma is "under good control" if the expectant mother is active without experiencing any asthma symptoms; sleeping through the night, and not waking due to asthma symptoms; and attaining her personal best peak flow number.

Avoid personal triggers (such as dust, smoke, cat hair) and talk to your doctor about the range of medications available. The risks of uncontrolled asthma far exceed the risks of most asthma medications.

resources

American Academy of Allergy Asthma & Immunology: aaaai.org

diabetes

PREEXISTING DIABETES (TYPE 1 AND TYPE 2)

Women with diabetes can have healthy, unproblematic pregnancies with proper blood sugar control throughout. A doctor or specialist can help develop a treatment plan for your pregnancy (this will change as your body changes).

GESTATIONAL DIABETES

Pregnant women are screened for gestational diabetes at 24 to 28 weeks. Women at higher risk may be screened earlier. About 4 percent of women develop gestational diabetes. Treatment involves changes to diet, exercise, and occasionally insulin, and is very effective in preventing any problems—short or long term.

breech babies

Babies in the breech position are head facing up; babies in the transverse position are lying sideways. Most babies are in a breech or transverse position earlier in pregnancy; about 3–4 percent remain that way until birth. Babies who are not head down are rarely born vaginally: the American College of Obstetricians and Gynecologists (ACOG) recommends C-section births for breech babies whenever possible. Widely accepted research has shown that for breech and transverse babies, planned C-sections are significantly less risky than planned vaginal births. Of breech babies, 90–95 percent are delivered by C-section; 100 percent of transverse babies are. It's the rare provider who will even attempt a vaginal delivery with a breech baby at this point, for liability reasons as well as dwindling expertise in this area. If your baby is breech and you're nearing your due date, talk to your doctor/midwife about your options; there are some ways to try to turn the baby before birth:

TECHNIQUES FOR TURNING BREECH BABIES
External Cephalic Version (ECV or sometimes just "Version")
The doctor or midwife physically turns the baby from the outside. The procedure is common, and a large majority of successfully verted babies deliver vaginally. The ACOG recommends that "all women near term with breech presentations should be offered a version attempt." ECV is often done after 37 weeks in a hospital and it can be painful: Some describe the pain as a feeling of "discomfort" or "moderate pain"; some say it "hurts like hell." A woman can request pain medication (such as a spinal block or an epidural) for a version. In some situations, ECV is not recommended due to slight risk factors (talk to your care provider to see if you're a good candidate for ECV).

Moxibustion
This technique comes from Chinese medicine and involves burning mugwort near a specific acupuncture point in the foot. It's unclear what the success rate is for moxibustion, but some studies suggest that it does in fact help move the baby (and reduce the need for an ECV). You'll need to find an experienced and licensed acupuncturist, which may or may not be easy depending on where you live. Acupuncture by itself is also an alternative (see Resources below).

Other Ideas
Some mothers report success with hypnosis, certain yoga positions, or other body movements. If you are interested in trying these, talk to your doctor first, and find a teacher who is experienced with pregnant women and breech babies.

resources
American Association of Oriental Medicine, aaom.org: Acupuncturists can be found through your state acupuncture association.

breechbabies.com: Resources and information for various alternatives for breech deliveries, including some on vaginal breech birth

spinningbabies.com: advice and information about fetal positioning

---

The American Diabetes Association recommends that pregnant women with any type of diabetes find:

- A doctor trained to care for people with diabetes
- An obstetrician who handles high-risk pregnancies and has experience with pregnant women with diabetes
- A pediatrician or neonatologist familiar with babies born to women with diabetes
- A registered dietitian who can help with diet during and after pregnancy
- A diabetes educator to help you manage diabetes during pregnancy

resources

Gestational Diabetes: What to Expect by the American Diabetes Association

American Diabetes Association: diabetes.org

ectopic pregnancy → See page 114.

epilepsy

Antiepileptic drugs are generally less dangerous than the risk of an uncontrolled seizure. But the question is complex: If your neurologist doesn't have extensive experience with pregnancy, talk to a specialist in maternal-fetal medicine.

fibroids

Fibroids are benign uterine growths. They are very common, especially among women over thirty-five, African-American women, and those with a family history. Many women don't know they have fibroids until they are discovered in an ultrasound or exam during pregnancy. A recent study found that women with fibroids were at higher risk for pregnancy complications: specifically, preterm labor, placenta previa, breech births, and other problems with positioning and presentation. Women with fibroids are also more likely to have C-sections and are at greater risk of severe postpartum bleeding. Most of the time, however, fibroids do not interfere with pregnancy, though they may cause some discomfort. The size and location of the fibroid make a big difference in whether or not it affects pregnancy or birth. Pregnancy can also affect fibroids, causing them to grow, shrink, or even degenerate. If you have fibroids, your care provider will determine whether or not they are a potential risk.

resources

The CDC Group B Strep Page: cdc.gov/groupbstrep

Group B Strep Association: GroupBstrep.org

group b strep

Group B strep is a bacteria that exists in about 20 to 40 percent of healthy pregnant women. It's not a problem for the carrier though it can be for a newborn, who may be exposed to it in the vagina during birth and become infected. Women are routinely screened for Group B strep at 35—37 weeks, so that the passing of bacteria can be prevented. Mothers who test positive will be given IV antibiotics during labor to help kill the strep bacteria. According to the U.S. Centers for Disease Control and Prevention (CDC), IV antibiotics during labor reduce risk of infection from 1:200 to 1:4,000.

herpes

Genital herpes can be passed to the baby through the birth canal (and in rare instances while in the womb). The risk of infection is greatest if a pregnant woman has her first herpes outbreak right before labor, since her body has not had time to produce antibodies that can help protect the baby. A baby born to a woman with a recurring herpes flare-up during labor has about a 3 percent chance of infection. If sores are present at the time of labor, a Cesarean section is recommended as the safest option. Since infection can pose serious health risks to the baby, it's important for mothers who have herpes or who have present or past partners with herpes (asymptomatic infections are possible) to discuss options and risk factors with their doctor or midwife.

high blood pressure

Treatment for blood pressure depends in part on the cause (diet, lifestyle, family history, etc.). Some blood-pressure drugs are safe in pregnancy; others are not. Because it can lead to serious complications, high blood pressure during pregnancy (whether it was a previous condition or not) is monitored and treated by physicians and midwives. → See Preeclampsia, Pregnancy-Induced Hypertension (PIH), or Toxemia, page 109.

infectious diseases (chicken pox, etc.)

Women who have not developed an immunity to diseases such as chicken pox, fifth disease, and cytomegalovirus may catch the diseases during pregnancy and infect the fetus. These diseases can cause various complications and may be very dangerous to a fetus in development. A blood test can let you know if you're immune to these diseases if you don't know whether you've had them. In some cases there is treatment available for pregnant women who become exposed during pregnancy, which can help prevent infection in the fetus.

Women who spend a lot of time with young children (their own or other people's) are at higher risk. Precautions include hand washing and not sharing utensils, as well as avoiding direct contact with saliva through kissing.

low birth weight

About one in every thirteen babies is born with a low birth weight (under 5 pounds, 8 ounces). A baby may have a low birth weight due to prematurity or may be "growth-restricted" (full term but underweight). Multiples are often low birth weight, even at term. Ultrasound can sometimes detect low fetal weight in utero, and in some cases the situation can be improved through care for the mother. Low-birth-weight babies are more likely to have health problems and require extended hospital care. → See Preterm Labor, page 110, and NICU, page 267.

molar pregnancy → see Loss, page 113.

multiples

About 3 percent of pregnant women discover they are carrying multiples—95 percent of the time these are twins. The rate of twin births has gone up about 74 percent since 1980. Part of the reason for this is that more women over thirty are having babies (and women over thirty are more likely to have multiples). Another major factor is the increased use of fertility drugs and assisted reproductive technology (ART). Recent revisions in ART procedure can minimize the chance of multiples.

Most twins are fraternal—two eggs fertilized by two sperm. Identical twins—a single fertilized egg split into two fetuses—are less common. About 95 percent of multiples are detected by the beginning of the second trimester via ultrasound. Ultrasounds may be able to detect whether twins are identical or fraternal (if there are two different sexes, for example). Other indications of twins are the size of the uterus, weight gain, and results of prenatal screening. The mother of multiples may also experience stronger versions of some normal early-pregnancy effects—nausea, heartburn, exhaustion, and insomnia. As the pregnancy progresses, breathlessness, backaches, abdominal pain, and pelvic pressure may be more intense than in single pregnancies. More weight gain is necessary, too—the numbers vary, and are something to discuss with a doctor. Substantial *early* weight gain is sometimes encouraged—partly because multiple pregnancies are most often delivered preterm, partly to help fuel healthy placental growth. Multiple pregnancies usually require extra prenatal care visits. The risk of certain pregnancy complications increases with multiple births, though good care can minimize or prevent some of them from happening. Here are some issues doctors look out for:

PRETERM LABOR: About 60 percent of twins are born before the due date (and about 90 percent of triplets). The average gestational age for twins is 37 weeks. Women with multiples are often asked to take it extra easy later in the pregnancy. This may involve bed rest. → See Preterm Labor, page 110.

PREECLAMPSIA AND DIABETES: Women carrying multiples have a higher risk. → See Preeclampsia, Pregnancy-Induced Hypertension (PIH), or Toxemia, page 109, and Diabetes, page 104.

TWIN-TO-TWIN TRANSFUSION SYNDROME (TTTS): This syndrome causes uneven distribution of blood flow between twins who share the same placenta. In utero treatment may be possible through amniocentesis or laser surgery. In some cases early delivery may be required.

VANISHING TWIN SYNDROME: Sometimes a twin will show up on an early ultrasound, then in a later screening, only one embryo or fetus is visible. In these cases, the pregnancy then proceeds as a single pregnancy. It is estimated that vanishing twin syndrome affects 21—30 percent of multiple pregnancies.

CONJOINED TWINS: This happens when there's an incomplete division of identical twins and it's very rare: about 1:100,000 births.

C-SECTIONS: About half of all twin births are vaginal births. C-sections are often recommended as the safest route for more than two babies. → See Birthing Multiples, page 129.
→ See Breastfeeding More Than One, page 292.
→ See Multiples, page 266.

resources

Everything You Need to Know to Have a Healthy Twin Pregnancy by Gila Leiter and Rachel Kranz

Expecting Twins, Triplets, and More: A Doctor's Guide to a Healthy and Happy Multiple Pregnancy by Rachel Franklin

The Multiple Pregnancy Sourcebook: Pregnancy and the First Days with Twins, Triplets, and More by Nancy Bowers

Twins!: Pregnancy, Birth and the First Year of Life by Connie Agnew and Alan Klein

Twins and Multiples by Cheryl Lage

Twinspiration: Real-Life Advice from Pregnancy Through the First Year for Parents of Twins and Multiples by Cheryl Lage

Your Pregnancy Quick Guide: Twins, Triplets, and More, the book you need to have when you're having more than one (Your Pregnancy Series) by Glade B. Curtis and Judith Schuler

Informative website from a mother of twins: elizabethlyons.com

Multiple Births, Prenatal Education & Bereavement Support: multiplebirthsfamilies.com

The National Organization of Mothers of Twins Clubs, Inc.: nomotc.org

The Twin to Twin Transfusion Syndrome Foundation: tttsfoundation.org

placental problems

PLACENTA PREVIA: This is when the placenta blocks part or all of the cervix. It occurs in about 1 of 200 pregnancies (in the second and third trimesters) and can be detected with ultrasound. Painless bleeding (especially from sex, coughing, or straining) can be a warning sign. Treatment includes bed rest. When placenta previa is present, a C-section delivery is necessary.
→ See Bed Rest, page III.

PLACENTA ACCRETA: In about 1 of 2,500 pregnancies, the placenta will attach too deeply into the wall of the uterus. Symptoms include vaginal bleeding in the third trimester. If diagnosed via ultrasound, surgical procedures (to remove the placenta after delivery) can be planned. Hysterectomy may be necessary if the condition is severe—this is something that should be discussed by patient and doctor beforehand, especially if there are other options and/or the mother wants to have more children.

PLACENTAL ABRUPTION: Placental abruption is a serious condition where the placenta separates from the uterine wall too soon. This can be very dangerous for the baby (who needs the placenta to live) and to the mother (who may hemorrhage). It happens in about 1 percent of pregnancies. Most of the time it happens late in the pregnancy. Warning signs include heavy bleeding, uterine pain, premature contractions, or back pain. Ultrasound can detect the problem; treatment includes monitoring, bed rest, emergency C-section, or induced labor. Mothers who smoke, use cocaine, have high blood pressure, and/or have had multiple children are at higher risk. → See Bed Rest, page III.

preeclampsia, pregnancy-induced hypertension (pih), or toxemia

In about 5—8 percent of pregnancies, a woman develops a condition characterized by high blood pressure and high levels of protein in the urine. It usually occurs after 28 weeks, though it can occur earlier or after delivery and is more common in first-time pregnancies. If untreated, preeclampsia can present serious health problems and may even be life threatening to mother and baby. Early diagnosis and good prenatal care can prevent or delay some of the effects of this serious condition. If preeclampsia occurs late in the pregnancy (after 36 weeks), the mother will probably be induced. If it happens well before the due date, doctors will take steps to lower the blood pressure and try to hold off labor for as long as is healthy. The only way to "cure" preeclampsia is to deliver the baby. HELLP syndrome and eclampsia are manifestations of preeclampsia. → See below and Bed Rest, page III.

Talk to your doctor if you have any risk factors or warning signs.

risk factors

- **History of preeclampsia (either your own or in family)**
- **History of chronic high blood pressure, diabetes, or kidney disorder**
- **First pregnancy or subsequent pregnancy with a new partner**

- Body mass index greater than 30 percent
- Pregnant with multiples
- African-American or Hispanic
- Over forty or under eighteen years old
- Polycystic ovarian syndrome
- Lupus or other autoimmune disorders (rheumatoid arthritis, sarcoidosis, MS)

warning signs

- Sudden weight gain
- Swelling of hands and feet
- High blood pressure
- Increased protein in urine
- Headaches
- Nausea, vomiting, abdominal pain in second or third trimester

HELLP SYNDROME: HELLP syndrome is a severe form of preeclampsia that affects 4—12 percent of women who have preeclampsia. (It stands for hemolysis, elevated liver enzymes, and lowered platelets.) HELLP syndrome can come on before any preeclampsia symptoms are detected, so it is sometimes misdiagnosed. Symptoms include stomach pain, headache, and pain in the upper right quadrant of the body. Because HELLP syndrome can be fatal to both mother and baby, it is essential that women with symptoms and risk factors for preeclampsia discuss them with their healthcare providers.

resources

Preeclampsia Foundation: preeclampsia.org

preterm labor

About 12 percent of births in the United States happen preterm or prematurely (before 37 weeks). Most of the time premature labor happens later in the pregnancy, between 29 and 37 weeks. Less frequently it occurs between 20 and 28 weeks. Some premature babies survive when born as early as 23 weeks, though the earlier a baby is born, the more severe the risk of health problems. No one knows exactly what causes premature birth. Sometimes identifying risk factors can help prevent (or at least prepare for) preterm birth.

some risk factors

- Previous preterm delivery (chance of recurring premature birth is about 17—37 percent)
- Over forty or under eighteen years old
- Premature rupture of the membranes
- Pregnant with multiples
- Prior second-trimester miscarriage(s)

- Smoking, illicit drug or alcohol use
- Lack of prenatal care
- Problems with uterus, including weakened cervix, and previous exposure to diethylstilbestrol (DES)
- Maternal complications or infections, or infections of membranes or amniotic fluid
- Fetal problems (including chromosomal abnormalities)
- Problems with the placenta
- Presence of an intrauterine device

signs of premature labor

- Contractions that happen about every 10 minutes (or 6 or more in an hour) and don't ease up. (These may feel strong and may or may not be painful.)
- A change in vaginal discharge—more mucus, blood, or watery fluid
- Pressure or pain in pelvic area, back, or abdomen
- Cramps
- Diarrhea and/or frequent urinating

Premature labor can be very obvious or subtle. If you suspect preterm labor, call your doctor or midwife right away. Depending on the situation, you may be asked to go to the hospital. There are ways to find out whether premature labor is under way and to check on the health and progress of the baby. There may also be ways to delay or prevent premature labor—including bed rest, fluids, and drugs. If premature birth seems inevitable, a doctor may recommend a steroid injection that can help speed up the baby's lung development in as few as 48 hours. Like any labor, a variety of procedures (induction, C-section, pain relief) are possible in premature births. (See "Birth Basics," page 120.) Preterm babies often require some length of care in a neonatal intensive care unit (NICU) since they have low birth weight and may have underdeveloped organs and/or immune systems, making them more vulnerable to infection. Advances in obstetrics and neonatology have improved chances of survival for even the smallest babies. → See NICU, page 267, and Preterm Babies, page 269.

bed rest

More than 700,000 pregnant women a year are put on bed rest at some point in their pregnancies. The reason varies with the complication, but most often bed rest is used to reduce stress on the body and pressure on the uterus/cervix. Although it is quite commonly prescribed (by this estimate, to about one in five pregnant women), bed rest is still somewhat controversial. Some question its benefits—it is difficult to prove whether a pregnancy would have had the same outcome regardless of the rest. Bed rest can also create problems, like low muscle tone and longer recovery periods. Bed rest for long periods of time can be hugely challenging, especially for women with jobs or other kids to deal with. There are several good resources out there by women who have experienced bed rest and have helpful ideas about how to make it more enjoyable (or at least less tedious).

resources

Case Western Reserve University Pregnancy Bed Rest site: fpb.cwru.edu/Bedrest

Days in Waiting: A Guide to Surviving Pregnancy Bedrest by Mary Ann McCann

The Pregnancy Bed Rest Book: A Survival Guide for Expectant Mothers and Their Families by Amy E. Tracy or pregnancybedrest.com

rh negative

Everyone has a certain blood type, which is either Rh positive or Rh negative. When a mom's blood is Rh negative (only 15 percent of moms are) and the baby's blood is Rh positive (due to an Rh-positive dad), there is an Rh incompatibility and the mother's immune system may start producing antibodies against the baby's blood. If this were to happen, subsequent pregnancies would be jeopardized, as the mother's body essentially fights the "allergen" fetus. This is very rare now due to RhoGAM, a shot given at 28 weeks gestation to prevent Rh incompatibility. If a blood test shows that the newborn is Rh positive, a second dose is administered within 72 hours of delivery. RhoGAM is safe for all pregnancies—Rh incompatible or not. RhoGAM is also administered at all times when fetal blood could mix with a mother's blood (after uterine bleeding, trauma during pregnancy, during CVS and amniocentesis). Some physicians and midwives recommend routine RhoGAM injections for all pregnant Rh-negative women regardless of the father's Rh type. This may be because paternity is not always certain. Others will test a father's blood type and then determine the need for RhoGAM.

weakened cervix (incompetent cervix)

This condition happens when the cervix becomes strained by the weight of the growing baby and opens too soon. It occurs in about 1 percent of all pregnancies and is responsible for about a quarter of all second-trimester miscarriages. Unfortunately, the condition is usually diagnosed after a miscarriage or premature labor. Treatment involves a procedure called cerclage (stitches are used to close the cervical opening). Talk to your ob-gyn if you have any of the following risk factors:

- **Previous surgery or trauma to cervix (such as D & C)**
- **Cervix damage from a previous difficult birth**
- **Malformed cervix or uterus (from birth defect)**
- **DES (diethylstilbestrol) exposure. (Between 1938 and 1971, about four million women took a synthetic estrogen, DES, while pregnant. Later it was discovered that this drug affected the reproductive organs of female fetuses and was banned.)** → See Loss, page 113.

loss

Early miscarriage (within the first 12 weeks) happens in about 10—20 percent of recognized pregnancies. The actual miscarriage rate may be much higher, but it's hard to say since many pregnancies end before a woman even knows she's pregnant. Most miscarriages take place during the first three weeks of pregnancy. The exact cause of a miscarriage is often unknown. Up to 70 percent of first-trimester miscarriages are the result of a random chromosomal anomaly. Even if the miscarriage takes place some weeks into the pregnancy, there's a good chance the cause was determined at conception.

Signs of miscarriage include cramps and bleeding, which sometimes don't start right away. Although many women experience early spotting, most of these women do not miscarry. If you start to bleed, call your doctor. A pelvic exam can indicate whether the cervix has opened and a miscarriage is happening. If not, an ultrasound can check for the fetal heartbeat. If the pregnancy is not viable, a doctor may recommend a procedure called dilation and curettage (D & C) to remove tissue from the uterus. Not all ob-gyns perform D & C, so you may have to go somewhere else for the procedure. Occasionally the word "abortion" is used to describe a miscarriage, which can make some women feel uncomfortable. But in this context it means the spontaneous, natural ending of a pregnancy.

An early miscarriage is most often regarded as a one-time occurrence. Women are usually given the go-ahead to try to get pregnant soon afterward—though some women may want to wait longer for a variety of reasons. (See "Coping with Loss," page 116.) It's only after multiple (or late) miscarriages have taken place that genetic tests are recommended to help pinpoint a cause and lead to the prevention of future miscarriages. The vast majority of women who have an early miscarriage go on to have a healthy pregnancy. And 60—70 percent of women who have experienced multiple miscarriages will go on to a successful pregnancy.

Late miscarriage (13—20 weeks) is significantly less common than early miscarriage. Around 20 to 25 percent of late miscarriages are caused by a weakened cervix or a problem with the placenta. In some cases the cause of a second-trimester miscarriage can be determined and steps can be taken to prevent another one.

→ See Preterm Labor, page 110, for signs and symptoms.

→ See Placental Problems, page 109.

→ See Weakened Cervix, page 112.

some factors that *may* contribute to miscarriage include:

- Age
- Hormonal problems
- Chronic health problems (poorly controlled diabetes, lupus, thyroid disease)
- Infections (listeriosis, mumps, measles, rubella, and gonorrhea)
- High fever

- Exposure to large doses of radiation or environmental toxins
- Cervical or uterine problems
- Immune problems
- STDs such as bacterial vaginosis, chlamydia, and HIV
- An IUD in place at conception
- Moderate to heavy smoking and drinking
- Illlicit drug use
- Heavy caffeine use
- Use of other drugs (including ibuprofen, aspirin, drugs to treat acne or cancer)

things that have *not* been found to cause miscarriage include:

- Exercise
- Sex
- Using a computer screen
- Carrying heavy objects or other children
- Working

anembryonic pregnancy

This phenomenon accounts for almost 50 percent of early miscarriages. The fertilized egg attaches to the uterine wall, but only the pregnancy sac, not the embryo, develops. It's sometimes called a blighted ovum or early pregnancy failure and is associated with a high incidence of chromosomal anomalies. Since the pregnancy hormone hCG is produced by an implanted and fertilized egg, the miscarriage may not be diagnosed until an ultrasound shows an empty sac. This kind of miscarriage rarely happens more than once.

ectopic pregnancy

In about 1 percent of pregnancies, a fertilized egg will attach itself somewhere other than the uterus: 95 percent of the time this happens in a fallopian tube (though it can also happen in the abdomen, ovary, or cervix). Early ultrasounds (as well as any symptoms below) can help detect ectopic pregnancies. Ectopic pregnancies require quick medical attention to prevent rupture of the fallopian tube (which can be dangerous, even life threatening). Unfortunately, an ectopic pregnancy cannot continue normally.

symptoms (may appear at some point between 4 and 10 weeks)

- Vaginal bleeding (often dark and watery)
- Abdominal pain (sudden or acute, may be on one side)
- Shoulder-tip pain
- Sickness, diarrhea, pain when moving bowels or emptying bladder
- Weakness, dizziness, fainting, weak or rapid pulse

resources

The Ectopic Pregnancy Trust: ectopic.org

molar pregnancy

In about 1:1,000 pregnancies, an abnormal tissue grows instead of a healthy embryo and placenta. If a molar pregnancy is detected by an early ultrasound, D & C (dilation and curettage) of the uterus is done to remove the tissue. The levels of the hormone hCG are monitored for 6 months or so to ensure that all the tissue has been removed. In rare cases, traces of the molar tissue can grow again throughout the body. In most cases, women who have had a molar pregnancy are advised not to get pregnant again within a year.

signs of molar pregnancy include:

- Vaginal bleeding
- Rapid uterus growth
- Enlarged ovaries
- High levels of hCG
- Severe nausea, vomiting, and/or high blood pressure

stillbirth

"Stillbirth" refers to a fetal death that occurs after 20 weeks of pregnancy. It happens in about 1 in 200 pregnancies. The major causes include malformations and genetic anomalies, placental problems (abruption, clots, malformations, and scarring), or bacterial or viral infections. (See "Placental Problems," page 109.) According to the International Stillbirth Alliance, umbilical cord problems account for 3—10 percent of stillbirths in developed countries. Blood loss and restricted growth are also factors. The majority (86 percent) of stillbirths occur before labor begins.

terminating a pregnancy

The decision of whether to terminate a pregnancy (due to abnormalities or other reasons) is often difficult and complicated. Even when the decision has been reached after much thought and all parties involved feel it is the right choice, it can still be an incredibly painful process. The subject of abortion is very controversial and largely taboo, so women do not often get the kind of support they need and may end up coping in isolation. Even women who feel quite comfortable with the idea of abortion in theory may find it hard to imagine talking to people they know about their experience. There can be a lot of guilt and shame involved. Though

I can't tell you the anguish some patients feel deciding about this, especially those who have experienced years of infertility and tremendous effort and expense to become pregnant. . . . However a patient decides to terminate (surgical vs. induction), the decision is a huge and invariably painful one, and how she does it becomes almost secondary to the very fact that she is doing it. She needs to have a good understanding with her partner and other important support people about what she might do, and if she does terminate that pregnancy, it is completely normal and appropriate to grieve the loss of that child, to be saddened by the change in expectation, and to be anxious about any subsequent pregnancies.

—Karlla Brigatti, M.S., C.G.C.

women sometimes receive counseling before and after terminating a pregnancy, it's often quite limited. There's not a lot of information available for patients. Even genetic counselors are given little training on the subject. Treatment through counseling and support groups has been proven to help. See Resources below.

After Valentine's Day, Rebekah and I returned to the hospital to attend a meeting of people who had "experienced perinatal loss"—miscarriages, stillbirths, accidents, babies with deformities so monstrous that the parents had elected to pull the plug. Under humming fluorescent lights was a conference table with coffee and untouched cookies, ringed by twenty or so frightened faces, one of which was flashing indignant looks and leaking angry tears. The woman said that she'd lost her girl and now everyone wanted her to pretend that her girl had never existed. The rest of the room seconded her complaint. We finished each other's sentences. At last we were among people who could understand us. Society was on trial and we were the jury. Everyone outside the room seemed to think that having another child would somehow erase the loss of this one, that death was some kind of math problem to be overcome by procreation. Everyone was supportive, but they were all secretly hoping that "it" would get better, that "things" would go back to normal, as if normal were an option, as if normal even existed. If one more person encouraged us to put it— it!—behind us, we might just lose *it*.

—Daniel Raeburn, "Vessels," *The New Yorker,* May 1, 2006

coping with **loss**

Whenever it happens, and whatever the cause, a miscarriage or stillbirth is a loss and it comes with grief. There's loss of life, of hope, of possibility and expectations. It can be hard to accept the fact that despite our world of research and technology, death is something over which we have little control.

In general, people can be very awkward when it comes to talking about loss: Doctors and nurses can be insensitive, friends may shy away, even family members might distance themselves from the sadness. Others may try to make you feel better with platitudes like "It's nature's way of telling you something was wrong," or, "Maybe it's for the best," or, "At least it was early," or, "It wasn't meant to be." These can be very disrespectful, as can the oft-heard "You can always try again." In reality this may or may not be true;

either way, pregnancies are not interchangeable. The potential for another one doesn't erase the pain of the one you've lost. People who have experienced a similar loss may be more sensitive or able to talk more honestly.

The experience of pregnancy loss can be very hard on relationships. Partners might respond to the loss in very different ways. One partner may want to start trying for another pregnancy right away; the other may need more time to grieve before even considering it. Sometimes one person retreats, while the other wants to talk it out. Supportive counseling—whether in a group, as a couple, or with an individual therapist—can be a crucial outlet for parents to express feelings of grief. → For more on postpartum depression, see Emotional Landscape of Parenthood, page 188, and Resources opposite.

resources

BOOKS

About What Was Lost: Twenty Writers on Miscarriage, Healing, and Hope edited by Jessica Berger Gross

Coming to Term: A Father's Story of Birth, Loss, and Survival by William H. Woodwell, Jr.

Coming to Term: Uncovering the Truth About Miscarriage by Jon Cohen and Sandra Ann Carson

Empty Cradle, Broken Heart: Surviving the Death of Your Baby by Deborah L. Davis

On Grief and Grieving: Finding the Meaning of Grief Through the Five Stages of Loss by Elisabeth Kübler-Ross and David Kessler

Inconceivable by Julia Indichova

Miscarriage: Why It Happens and How Best to Reduce Your Risks—A Doctor's Guide to the Facts by Henry M. Lerner, M.D., and Alice D. Domar

Motherhood Lost: A Feminist Account of Pregnancy Loss in America by Linda L. Layne

Pregnancy After a Loss by Carol Cirulli Lanham (recommended for parents of stillborn babies)

A Silent Sorrow: Pregnancy Loss—Guidance and Support for You and Your Family by Ingrid Kohn, Perry-Lynn Moffitt, and Isabelle A. Wilkins

Trying Again: A Guide to Pregnancy After Miscarriage, Stillbirth, and Infant Loss by Ann Douglas, John R. Sussman, and Deborah L. Davis

WEBSITES

Babyfruit Miscarriage, Pregnancy and Baby Blog: babyfruit.typepad.com

Center for Loss in Multiple Birth: climb-support.org

Fertility Plus: fertilityplus.org/faq/miscarriage/resources.html

Hand of the Peninsula/Helping After Neonatal Death: handsupport.org

Resources and stories about terminating pregnancy: aheartbreakingchoice.com

Discussion of postpartum depression and pregnancy loss: bornangels.com/ppd.htm

Blog about infertility, loss, and pregnancy: georgia.typepad.com

"How to be Good Friends with an Infertile": tertia.typepad.com/so_close/2004/05/how_to_be_good_.html

International Council of Infertility Information Dissemination: inciid.org (includes Elizabeth Carney's essay "The Miscarriage Manual: Coping with the Emotional Aspects of Pregnancy Loss")

International Stillbirth Alliance: stillbirthalliance.org (stillbirth information and support)

The Miscarriage Association (UK): miscarriageassociation.org.uk

Postpartum Stress Center: postpartumstress.com

Recurrent Miscarriages Info Center: recurrentmiscarriages.com

Share: Pregnancy and Infancy Loss Support, Inc.: nationalshareoffice.com

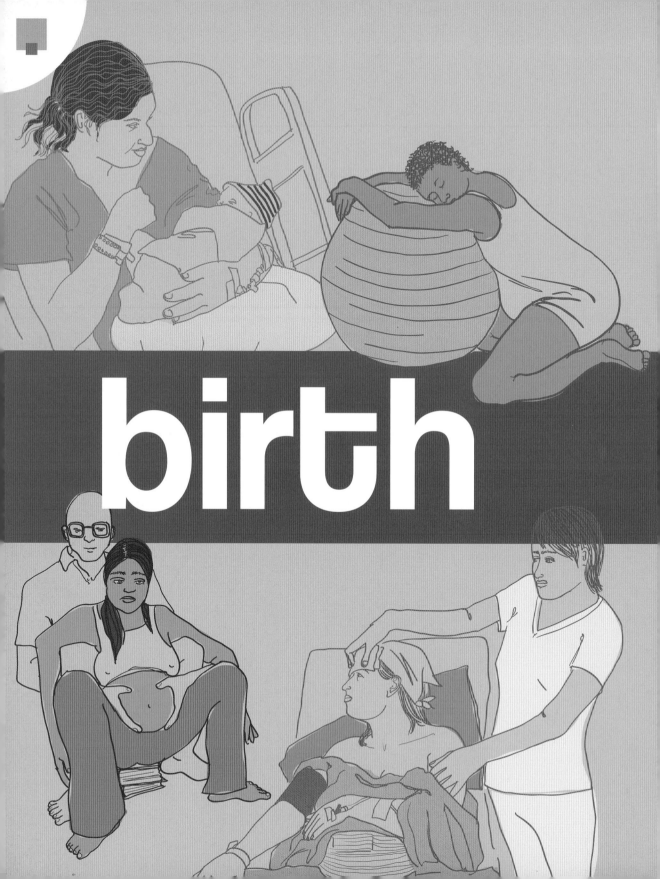

birth

Once we'd reached a certain point in pregnancy, it seemed everyone had something to say about birth. Random women would tell us how awful it was, or how they felt connected to the universe, or how they puked on their husbands. We took the classes and learned about the ten million different ways the birth could pan out. We saw the videos of women with odd hairstyles groaning inhuman groans. We read about nightmare births, average births, ecstatic births, and wondered what was in store for us. We got speeches about the importance of unmedicated childbirth in one ear and "Dude, you've gotta get the epidural!" in the other. We devised loose (but thoughtful) birth plans. And then it happened. And a lot of what we'd heard was true: Birth did touch on the profound as well as the banal. We both, despite our grounded, realistic expectations, felt a little disappointed when events pushed our births in directions we hadn't planned for. As much as we knew we had to keep an open mind, it was hard not to harbor a few hopes.

So much of what people say about birth is about control. The messages can be confusing: *"Don't let them limit your options!" "Just give up! You don't have any say over what happens anyway!"* In our own experiences, birth was less about having control than figuring out how to let go of it when necessary. Finding that balance was one of the biggest challenges (though the pain and the pushing were pretty damn challenging). This part of the book will introduce you to the different kinds of things that can happen during labor and birth, both in your body and in the birth environment. We'll talk about the many ways women prepare for labor and cope with pain. We'll also delve into ideas and opinions that may affect your birth experience, as well as the mix of feelings that can come up before, during, and after.

birth basics

The basic, average birth can be easily defined on paper, but it's not often experienced in life. Very few women actually give birth on their due date. A full-term birth can happen as early as 3 weeks before the date you're due and as much as 2 weeks afterward. Likewise, the average first labor is said to be 12—14 hours, but many first labors vary dramatically from that number. The experience of labor is dependent on so many factors: position of the baby, where you are, whether or not you're in pain, whether this is your first baby, who is helping you, how many babies you are carrying. It's useful to learn about stages and symptoms so you can know what's going on when it happens, but try not to get too bogged down in numbers or ideas about how things should be going. A few conversations with women who have given birth will reveal the immense variation in childbirth experiences, basic and otherwise.

early signs of labor

Here are some of the things you might feel in the weeks, days, or hours before your baby is born. Some signs of pre- or early labor are glaringly obvious; some are much less so—you may not even notice them happening.

LIGHTENING/ENGAGEMENT: This is when the baby's head moves or "drops" down into the pelvis in preparation for birth. It happens in stages or "stations," usually starting about 2—4 weeks before labor. Women who have previously given birth are more likely to drop much closer to, or during, labor. Lightening can be a big (or at least partial) relief to anyone who has been feeling a lot of discomfort up around the ribs; the lowered baby can make it easier to eat a normal-sized meal and breathe deeply. The discomfort tends to move downward, however, putting pressure on the pelvic area and bladder. Some women notice a big change when the baby drops; others find out the baby is engaged only during a pelvic exam.

MUCUS PLUG/BLOODY SHOW: During pregnancy the cervical canal is sealed with a plug of thick mucus. As the cervix begins to efface and dilate, the plug loosens and comes out. This is an indication that your body is preparing for labor (though labor can be anywhere from hours to weeks away). Some women notice a reddish, pinkish, or brownish discharge; others never see it.

> To be honest, I've forgotten the actual pain, but I seem to remember comparing it to having someone tie your intestines in knots.
> —anonymom

> I remember when I was a teenager with really bad period pain and asking my mother, "Is this what it's like having a baby?" and she said, "It's the same sort of pain but much, much worse because it's stronger and longer" (in fact my experience was that the period pain I'd had was actually worse because it didn't come and go rhythmically like labor!).
> —anonymom

> It's like a giant hand is putting your midsection through an orange juicer.
> —anonymom

CONTRACTIONS: The uterus muscle tightens, contracts, and releases in order to open the cervix and prepare to push the baby out. The break between contractions can be anywhere from a half hour to seconds depending on where you are in the labor process. The intensity varies widely—like the flexing of any muscle, the longer the flex, the shorter the break, the harder the work out. Early or prelabor contractions may be intense but aren't always described as painful. As labor progresses, contractions can feel overwhelmingly strong and painful (you may not be able to talk through them).

Pregnant women, especially those experiencing heavy Braxton Hicks contractions, may feel on guard, wondering Is this it? on a pretty regular basis leading up to the birth. → See Braxton Hicks Contractions, page 51.

some ways to identify actual labor contractions

- They become progressively stronger and more frequent, lasting about 30–70 seconds.
- They do not go away when you move around or drink water.
- The sensation may be in only the back or start at the back and move to the front.
- The cervix is dilating (this is something a doctor or midwife can determine with a pelvic exam).

A contraction is a menstrual cramp from hell. It is tight and wrenching.
—anonymom

Like a boa constrictor around my abdomen and back.
—anonymom

In early labor ... like one of the worst menstrual cramps I had ever had. Later on it felt like all of my insides were one giant washcloth ... and it was being wrung out over and over again.
—anonymom

All the pain and pressure were in my rectum and perineum. It feels like you have to go number two really really bad—but nothing will come out and the sensation won't go away until the contraction ends.
—anonymom

Extremely powerful. Your body just does it. It's like some demon or angel takes over and you have only a certain amount of control. It is very inward. You can handle it if you have support and you make some progress.
—anonymom

You know the way your stomach contracts to puke? Well, it's sort of like that but way stronger *and* I was also puking, so I had an immediate compare/contrast situation.
—anonymom

It's a wave. A painful orgasm. It builds and builds, inside of you, very deep inside. You shudder. It is like a thunderbolt; huge. Resonating all through you. Once you peak, the descending pain is a relief.
—anonymom

I was surprised at how amazingly physical the contractions were; every moment my entire being was caught up in what was happening to my body. For me, I would feel the contraction coming on like a wave of a large muscle spasm in my abdomen. It would begin and squeeze, Squeeze, Squeeze, SQUEEZE ... then start to subside. For me the pain would become the worst right after the top of the contraction as it started to back down. It was painful for me, but it was also very focused pain.
—anonymom

back labor

Labor and birth are affected by the position of the baby's body in the uterus. When a baby is facing "sunny-side up" (posterior position), his back may press against the laboring woman's spine. This is known as back labor, and it can be extremely painful. Babies in a posterior position are sometimes harder to push out. Back pain in labor may be due to other causes (tension among them). Changing positions can help (getting on all fours or a birthing ball), as can counterpressure on your back (from hands, warm water, a tennis ball, etc.). For more info on how to encourage optimal fetal position, see spinningbabies.com.

If pregnancy was a book, they would cut the last two chapters.

—Nora Ephron

I don't know if it's the heat or just being huge or some combo thereof but I am really quite cranky and miserable. I know you're supposed to "savor" this last time of non-mommyness but mostly I feel compelled to sit around and stew in my big fat juices.

—anonymom

Some people act exasperated that I haven't given birth yet, like I'm holding them up for something! Ridiculous.

—anonymom

the waiting

The average first-time birth takes place a full week (and a day) after the 40-week estimated due date. A pregnancy is not even technically "post-term" until 42 weeks. But if you're into your tenth month of pregnancy, chances are you're pretty tapped out in the patience and stamina departments. And with each passing day, this tedious limbo, this anticlimax created by a false deadline, gets more intolerable.

Since your due date is determined so early on, it can be hard not to get attached. Even if you continually remind yourself that it is only an estimate, others tend to cling to the numbers. You may be tempted to stop answering your phone to avoid the expectant voices. "Are you *still* there?" If you're taking maternity leave, colleagues may plan on your absence by the due date or even have a temporary replacement on board. If you were told you might go into labor early (or prescribed bed rest), you may feel hopelessly sluggish when you hit 39 weeks, let alone 41. People in your life, including professionals, can sometimes play a hand in the waiting game by noting signs of impending labor with a bit too much cheer: "You're one centimeter dilated? Any day now!" But women can walk around dilated for weeks. You may also be told to keep an eye out for some nonphysical signs of labor, such as nesting or feeling less social. But those signs are highly personal and not always reliable.

If you are feeling the pressure of the waiting game, it might help to remember that every gestation has its own clock—passing the somewhat arbitrary due date is not a sign of anything . . . except that due dates themselves are simply educated guesses.

WATER BREAKING: The membranes around the amniotic fluid can break before or during labor (babies can even be born with membranes intact). Sometimes a doctor or midwife will manually rupture the membranes as an effort to speed up labor, to prepare for an assisted delivery, or for other reasons. If your membranes (or "waters") break before labor, you may feel a gush or trickle of liquid or hardly anything but a wet spot on your sheets or underwear. The flow of fluid depends on a number of factors, including where the membranes ruptured and the position you are in. Lying down may increase the flow while standing up can slow it down (the baby's head can block the opening of the cervix).

If your waters break, call your doctor or midwife. Since the risk of infection goes up once the membranes have ruptured, it's important to not put anything in your vagina (finger, tampon, penis, etc.). Most of the time contractions begin within 6 to 24 hours of the water breaking. If labor doesn't start on its own, you may be induced to prevent the risk of infection. Opinions vary widely about how long is too long to wait.

Occasionally, amniotic fluid is tinged with a yellow, green, or greenish brown color. This indicates that the baby has passed meconium (the first bowel movement). Meconium is more likely to be present when a baby is past due; it can also suggest the possibility that the baby is in distress. By itself, meconium is not a sign that the baby is in any danger; however, fetal monitoring is often recommended to make sure there are no other indications of problems.

> If you are Strep B positive and your water breaks, you have to get to the hospital a bit early, so when you first call, make sure you know your status or get there sooner if you never had this test done. I think the whole thing is downplayed too much considering the risks.
> —anonymom

> My body is not my own.... I want out! I want my body back!!! Can't go out for long walks, can't fly, I have to pee all the time. Everything is affected. The daily routines have stopped and made way for a new lying-on-the-couch routine.
> —anonymom

when is it time to go?

Women are often instructed to start timing contractions if they suspect labor has started and to call their doctor or midwife when the contractions are between 5 and 10 minutes apart for some period of time (maybe an hour or two). Deciding when to "go in" (if you are not birthing at home) depends on many variables. If you are interested in a drug-free or natural birth, some suggest laboring at home for as long as possible—maybe until you can "no longer talk" through the contractions. This allows you to enjoy your own environment for what may be a very gradual, long early labor, sometimes lasting days. It can also help you avoid any early and possibly unnecessary interventions. Every situation has its own set of circumstances, however. Call your practitioner and tell them what's going on; and you can decide together what to do and when. → See Interventions, page 126, and Taxi!, page 151.

stages of labor

prelabor (days leading up to birth)

- May include loose bowel movements, low back-ache, bloody show, lightening, thinning of cervix, increased Braxton Hicks

first stage

The first stage can last hours or days, depending.

1. early labor

- Cervix effaces and opens to about 4 centimeters.

- Contractions are usually 30—45 seconds long and 5—30 minutes apart (increasing in frequency and intensity over time).

- Some women have mild contractions for a long time (days) before the cervix dilates. For others, early labor accelerates relatively fast (within hours). Your water may break, you may notice the bloody show, contractions can feel like cramps or like Braxton Hicks contractions.

- May include backache, menstrual-like cramps, indigestion, nausea, diarrhea.

2. active labor

- Cervix effaces and dilates to 7 centimeters.

- Contractions are about 45—60 seconds long, about every 3—5 minutes.

- On average this phase lasts 3—5 hours.

- As it progresses, you may be unable to talk through contractions, vomit, feel tired, have backache, pressure, or leg discomfort. Membranes may break now if they have not.

- Active labor is usually the time to move to the birth setting if you're not already there. ➜ See When Is It Time to Go, page 123.

3. transition (or hard labor)

- Cervix opens from 7 to 10 centimeters (fully opened).

- Contractions are 60—90 seconds long, every 2—3 minutes. Usually the shortest, most intense phase of labor, transition generally lasts between 15 minutes and 2 hours, though maybe longer. The contractions can feel almost nonstop, since there is very little time between them. Membranes can break, if they haven't. Some women feel the urge to push during transition; others don't. At the end of transition there can be a break where contractions do not feel as strong.

10 cm
actual size

10 cm =
full dilation =
size of average
gerber daisy

> I got an epidural and basically slept through the transition!
> —anonymom

> Transition was the hardest part. I wanted to leave my body. Run away. I did hypnobirthing, but it still hurt. It helped me rest in between contractions. Pushing was even more intense. Not more painful, until the end when you stretch. Pushing was more focused. It was tiring. It took it out of me, all of it.
> —anonymom

The transition time was definitely the hardest. The waves of contractions were coming so quickly and behind them an urge to push. I kept visualizing a river flooding and the flood was the pain, my body the poor overwhelmed riverbanks. I just kept imaging the water flowing (and the floodwaters taking with it houses and cars and everything else in its wake). In the end, nothing could stop my natural urge to push. My body had totally taken over the process and the baby slid out fairly easily with very little pain and to my total relief.

—anonymom

I knew I was in transition because the contractions changed very abruptly. The pain increased a lot during transition and in my mind I knew the pushing was only moments away. The pushing, for me, was a relief. I had a second wind that kept me going, and I knew it was nearly over.

—anonymom

Transition was intense—felt like my body was turning inside out. Pushing was a relief but really just amazing—the force of the urge. I was alone with my partner and was trying not to push, waiting for the midwife . . . when the midwife finally came and said to follow my body's signals, I pushed with everything I had and my daughter was born in eight minutes.

—anonymom

My transition lasted nearly two hours, with a long series of camelback contractions lasting as long as two minutes at a time. After all that time, I still hadn't dilated any further, so I finally had an epidural, and couldn't feel a thing after that. Transition was amazingly, awe-inspiringly powerful—literally awful.

—anonymom

- May include nausea and vomiting, shaking, cramping legs, pressure on lower back or rectum, sweating, shivering, and intense fatigue (some women fall asleep between contractions even if just for a minute).

second stage

- Contractions are 60—90 seconds and about 2—4 minutes apart. (This is the time when women push—timing depends on contractions.)
- Usually lasts from about 20 minutes to 2 hours, sometimes longer.
- May feel intense pressure on rectum, burning, or stinging around vagina.
- The baby is born.

third stage

- Delivery of placenta or afterbirth (usually within 20 minutes after baby is born).
- May be asked to push.
- In multiple pregnancies, there can be more than one placenta. → See Birthing Multiples, page 129.

Pushing is not an *urge*, it is a demand backed up by all the violence your body, suddenly turned into an enemy, has at its command.

—Jane Lazarre, *The Mother Knot*

The pushing was the most difficult part for me. I felt like these sounds were coming out of me that I didn't know were in me. It was like someone else was making these sounds.

—anonymom

It was far more doable than I'd thought it would be. . . . That said, it was an intense marathon. Mercifully, you're not in your right mind, so you don't comprehend the pain in your normal way.

—anonymom

125

procedures and possibilities

Depending on what happens and how your caregivers respond to it, your birth may involve any number of medical procedures. (Many of these are more likely in hospital births.) Here's a list of some of the more common things that may happen on the way to a baby. You may have some input into the situation if you want it. → See What You Can Control and What You Can't, page 146.

fetal monitoring

A fetal monitor measures the baby's heart rate. It is often used in conjunction with a monitor that reads the length and intensity of the mother's contractions. With continuous fetal monitoring, a monitor is affixed with a belt to the pregnant woman's stomach and remains there during labor. Intermittent monitoring is done at intervals throughout. Internal fetal monitoring, in which an electrode is attached directly to the fetal scalp through the cervix, may be used in some situations. Once the electrode is in place, it's there until the baby is born.

Continuous monitoring has been the norm in hospital births since the 1960s or '70s because doctors thought that reading the baby's heart rate would lower the chances of neurological or other problems. More recent research suggests that continuous fetal monitoring doesn't seem to decrease the chances of most complications. Continuous monitoring does, however, increase the chances of a C-section for a variety of reasons. Many relate to technical issues and interpretations of data. Continuous monitoring also means impaired mobility, limiting positions that can encourage labor.

It may be possible to move around as long as the monitor stays steady (no easy feat during major contractions). A slip of the monitor can cause a lot of panic because a pause in the information can be interpreted as a dip in the baby's heart rate. This may cause the nurse to ask you to stay put so the monitor does the same. Most hospitals will use continuous monitoring by default unless the parents request otherwise (they may or may not allow intermittent monitoring upon request, depending on policy and the situation). This is partly a result of the use of pain medication, which may affect the fetus and thus requires monitoring. Also, since births are no longer continuously monitored by

interventions

The word "interventions" is used in childbirth lingo to describe medical procedures used in birth. Procedures can range from monitoring the baby's heartbeat throughout labor to inducing labor with drugs, or using drugs for pain relief. Some natural childbirth advocates see interventions as unnecessary and potentially dangerous, easily spiraling into a birth in which the mother is totally out of control. Doctors and/or nurses are more likely to see them as vital cautionary measures for a safe birth.
→ See Natural vs. Medical Childbirth: Either/Or?, page 141.

staff (generally there are fewer nurses on duty than patients in labor), they are continuously monitored by machines. Continuous monitoring means fewer visits to the room to reaffix the monitor, no need to keep track of timing intervals, and a printed record for legal protection. Continuous monitoring is generally not used in birth centers; intermittent use is more likely.

restrictions on food and drink

Some hospitals require that women stop eating and drinking when they are admitted to the labor and delivery floor. The purpose of this is to keep stomachs empty in the rare case that general anesthesia is necessary for an emergency C-section. The risk of aspiration while under general anesthetic is very small (some say purely theoretical). Many are critical of this restriction policy, suggesting it results in decreased energy to handle contractions and pushing. Talk to your care provider to see how she feels about food and drink; there may be some flexibility. If you're going to eat, you may want to be discreet about it as hospital policy probably dictates otherwise.

inducing labor

There are a lot of ways to instigate or augment labor, and a lot of reasons for inducing. Some are nonmedical techniques (such as nipple stimulation). Others involve drugs that simulate labor hormones. Sometimes one method is enough to kick labor into gear on its own; sometimes it takes the whole package to get things going. In some cases even a full-steam induction doesn't work and a surgical birth is the only option. Many factors contribute to the reasons for induction and the manner chosen, as well as how effective they are.

some reasons labor is induced

- Waters have broken but labor isn't moving forward.
- Pregnancy is overdue (up to 42 weeks is usually considered safe, depending on various factors and your doctor's or midwife's opinion).
- Mother's or baby's health requires delivery (as in uterine infection, preeclampsia, placental or amniotic fluid problems, and other situations where one or both are in danger).
- Logistics (such as distance between home and hospital).
- Labor starts but stalls or slows down. (Induction techniques may be used to augment labor in this case.)

NONMEDICAL INDUCTION: Nonmedical induction techniques are pretty straightforward and can be done at home. (If your waters have broken, don't try any inducing method that requires putting something in your vagina or that involves immersing yourself in water.) These maneuvers may or may not get labor going. They are often used by women who are past their due dates or are trying to get labor started themselves in order to avoid a medical induction. Much of the evidence supporting their effectiveness is anecdotal rather than scientific.

> I made the mistake of not eating something before going to the hospital before my twelve hours of labor. I get low blood sugar and migraines if I don't eat regularly, so I should have eaten and risked throwing up rather than feeling horrible from not eating.
> —anonymom

some techniques

- *Nipple stimulation:* This can trigger the release of oxytocin (a labor hormone, also released in breastfeeding). You can tweak nipples by yourself, with assistance, or even with a breast pump. Most suggest this needs to be done very frequently to be effective. Stop stimulating during contractions, resume between them.

- *Sex and/or orgasm:* Semen contains prostaglandins that may trigger labor. Orgasm releases oxytocin and contracts the uterus.

- *Herbs:* Applying evening primrose oil to the cervix may soften it. This can also be taken orally. Black haw, black and blue cohosh, and red raspberry leaf tea are also used occasionally. Only use these under guidance of your healthcare provider and someone experienced with herbal remedies.

- *Castor oil:* This old-school (and possibly quite unpleasant) labor-inducing elixir often causes diarrhea and vomiting, which might bring on labor. Small doses are recommended, if used. And lots of water can stave off any dehydration (which is not good for a laboring woman). Talk to your doctor or midwife before trying this.*

- *Walking around.*

- *Enema:* Flushing out the bowels may trigger labor. Because there is some risk of dehydration, drink lots of fluids.*

- *Acupressure/acupuncture:* A trained acupuncturist, midwife, or doula may be able to manipulate some pressure points that can instigate labor. Transcutaneous nerve stimulation (TENS) is also sometimes used.

*Castor oil and enemas are not recommended if your cervix is not ripe, so it's especially important to check with your doctor or midwife before trying them.

MEDICAL INDUCTION: Medically induced labor may involve sweeping or rupturing membranes and/or some combination of synthetic hormones: prostaglandins (for cervical ripening) and/or Pitocin (for dilating/contractions). Labor that is induced by synthetic hormones requires continuous electronic fetal monitoring, and it is realistic to think you may need an epidural. Induced labor can bring on stronger contractions than labor without induction. But the intensity of labor, length of contractions, and effectiveness vary tremendously from woman to woman. In some cases medical induction reduces the chances of a C-section (if it works, and your labor progresses as planned). In other cases, it makes a C-section more likely—if labor is induced and your body (or your baby) doesn't respond, you'll probably have a surgical birth. The latter scenario is more likely if you have no physical indications of being ready to go into labor.

some ways a doctor or midwife may induce labor

- *Sweeping membranes:* The midwife or doctor may try "sweeping the membranes" (sometimes called stripping or stretching). She inserts a finger through the opening of the cervix and gently "sweeps" the membranes to separate the amniotic sac from the cervical wall, thus releasing prostaglandins (which may help trigger labor). This can only be done if the cervix has dilated wide enough to fit a finger. It's a short procedure that can be done in a doctor's office, but it does cause some discomfort (or even pain) and may not make much of a difference in terms of when labor starts or how it progresses.

- **Rupturing membranes:** A midwife or doctor may opt to artificially rupture the membranes. The idea is that this will cause prostaglandins to enter the mother's bloodstream. This is considered a better option for speeding up labor than starting it from scratch. If labor doesn't start from this method, time pressure increases.
  → See Water Breaking, page 123.

- **Cervical ripeners:** To ripen, soften, and open the cervix, your doctor or midwife may apply a form of synthetic prostaglandin to it (the prostaglandin comes in a vaginal gel, tablet, or suppository).

- **Synthetic oxytocin:** To stimulate contractions (or make them stronger), synthetic oxytocin (Pitocin) can be given intravenously. Pitocin is usually started once the cervix has softened (either on its own or from synthetic prostaglandins).

the cytotec controversy

There are two kinds of synthetic prostaglandins (the kind used to ripen the cervix): Cervidil/Prepidil (dinoprostone) or Cytotec (misoprostol). They are equally effective at ripening the cervix for an induction. Studies have shown that Cytotec is effective and safe when used at the right time and in the right dose for women with no prior uterine surgery. In fact, while women who are given Cervidil almost always need to follow up with Pitocin, Cytotec is more likely to get labor going on its own. However, in high doses, Cytotec can cause very strong, long, and potentially harmful contractions. It can also cause uterine rupture in women who have had previous uterine surgery. It has been FDA approved only for the prevention of stomach ulcers, not for inducing labor. For this reason, some consider Cytotec use a controversial and unregulated experiment. It is also much, much less expensive than the alternatives, making it desirable from the hospital's point of view (and possibly more suspicious from the laboring woman's point of view). In recent years, doctors have developed a greater understanding of the drug and how to use it safely. Which is a good thing, because hospitals usually don't give patients a choice about which drug they will be given.

birthing multiples

Multiple pregnancies generally are at greater risk of birth complications. The more babies you're carrying, the more likely they will be born preterm and with a low birth weight.

THE AVERAGE GESTATION FOR MULTIPLES:
- Twins: 36 weeks
- Triplets: 32 weeks
- Quadruplets: 30 weeks

Bed rest is more common in multiple pregnancies because of the frequency of preterm labor.
  See Bed Rest, page 111, and Preterm Labor, page 110.
  Most triplets and just about all quadruplets are born via C-section. Vaginal birth is more common for twins—about half of all twin births are vaginal. The position of the babies often dictates how they will be born. In a twin birth, when both babies are facing head down (about 40 percent are) and there are no risk factors, a vaginal birth is pretty likely. If the first baby (the one closest to the birth canal) is breech or transverse, however, a C-section will probably be planned. If the first baby is facing down but the other one is not, your doctor or midwife can talk to you about your options. Sometimes the second baby is born feet first, or turned to a downward-facing position manually after the first baby has been born. In about 10 percent of twin births, the first baby is born vaginally and the second by C-section—this is more likely if the second baby is breech or transverse, though other factors may contribute.

episiotomies

An episiotomy is a 1- to 2-inch incision made in the perineum—the area between the vagina and the anus—to increase the size of the vaginal opening. For much of the last century, episiotomies were a routine part of hospital births. The smooth cut of the incision was considered easier to repair than the jagged edges of a tear. The cut was supposed to help women heal more easily, endure less urinary incontinence, and enjoy a better sex life (possibly due to the anecdotally popular phenomenon known as the husband stitch, in which the doctor sews a woman up extra tight for her man's pleasure). But recent research implies that these benefits do not exist. According to a 2005 study, routine episiotomies did not improve recovery times or lessen a mother's pain after childbirth. In fact, the opposite was often true. Episiotomies can lead to larger and deeper tears—just like a snip on the edge of a cloth can make it rip more easily. ACOG practice guidelines discourage the use of routine episiotomies in childbirth and suggest limited use where the physician deems the cut necessary. In cases of fetal distress, episiotomies can help speed delivery. Though cutting is becoming less common, it is still used in a fair number of vaginal births (33 percent in 2000). You can talk to your provider beforehand to find out how she feels about episiotomies and when she performs them. You can also ask her about the techniques below if you'd like to take steps to reduce your risk. Some of these can be done at home, others require the cooperation of your doctor or midwife.

things that may help you avoid an episiotomy

- *A provider who does not routinely perform episiotomies.*

- *Perineal massage:* regularly massaging the perineal area with warm oil toward the end of the third trimester of pregnancy. (This is hardcore painful stretching, not foreplay.) Some studies suggest this will reduce the chances of episiotomy, especially for first-time mothers. Other studies say it's useless.

- *Slow second-stage labor:* This may or may not be something you can control, but you can ask your doctor or midwife to help moderate your pushing if circumstances permit. Kegel exercises during pregnancy can help you learn how to relax your pelvic floor muscles during birth, which can help the baby out more easily.

- *Massage and compresses while pushing:* Massaging the perineum with warm oil or applying warm compresses may make the skin more flexible. Your doctor, midwife, or a nurse can do this during second-stage labor.

assisted vaginal delivery: forceps or vacuum extraction

Assisted delivery is used when the attending physician or midwife believes that the baby needs help getting out of the birth canal. This can happen for many reasons. If doctors or midwives think that the mother may be unable to push out the baby, or there is concern about the fetal heart rate, they may opt to use a tool (forceps or vacuum) to try to get the baby out faster. The two means of extraction have pros and cons and many doctors have a preferred method. Vacuums often cause less trauma to the mother's body and are easier for the physician to master, but they have a lower rate of successful vaginal delivery than forceps. Both methods can cause injuries to the newborn (most often minor—such as marks on the head or face). Assisted deliveries may require a large episiotomy and have longer recovery times than unassisted ones, with a higher risk of some postpartum complications.

c-section births

A Cesarean or C-section is a surgical birth in which the baby is removed from the mother's uterus through an incision in her abdomen. The name is commonly thought to be derived from the birth of Julius Caesar, but history actually indicates otherwise (Caesar was born vaginally). The rate of C-sections in this country has been increasing steadily in recent years. In 2004, 29.1 percent of births were by Cesarean, a 40 percent increase since 1996.

some possible reasons for an increase in c-sections

- More older mothers/obesity/high-risk pregnancies
- More multiple births
- Liability issues
- Society's increasing comfort with surgery leads to more elective C-sections
- Fewer VBACs (vaginal birth after Cesareans)

some situations that may lead to a c-section (Having one of these conditions does not mean a c-section is obligatory. Talk to your doctor to see what your options are.)

- Position of the baby (10—15 percent of C-sections are due to breech or transverse babies)
- Abnormal heart rate for baby
- Developmental abnormalities with baby (such as neural tube defects)
- Multiple babies (triplets, twins sometimes)
- Umbilical cord prolapse (a rare emergency when cord slips out before baby)

> The C-section was my first surgery so I kept my eyes closed as ten healthcare professionals were surrounding me. My husband was right beside me watching the whole thing, fascinated.
> —anonymom

- Placenta previa or other placental problems → See Placental Problems, page 109.
- Prolonged or arrested labor
- Too large of a head to fit though the mother's pelvis (clinically happens less than 1 percent of the time, but is often given as a reason after the fact)
- Infectious disease (HIV, active herpes)
- Previous uterine surgery → See VBAC, page 133.
- Severe illness, such as preeclampsia

Okay, I had a C-section, no need to get the bottle of water and squirt me down there—but yes, they do. And it tickles, so you jump and that of course hurts your stomach from the C-section. And then when you go to the bathroom for the first time, they squirt water to wash you off down there and again, it tickles and you jump and hurt your stomach. I swear, I wanted to slap those nurses across their face for doing that.

—anonymom

I had always thought that C-sections were not a big deal—they tend to be downplayed and have sort of a cute name, but the fact is that it is pretty significant surgery, and I think downplaying it sort of does women a disservice. Here's what no one told me about C-sections: (1) you have to lie at a weird angle, which was disorienting; and (2) they take a really long time to stitch you up after the baby is out. Midway through mine, I started to lose a ton of blood. I started to get really faint, and my husband (who is clearly not a medical sort of person) was convinced that I was dying. It was very traumatizing for him because he could tell that there was a problem and no one was telling him what was going on. He responded to this by getting very close to my face and repeatedly telling me to "look into his eyes," which, frankly, was the last thing I wanted to do at that point. It was rather comical in retrospect; bless his heart, though—after we were in the recovery room for a while, I kicked him out to go tell our moms that the baby was here in one piece and was great. He held his composure until he saw his mom and then dissolved into a gigantic pile of tears.

—anonymom

While the baby is still in the room, that's all you can concentrate on and you don't realize anything else. But once the baby leaves and they finish you up, everything hits you like a ton of bricks. All I wanted to do was sit up. I did not want to lie down anymore, but they wouldn't let me. I felt like I was going to die. I could hardly breathe and they said that was normal because sometimes air gets pushed up when they are doing all that pushing and tugging. Finally I was all stitched up and then they had to clean me. That was a weird feeling. They roll you from side to side and you feel like you're going to fall off the tiny table you're on. Then my leg kept falling off the table—but I couldn't feel it because of the epidural. But it just kept falling off and someone actually had to hold it on the table. Haha. Then we went to the recovery room, where they only let me sit up halfway because my blood pressure was so low. I remember being so weak from that, that I actually had to keep my eyes closed and I couldn't even hold my own son!!

—anonymom

For me, the baby was still high up there so they had to reach up high and really pull and push and tug. At one point the one nurse was completely on top of my stomach pushing down with her elbow to get the baby out. That pushing/tugging and pulling was enough to make me say "Oh my god" while I could hardly breathe through it.

—anonymom

c-section risks?

C-section births are generally very safe but do have different risks than vaginal births. Where a choice is possible, the risks should be considered carefully:

- **Maternal infection is much more likely than in vaginal birth.**

- **Twice as many women need rehospitalization after C-sections than after vaginal births.**

- **Risk of maternal death, while still low, is five to seven times higher than in vaginal birth.**

- **Higher risk of heavy bleeding or hemorrhaging (this is more of an issue with unplanned C-sections).**

- **Some mothers react adversely to anesthetic.**

- **Respiratory problems for the infant are more common in C-sections (these are more likely with younger gestational age).**

- **The risk of future placental problems rises with each C-section; elective C-section is not recommended for women who want more than two children.** → See Placental Problems, page 109.

planned c-sections

A C-section can be scheduled for any number of reasons. Physical issues may prevent or discourage a vaginal birth. All babies who are transverse, and almost all who are breech, are born via Cesarean. The position of the placenta can also necessitate C-section, as in placenta previa, in which the placenta grows over the cervix. C-sections are common with multiple births. And many high-risk pregnancy conditions lead to scheduled C-sections. If your doctor suggests you schedule a C-section and you feel strongly about trying to give birth vaginally, you can ask him whether or not there are any alternatives. Some of these situations are not negotiable. It is impossible to do a vaginal delivery with placenta previa, and in most places it would be difficult to find a provider willing to take on the liability of delivering a breech baby vaginally. → See Breech Babies, page 105.

A surgical birth can also be requested by the mother, with her doctor's permission. Women who have had C-sections in the past might decide to have another because it's familiar, or because they want to circumvent the small risk of uterine rupture. (See VBAC, right.) Likewise, women who have had scary or difficult vaginal births may opt for a C-section to avoid anxiety about a repeat performance (however unlikely). Women may schedule C-sections simply because the operating room gives them the illusion of control while labor feels unpredictable. In our surgery-friendly

vbac

Although the majority (75 percent according to a 2004 study) of women who try for a VBAC—vaginal birth after a previous C-section—are successful, fewer and fewer women have been attempting this procedure. In the mid-1990s, more than 25 percent of women tried for VBACs. In 2004, that number was less than 10 percent. This dramatic dip may be partially a backlash against a policy set in the nineties in which insurance companies, trying to cut costs, mandated labor trials for women who had had previous surgical births. This indiscriminate policy led to a lot of complications, and a lot of lawsuits. Subsequently, to avoid potential liability, many hospitals stopped allowing VBACs.

society, it may be easier to conceive of the risks and recovery of an operation than the mysterious pain of old-school childbirth. Some women have C-sections because they've heard they'll have less pelvic floor damage. Studies have shown no long-term difference in pelvic floor function.

unplanned c-sections

If your provider determines that you and/or your baby would be safer if the baby was out of your body rather than in it (and that's not possible vaginally for whatever reason), she may decide on the spot to give you a C-section. This can happen at any point during labor, or before labor even happens. The level of urgency depends on the situation. An unplanned C-section can be more stressful than a planned one for many reasons. A change in plan can be upsetting, and you may have to make decisions while in labor. Since you're not necessarily prepared for this kind of birth emotionally, you may be dealing with shock and disappointment in addition to anxiety about everyone's welfare. If you have a C-section after a long labor, your body will have some extra recovering to do, too.

→ See Dealing with Disappointment, page 167.

→ See Dealing with Disappointment, page 167.

resources

Cesarean Section: Understanding and Celebrating Your Baby's Birth by Michele C. Moore and Caroline M. de Costa

The Essential C-Section Guide: Pain Control, Healing at Home, Getting Your Body Back and Everything Else You Need to Know About a Cesarean Birth by Maureen Connolly and Dana Sullivan

What if I Have a C-section? by Mark Landon and Rita Rubin

"A Balanced View of Cesareans": csections.org

The Coalition for Improving Maternity Services website: motherfriendly.org

pain relief

There are lots of ways of dealing with pain in childbirth. Sometimes women pick a particular pain strategy and try to stick with it; others like to familiarize themselves with various methods and medications so that they have some options once the pain begins. Many of the techniques below are taught in childbirth classes or described in birthing books. You might also get tips from your friends or caregiver that can help. Here are some things you may or may not find effective, in alphabetical order.

AROMATHERAPY: Aromatherapy can be great during labor for people who like it. There are aromas that are said to calm, invigorate, and inspire confidence, among other things. Lavender oil is often recommended, sometimes in combination with other scents and especially in early labor. An expert on aromatherapy or some books on the subject can give you more ideas. Since you don't know how you'll react to smells during labor, it's a good idea to keep aromas somewhat contained in case you find them unexpectedly repellent!

BREATHING: Breath is linked to both mental and physical health, and especially to relaxation. So it

> For most of my labor, I would lean on my husband and we would breathe together while our doula massaged my lower back and offered encouragement. At one point I had to lie on my back while they checked out the baby's condition and that was by far the most painful time.
> —anonymom

> The pain was extreme but always bearable if I knew how to handle it. . . . I used meditation, hypnosis, massage, deep breathing, and water therapy. They all worked amazingly well. Especially the water therapy. The second I got into the tub, my contractions went away instantly. We took Bradley and hypnobirthing classes.
> —anonymom

makes sense that focusing on and/or controlling the breath is a big part of so many pain-relief techniques, official and otherwise. There are many different takes on how breathing can make birth pains easier. Prenatal yoga classes can also be a good place to learn about using breath in labor. ➔ See Birthing Techniques, page 136, for more information on some of the leading breath-oriented methods.

MASSAGE: If you like massage in general, you might find it soothing during your birth. Then again, you might not. Pain can alter your perception of (and desire for) touch. You may want to be rubbed constantly, or be surprised to find that despite your partner's massage expertise, you can't stand being touched at all. Long, downward strokes and continuity of touch can be soothing. Poking and tickling are usually not. Pressure on the lower back can be particularly helpful for back labor.

MOVEMENT AND POSITIONING: Changing positions may ease contraction pain and also give you the feeling that you are actively doing something to improve the situation. Many women find moving around during labor lessens the pain or makes it easier to deal with. Different positions can also make use of gravity. Rhythmic motion can be comforting and distracting; props like balls or rocking chairs can help facilitate this, but you can also do it on your own. Any position that feels like it might take the edge off is worth trying.

MUSIC: The right song can relax you, distract you, or give you a boost of energy. For people who respond to music, a set of headphones (or a birth situation that allows you to turn up the volume) can be a great help in labor.

PROPS: Some props, like the birthing stool and squat bar, are specifically designed to make birth easier, though not necessarily less painful. Birthing balls (also used for general exercise) can help a woman find comfortable positions during labor and move in a way that takes the pressure off. Anything you find soothing or helpful can be a pain-relieving prop during birth: a cold pack for your forehead; an eye mask to shut out the light; familiar or comforting things to touch, hold, or smell.

SELF-HYPNOSIS: Some women are able to put themselves into a hyperrelaxed trance state, with training. Hypnosis is becoming an increasingly popular tool for labor pain management. Being willing and able to put faith in the method is important to its success. Hypnosis can be especially helpful for people who are very afraid of labor. Classes in hypnosis for birth teach the required techniques.

WATER: Many women find that being immersed in water relieves contraction pain. The warm water can relax muscles and improve circulation, while the buoyancy provided by the water can reduce the stress of

> I moved around in all different ways. I invited the pain so that the contractions would be more efficient, like sitting on the toilet to relax the perineum more.
> —anonymom

> In transition I actually got out of bed and squatted to get her down more and get to the pushing stage. That was very helpful.
> —anonymom

> The birthing ball was the most effective, particularly in active labor because it seemed to help the baby drop.
> —anonymom

labor and take the pressure off your abdomen and back. Depending on where you are in labor, immersion in water may be discouraged. Birthing centers are more likely than hospitals to have tubs. The warmth of a shower can also be soothing. Many women who give birth in rooms without baths spend much of their labor in the shower. You can rent a tub for use at home. ➔ See Water Birth, page 156.

> I tried the tub. It didn't work. I tried the bouncy balls. They didn't help the pain in my back. I tried sitting in a beanbag chair, which helped the pain in my back but increased the pain in my abdomen. Standing and leaning forward clutching the edge of a table helped, but my legs were so exhausted they were shaking. It's what climbers call "sewing machine leg."
> —anonymom

> The only thing that seemed to distract me enough and feel okay was a hot shower. If I was in a birthing center, I would have loved to try that whole water-birth thing. It felt so good. Well, as good as it could have felt.
> —anonymom

birthing techniques

LAMAZE The Lamaze method was developed in France in the 1950s, and caught on in the United States around ten years later. The method, based on Pavlovian conditioning, uses stylized, shallow breathing and visual concentration to help a mother develop an automatic learned response. She trains herself to become relaxed by the breath and then uses this technique in labor. Lamaze classes became so popular in the following decades that members of the sixties generation often use the word "Lamaze" to describe any kind of childbirth preparation.

BRADLEY In 1960, the Bradley method was developed by an American pediatrician who felt that labor should be a partner effort. He emphasized the father's role in coaching the mother and supporting her throughout the birth. The Bradley method discourages medical intervention in the natural process of birth. Women are encouraged to labor in a quiet, dark, and comfortable environment, using slow, deep breathing and taking their time as needed.

These two methods are the most popular, but there are lots of other organized approaches to childbirth preparation. Combining aspects of different methods is also an option. Childbirth classes can give you a general overview as well as some information about specific techniques. ➔ See page 149 for info on childbirth classes. See the list of birth books, page 142, for more resources; many describe explicit techniques for handling the pain of labor.

resources

Husband-Coached Childbirth: The Bradley Method of Natural Childbirth by Robert A. Bradley

Natural Childbirth the Bradley Way: Revised Edition by Susan McCutcheon-Rosegg

The Official Lamaze Guide: Giving Birth with Confidence by Judith Lothian, Charlotte DeVries

Preparation for Birth: The Complete Guide to the Lamaze Method by Beverly Savage, Diana Simkin

The Bradley Method® website: bradleybirth.com

The Lamaze® International website: lamaze.org

pain medication

ANALGESICS AND NARCOTICS: These kinds of medications (including Demerol, Stadol, and fentanyl) are sometimes given to laboring mothers— usually earlier on in labor, and sometimes in conjunction with an epidural. They may not take away much of the pain, but they do tend to relax women or make pain more bearable (they can make you feel high and/or sleepy). Narcotics do not numb the body, so moving around is still possible. Some common side effects for the mother may include nausea, itching, vomiting, sleepiness, sluggish bowels, a drop in blood pressure, and respiratory depression. Since these drugs enter the bloodstream, they may affect the baby, possibly causing an inability to regulate body temperature, breathing difficulties, and a general drowsiness that can interfere with initial breastfeeding. Exposed newborns may be given a drug to counter effects and taken to the NICU. Mothers may also be given an additional drug to counter any related nausea. To keep side effects to a minimum, narcotics are generally given in small doses in early labor. Narcotics can be given via IV, a one-time injection into the spinal column, or injection into the muscle.

TRANQUILIZERS OR BARBITURATES: In small doses, tranquilizers or barbiturates may help a woman feel more relaxed and less anxious—they can, however, cause intense drowsiness and pose some risks to the baby (such as decrease in muscle tone and movement at birth). They do not actually reduce pain and are rarely used.

epidural anesthesia

An epidural block is the most commonly used anesthetic for labor. It involves blocking the nerves (and accompanying sensation) to only the lower part of the body so that a laboring woman can be relatively pain-free and alert as the labor progresses and the baby is born. In some cases, removing the pain can relax a woman and help her labor progress. Others suggest that epidurals given too early may slow down labor. There are different kinds of epidurals, including "spinal epidural," "narcotic epidural," and "walking epidural" (this is just a lower dose, but not usually low enough to allow for easy walking). These are often lumped together and discussed simply as an "epidural." All use some form of drugs in addition to

> When you're in that much pain, the epidural feels like a tickle!!
> —anonymom

> I hadn't dilated after an hour or two of labor; I got the epidural and went from four centimeters to ten centimeters in forty-five minutes. It helped me to relax, which did the trick. It felt strange; I could move my legs but felt nothing.
> —anonymom

the nerve block, but the exact cocktail varies by hospital. You may also be offered antinausea medication to combat any side effects from the narcotics. Spinal blocks are inserted into a different part of the body than an epidural. You can talk to your doctor about the various options beforehand (even if you plan to avoid medication), but you may not have much say over which kind of epidural will be available.

PROCEDURE: An anesthesiologist, or anesthetist, numbs the area, then inserts a needle into the epidural space in the spine. A catheter is then inserted into that space, and some combination of anesthetic and/or narcotics is administered. Some feel a tingling or pressure or a short, shooting pain. The numbing effects start within minutes. Epidural medication can be on a continuous flow, topped up, or increased over time. It can also be decreased or removed. If a C-section becomes necessary, the epidural is already in place and the level of anesthetic is increased. (Epidurals are the primary anesthetic for a C-section; a general anesthetic is used only rarely.) A spinal is a one-time injection that takes effect very quickly but cannot be topped up over time (which is why it is sometimes combined with an epidural). It may take a while for the anesthesiologist to arrive once called, and visits may be rushed. If you have a lot of questions about the epidural, or any back issues that could complicate the process, you may want to ask for an early consult with an anesthesiologist.

> Everyone says "Get an epidural" so you won't have any pain... to some degree this is true ... you may not have any pain but no one said you won't have pressure. If you think pressure can't be painful... imagine a full-grown elephant sitting on your pelvis for, say, twenty-six hours—might sound a bit uncomfortable, huh?
> —anonymom

> When I reached stage two of my labor... I knew there was no way I was going to give birth without an epidural. I was two centimeters dilated, and the baby's head was pushing down on the birth canal. I could hardly walk to the car. I was hyperventilating and howling like a wolf. I cannot even fathom a natural birth. The excruciating pain would have ruined the experience for me, which turned out to be the most wonderful experience of my life.
> —anonymom

SIDE EFFECTS: Though major side effects are uncommon, there are some common and sometimes very unpleasant minor ones: An epidural can make a woman feel very itchy and cause shivering or shaking. The drugs can cause nausea and vomiting. A small percentage of women experience an incapacitating headache afterward (this is more common with a spinal block, and it can usually be treated). In some cases, epidural use (especially if in place for more than five hours) can lead to a fever during labor, which can be dangerous for the baby. The laboring woman is also unable to move around, thus limiting the variety of birthing positions. She may get into a weird position and be too numb to realize it, causing back pain or other muscle aches after the birth. The injection site can also be achy or tender. Epidurals require IV fluids (as well as any additional medication if needed), continuous electronic fetal monitoring, a bladder catheter, and more frequent blood pressure monitoring. Since epidurals can prolong the length of labor, they are associated with increased use of Pitocin and assisted delivery (vacuum/forceps). Occasionally the epidural will numb only part or one side of the body, or not work at all. Rarely, a woman will experience an allergic reaction. More serious or lasting side effects, such as neurological and back problems, are extremely rare.

> It felt like the smallest of bee stings and then like a rush of ice water right down my spine. I had actually been more afraid of the shot than of the birth itself . . . but it was given during a contraction and was so needed that I hardly felt a thing.
> —anonymom

> It hurt like hell going in, but helped the pain immediately. I had hoped not to have to get one. I'm not sure how I feel about it now. I think it made pushing harder for me, since I couldn't feel what I was doing. Also, because of all the fluids they were pumping in me, I was horribly swollen for about a week afterward. But at the time, I couldn't have been happier.
> —anonymom

> I already had the epidural in, so all they needed to do was put in more numbing medication to fully numb me for the C-section. It was sooo cold going down my back, but at the same time it felt really good and refreshing.
> —anonymom

> I had a blinding epidural headache after the birth. It was worse than labor!! I could not even sit up, let alone stand up. I was totally drugged up on codeine, which then made me so constipated I had to do an enema! Never, never again for me (though I know the chances are only like 1 in 100).
> —anonymom

epidurals and c-sections?

Does an epidural make it more or less likely that a woman will have a C-section? Studies haven't been able to prove anything either way. For some women the epidural provides the relief they need to relax and dilate, allowing for a vaginal birth. For others it may prolong or stall labor, leading to a surgical birth. Some studies have indicated that the timing of an epidural may affect birth outcome—with early epidurals associated with more C-sections. In the 2005 *New England Journal of Medicine,* a controversial study concluded that the timing of an epidural did not affect the likelihood of a C-section. The American College of Obstetricians and Gynecologists recently dropped its recommendation that epidurals be postponed until a woman has reached 4–5 centimeters. The decision about when to start an epidural often involves taking into account how the labor is progressing. Talk to your caregiver about timing and epidurals; every situation is unique.

> I had an epidural and even though you do hear in rare cases there are side effects, no one really said I would have pain in the same spot they put the needle in. There is no mark or sign that a needle was put in but when I lie back, I can feel that same spot very tender and achy. It's been over eight weeks!
> —anonymom

> For months afterward if I lay the wrong way or sat the wrong way or something like that, I had a cold-water feeling go up my back from where the epidural went in all the way up to my right shoulder. That doesn't happen anymore and it's been almost ten months.
> —anonymom

There is little conclusive data on the effects of epidurals on babies. Dosage and length of labor are variable and babies respond to the medications differently. Some potential problems that have been cited include lethargy (which can affect positioning and progress of birth), heart rate fluctuations, and difficulty with breastfeeding.

local anesthetic

Sometimes a local anesthetic is injected into the vaginal area before the birth of the baby to temporarily numb the area. There are two options: a pudendal block (used on the vaginal wall) or local infiltration anesthetic (used on the vaginal tissue). A pudendal block is often used in conjunction with a forceps- or vacuum-assisted birth and/or an episiotomy. A local infiltration anesthetic may be used to repair a tear. Since they are local anesthetics, the repercussions tend to be minimal (no pain relief from contractions but few known side effects).

> In my first birth I had an epidural after a long eighteen hours of unmedicated labor. It totally relaxed me, and I dilated seven centimeters in, like, an hour. I loved it so much that in my second birth I got one at the first opportunity. But this time IT WAS THE WORST: I was totally dead from the abdomen down and had major paralysis anxiety. I was dry-heaving and shaking like a junkie in withdrawal. The epidural side effects were probably the worst part of the whole birth!
> —anonymom

preparing yourself

There are lots of ways to get ready for birth: Classes and books to gain knowledge. Physical exercise to build endurance. Emotional and spiritual centering techniques. Creative expression to articulate hopes and fears. Sublimating it all into the mad cleaning frenzy known as nesting. Some people don't do much conscious preparation at all, which is a perfectly valid plan if you're not inclined. Physical, mental, and logistical legwork (like touring a hospital and practicing breathing) can give you a feeling of being prepared, whether or not you end up using what you know.

expectations, fantasies, and fears

When it comes to birth, it's hard to know what to expect. You hear stories that sound like horror-tinged science fiction. ("Why kid yourself? It's gonna be torture.") Your prenatal yoga teacher preaches positive thinking to encourage a positive outcome. ("Don't listen to those undermining scare tactics!") Meanwhile, your birthing class instructor tells you not to have any expectations at all. ("You never know what could happen!") While it's true that birth is not a predictable experience, it's also perfectly reasonable to imagine how yours is going to play out, and nearly impossible to avoid some kind of preconceived notions. The real task is to inform yourself without cornering yourself: to keep an open mind, staying aware of how information is being framed.

It's normal to have hopes and wishes for a particular unfolding of events, but if your birth fantasy runs too deep, you may be more disappointed if the reality doesn't measure up. Learn whatever techniques you want and imagine away—but then be willing to toss those ideas (and possibly ideals) out the window if things take a new and unpredictable turn.

natural vs. medical childbirth: either/or?

The expression "natural childbirth" can refer to anything from home birthing with a midwife to giving birth in a hospital with an obstetrician, but without any pain relief or other interventions. If a pregnant woman feels inclined toward this kind of birth, she may find it helpful to prepare with classes and books that highlight the power of natural birth—and the potential dangers of "medicalized" birth. Some natural childbirth literature suggests that women intuitively know how to give birth and go further to claim that medicine can only serve to obscure this power and bungle our births. This idea can serve as a great motivator for women who want to birth without intervention.

It may well be true that you have the resources within yourself to birth a baby without the help of medicine or monitors. It is a fact that drugs, tubes, and monitors affect your labor and restrict your movement. But it is not a fact that all medical assistances to childbirth are tools of the male establishment and will almost definitely put you on the path to a C-section in order to give your OB more time to play golf.

Childbirth is not always within our control. We can choose our caregivers (or at least the ones we hope will be on duty when we go into labor). We can choose our birthing locations and hope all goes smoothly. But if you find yourself hooked up to a fetal monitor, which limits your movement, which limits your pain relief options, which leads you to ask for an epidural, you are not giving up your awesome power to the oppression of The Man. If interventions enter the picture, you're just letting an inherently unpredictable event unfold in a way that makes most sense at the time. This is not to imply that a medical birth is the wisest choice, either. It isn't. Statistically, neither scenario is more or less risky. Both sides just look at the statistics differently.

The question for us is, Why must things be so polarized? A hospital birth promises access to medicine, but a lack of control. A home or birth-center birth promises a natural experience, but there's no access to pain medication, and you'll probably be warned of the dangers of hospital births. Why do women who want the option of pain relief have to be denied freedom of movement in labor before they even decide whether or not to be medicated? Why do women who want to learn about natural childbirth have to hear every horror story associated with procedures they may not ultimately be able to avoid? In the words of one woman who'd recently had a hospital birth, "Why can't we have the massage, the fresh-baked bread, the warm bath . . . and then the epidural if we want one?" It's as if natural birth and medical birth are opposing teams, and you've got to pick a side and stick with it. This isn't true everywhere; there are places (not many in the United States, unfortunately) where it's possible to have a more integrated experience. And there are ways of cobbling together your own hodgepodge of natural and medical birth techniques; hiring a doula to help support natural pain relief during a hospital birth is one example. → See Professional Support: Birth Doulas, page 160, Interventions, page 126, and Birth Center, page 154.

resources

Birthing from Within: An Extra-Ordinary Guide to Childbirth Preparation by Pam England, Rob Horowitz, birthingfromwithin.com. *Birthing from Within*'s creative birth prep techniques, designed by artist/midwife Pam England, include breathing awareness, self-hypnosis, and visualization, as well as a lot of arts and crafts.

The Birth Partner by Penny Simkin. Penny Simkin's classic focuses on the partner's role in childbirth (whether that's the baby's father or someone else who will attend the birth). Though the book leans toward unmedicated birth, much of it applies to childbirth in general.

The Birth That's Right for You by Amen Ness, Lisa Gould Rubin, Jackie Frederick Berner. In an unusually bipartisan effort, an ob-gyn and doula join forces, encouraging readers to do what feels right to them. Hospital birth and medical pain relief options are discussed nonjudgmentally.

The Complete Book of Pregnancy and Childbirth by Sheila Kitzinger, sheilakitzinger.com. British grand dame of natural childbirth Sheila Kitzinger has written and taught for decades on woman-centered birthing practices. She delivers straightforward information and progressive ideas with a direct, friendly approach.

Ina May's Guide to Childbirth by Ina May Gaskin, inamay.com. Ina May Gaskin has been credited with single-handedly reviving both home birth and the midwifery movement in America. Her book focuses on the power of the body in birth, using personal stories to build women's confidence.

fear of death

The maternal mortality rate is now very low, but historically, childbearing has been pretty risky business. This was mostly due to maternal infections in the days before antibiotics. However, the fear of dying in childbirth still looms for many women. As of 2001, only about 9 in 100,000 births (adjusted across age and race) resulted in death for the mother in the United States. To put this into perspective, your odds of dying in a transportation accident are almost double that in any given year.

fear of grossing people out

Birth is not pretty, at least not by the usual standards. Worry about looking disgusting during the process is a big deal for many women. Although birth can involve a certain amount of blood and guts and gore, for most people the beauty and/or pain of the moment transcends or even obliterates the icky stuff . . . including the dreaded poop that might get pushed out in the process of pushing out the baby. It's best not to dwell on this stuff too much—there's little chance that anyone around you will be giving it a second thought.

→ See Partner Positioning, page 158.

fear of pain

Cultures all over the world and throughout history have assigned various meanings to the pain of birth: The Bible says it's woman's punishment for Eve's sins. There are somewhat more pleasant connections, too; i.e., labor as an exalted (if brutal) physical state that has the power to connect all women in a kind of cosmic and heroic unity.

As you prepare for birth, the fear of pain may be more or less at the front of your mind. There are lots of strategies for pain relief (see "Pain Relief" on page 134). One way of dealing with pain is thinking about how you want to address it before you're actually in the painful situation. Everyone has a different way of putting the fear of pain into perspective: Some like to pump themselves up, others like to focus on the mind-body connection and try to control the perception of pain. And a lot of people just count on advances in science to make the pain go away.

positions on pain

GET TOUGH! BIRTH AS BATTLE: *A birthing woman should be strong or stoic enough to go beyond her limits in order to reach glory. The reward for sacrifice is knowing you kicked ass for the good of your baby. And maybe a bonus for you, too: Just as a marathon runner experiences a flood of endorphins after some substantial amount of physical strife, a woman in labor can get to that natural ecstasy if she toughs it out without medication.*

The birth-as-battlefield/Olympic field metaphor may feel like a useful tool, or an unnecessary challenge. If the "no pain, no gain" equation inspires you, thinking of labor as a kind of marathon may give you confidence. But you don't have the benefit of knowing what your labor will be like, so you can't exactly train like a marathon runner by slowly building up to what you'll need to handle. If the pump-up, GI Jane attitude feels like a lot of pressure, keep in mind: You are a warrior and a winner no matter what happens in your birth. Don't feel compelled to endure anything you don't have to . . . unless you want to.

WHY SUFFER NEEDLESSLY? *Romanticizing labor is unwise and unfair. Labor drugs are a feminist choice— the epidural would probably have been invented sooner if more women had been allowed in medical school! Endurance of pain is hardly heroic. It's cruel. And, given the excellent medical pain-relief options available, completely illogical. Would you have a root canal without anesthetic?*

The early-twentieth-century labor pain relief known as Twilight Sleep is often used as an example of the subjugation of laboring women to the oppressive male medical regime. But it was actually championed by the suffragettes as emancipating! The return-to-nature childbirth movement was largely a reaction to various practices of drugging women and then bringing them their babies at some later point. These days we have much, much safer and more humane methods of medical pain relief, and many people think that turning down these options is just plain masochistic.

Women have been known to write on their birth plans "Do not let me have drugs, even if I beg." Is the decision made before knowing what labor feels like really more valid than the one that's made in the throes of pain? If you feel that drugs may help you, there's no reason to feel guilty— or to feel that your birth will be less authentic or triumphant than if you went without. As with all pain-relief strategies, it's worth keeping an open mind about medication. Fantasizing about an epidural for nine months can put some pressure on, too: What if there's a logistical snafu— they do happen—and you can't get one? What if, for whatever reason, it doesn't work? Addressing the physical challenges ahead with more than just an eye for the catheter can give you additional resources for unexpected or lingering pain.

Twilight Sleep was also called scopolamine (the same stuff used for motion sickness) and made you feel in a fog and powerless while you still had pain. Believe me, I had it and it was a Twilight Nightmare.
—anonygrandmom

There's a good case to be made that frightening women makes them anxious and tense, which actually adds to the pain because they are therefore unable to relax mentally and physically enough to have any control. On the other side, if you're expecting a lyrical experience in which any pain can be avoided if you simply follow a breathing pattern, you can get really frightened if there's pain and you assume something's very wrong or you're a failure.
—anonymom

PAIN IS IN THE EYE OF THE BEHOLDER: *Pain is a state of mind as well as body. The more we conceive of birth as normal and natural, the less likely we are to feel pain. Hospitals and doctors (among other influences) contribute to a hyped-up sense of sickness and death that inform our perceptions. Birth can even be pleasurable if we let go of the fear.*

In his widely read *Childbirth Without Fear,* Grantly Dick-Read, father of "natural childbirth," described "primitive" women who did not feel any birthing pain. He wrote about societies where birth was not considered an urgent matter requiring doctors and/or hospital care, and where women did not feel as much, if any, agony. More contemporary natural childbirth gurus tell stories of animals who actually seize up and stop laboring when they sense danger. For us human animals, the theory goes, it's the hospital that's scary and dangerous. In the absence of alarming machines that go "bing," and a distracted hospital staff, women may be less uptight (emotionally, and literally, as in uptight in the cervix) and less likely to feel any pain. Once the fear has lifted, women are free to explore and even enjoy the power of their bodies in birth—maybe even to the point of pleasure. Legendary midwife Ina May Gaskin contends that one in four of her fellow Farm midwives has assisted in an orgasmic birth.

Remembering that labor is a part of life (rather than a part of sickness and death) can go a long way toward reducing panic. And positive thoughts can encourage positive feelings. But putting too much emphasis on your positive attitude can add a ton of pressure—a painful labor becomes the result of your failure to think good thoughts instead of just a difficult experience. Reading about the possibility of an orgasmic birth can give you hope or make you feel like you've failed if yours is nowhere near euphoric. Many examples of pain- and fear-free births seem to take place in insulated environments where natural childbirth is entirely supported logistically and emotionally. Not everyone has the opportunity (or proclivity) to give birth in a commune run by world-class midwives. Trying to carve out a childbirth free from doctors and hospitals in a world that reveres medicine is a much different task. If you are drawn to the idea of the mind-body connection, do what you can to absorb the positive vibes and avoid things that make you feel scared or stressed. Viewing birth as normal and healthy may not eliminate pain, but it may simply make you feel more game about coping with it.

> We all hear horror stories, the pain is so bad, etc. But it's not until going through it that any of us realize the reality.... "Anticipating" the excruciating pain of labor is just not enough. Not until you "experience" that pain are you able to fully comprehend it. *Then* you can decide about pain control.
> —anonymom

resources

Birth: The Surprising History of How We Are Born by Tina Cassidy

Deliver This! Make the Childbirth Choice That's Right for You ... No Matter What Everyone Else Thinks by Marisa Cohen

what you can control
and what you can't

If this is your first baby, labor is an entirely unknown quantity. Other people's descriptions of birth may not do much to help you understand how it feels—unless you've pushed an eggplant out your nose or a basketball out your butt, those analogies are good for nothing but comic relief. Toward the end of pregnancy the labor can seem like a light at the end of the tunnel with a big blinking question mark hanging over it. Though you can't predict how your baby's birth will unfold, there are some things you can do to make it more likely that you'll have a birth you feel good about.

talk about what scares you

Everyone has different kinds of anxiety about birth—some worry more about the physical stuff (like pain, scars, bruising) and some, the psychological stuff (confidence, happiness, bonding). Trying to keep a stiff upper lip about certain fears you have may prevent you from seeking out the right kind of pain relief techniques and supportive environment that can help you. The more open you are with yourself and your support team about your specific concerns, the more likely you are to develop some good coping strategies that you'll be able to use when the time comes.

tune out the noise

One day you may be completely won over by one theory, the next you're swayed by an opposing approach. When you meet a woman at a party and become fast friends, and she says "You know I'm getting that epidural!" it can be hard not to let that reflect on your own ideas about birth: Is she right? What does getting an epidural say about a woman? Sometimes decisions about birthing can be presented to you as political platforms to rally behind: Do you "believe" in natural childbirth? What's your take on medication? Your birth can seem more about your values than the impossible-to-predict contingencies of labor. If you feel like you're getting swamped by too many agendas and it's stressing you out, try to peel away the stereotypes and schools of thought and focus on what makes you comfortable. You may, in principle, object to the "medicalization" of birth, but feel more relaxed with an expert obstetric team down the hallway. You may love the idea of pain medication but feel driven to try natural birth. There are many roads to childbirth. Yours might not be a straight line.

my birth, myself

Oh, you're a yoga fanatic? Well, you'll doubtless be laboring in goddess pose, chanting your way through contractions. You're a party girl? Order the drugs on the way to the hospital. You're a whip-cracker at work? You'll surely be calling the shots in the delivery room. Or not. Your personality does play a role in your birth but it doesn't define it. Don't let other people's perceptions

> Do not bother with a birth plan—it never turns out the way you envision!
> —anonymom

> I had a plan ...and none of it happened like I had "planned." I gave birth three weeks premature and was so swollen with water retention I didn't care how things happened ...just that I was finally going to have this baby!
> —anonymom

of who you are, or even things you know about yourself, push you in directions you don't feel good about when it comes to birth. You're probably a lot more complicated than any one trait, no matter how easily it lends itself to a birth stereotype. You get to define the kind of person you want to be in the birth room, whether or not it's who you are at work, working out, or wherever.

keep an open birth plan

Birth plans have been a popular way for women who want to have some level of control in a hospital birth to communicate their priorities to the staff. A birth plan can be a useful tool to help you articulate your wishes. But the word "plan" can be misleading: The idea that you can map out a birth is questionable (some, in retrospect, say laughable). Sometimes they are called wish lists or preference sheets. Some suggest you bypass a list altogether and go directly to the nurses and doctor/midwife about your desires, either in writing or in person. However you decide to go about the process, keep in mind that what you're doing is talking about what you want, not what you absolutely must have. Birth rarely follows a plan. So you'll need to be flexible, even if that means throwing your whole plan out the window when you get off-course.

For me, my birth plan [was] absolutely worthless. In fact, my ob-gyn laughed at me when I had one. I had a very high-risk pregnancy, and it was my first pregnancy, and they didn't inform me that a birth plan was out of the question since they had to follow certain procedures in order to bring my son into the world safely and keep me safe, too. But I was upset that my ob-gyn treated my birth plan that way since she never discussed with me that I would be stuck in bed (one thing I wanted was to be able to walk around while I was laboring).
—anonymom

And what advice would I give? Just for new moms to know that, look, not everything is going to go according to plan because, frankly, there's a lot of stuff you can't control. Be careful about making sweeping proclamations about what you plan to do—it's far better to have an idea, but be flexible based on your health needs and the needs of your baby. It's not a contest, so just do what feels right and is medically necessary.
—anonymom

My birth plan bore no resemblance to how I gave birth. I did not want the EFM; I did not want the epidural; I certainly did not plan on the premature labor! . . . I'm still not happy with how the delivery went, but I have a beautiful, healthy little girl, so the end result was worth it.
—anonymom

If it makes you feel better about a situation that, let's face it, is out of control, then do it. . . . It [a birth plan] gave me such a positive experience even though everything about the birth flip-flopped around. . . . The underlying theme of the room was positive and superconfident that I could do it.
—anonymom

I am a planner by profession. A plan is a goal. Write down your thoughts about want you want, but be prepared to take other paths without regret. A plan will help you and your partner communicate with staff, but don't let it set you up. Have your partner or someone from your team help you communicate. You really need support.
—anonymom

My birth plan was to go into labor and do the whole thing naturally. Ha! Yeah, right. I was induced, had an epidural, and I don't regret it at all. All that worry and it was just one day in my life, as opposed to the rest of my daughter's life, which I remember much more clearly than my labor to deliver her.

—**anonymom**

My birth plan was, in essence: (1) go into labor on my due date; (2) go to the hospital; (3) change into cute clothing; (4) have an epidural from the minute I got there; (5) rest comfortably (perhaps chatting with girlfriends on the phone) until it was time to push; (6) quickly have a vaginal delivery; and (7) produce a great baby for the world to see. I think I thought the experience would be somewhat akin to going to a day spa, with some minor discomfort, but nothing too crazy because, after all, I would have an epidural. Here's what happened instead: (1) Ten days into "overtime"—past my due date—my husband and I drove to the hospital to be induced; (2) the drug I received to make the induction process better made me really sick to my stomach and sort of gross feeling, so there was no chitchatting to be had; (3) I received an epidural (which was great—but my mom is an anesthesiologist, so I'm biased), but still had a significant amount of cramping because the Pitocin was turned up so high (I am sure that it was much better than the real thing); and (4) after seventeen hours of labor, I was stuck at six centimeters and not progressing. Granted, it was a Friday night at about 8:00. And was my doctor's b-day, but I was also running a slight fever and my water had been broken for too long—it was time to throw in the towel and have a C-section. Oh—and by the way, during this entire process, I was wearing a slightly greenish hospital gown, which I was instructed to wear from the first nurse who prepared the induction.

—**anonymom**

As a mom and a labor and delivery nurse, I find the birth plans to be absolutely useless. We are in a world of control. I see a lot of couples come into the hospital expecting "the perfect delivery" . . . whatever that might be. They hand off their nicely typewritten birth plan to the nurse and expect everything to go that way. Reality check to all the expecting moms out there . . . you have *no* control over what happens. So just let it go and focus on what really matters . . . you are giving birth to your new healthy baby boy or girl. Stop trying to control everything! If you want your lights dimmed, just ask at that moment (you might be in pain but you can still talk).

—**anonymom**

I planned on having the baby delivered by a midwife in a birthing center in Houston. Then Hurricane Rita came through and I was forced to leave my city, which stressed me out so much that I lost amniotic fluid, causing them to induce me before my time, which brought on an extremely long thirty-six-hour labor. This in turn allowed me to buckle enough to beg for an epidural. Also not in the plan. I guess you just can't plan this stuff.

—**anonymom**

I had a doula. I wanted to try for natural—no drugs. No induction, etc. *None* of that worked out as I'd planned. Alas . . . I was induced . . . I labored for seven hours without drugs, seven more with drugs, and I highly recommend the drugs. It was not nearly as bad as I'd imagined, although the major abdominal surgery was not something I'd planned for. . . . I had a plan and it went horribly awry. *Nothing* worked out as I had planned, a good lesson for parenthood, I suppose.

—**anonymom**

prep and logistics
birth classes

Birth education and prep classes have one thing in common: They all teach you about childbirth. But exactly what you'll learn varies hugely from class to class. Some classes teach specific breathing and pain-relief techniques, such as Bradley or Lamaze. (See "Pain Relief," page 134.) Some focus on how to make choices during labor. A class given by a nurse at a hospital may focus mostly on hospital policy. A natural childbirth class may discourage the use of drugs in labor and strongly suggest resisting hospital policy. It can be hard to find a class that gives a broad, nonjudgmental overview of the possibilities you may come across. This is partly because there are so many possibilities, and partly because the people giving the classes have their own ideas about what makes a good birth.

Birth classes can be a great way to familiarize yourself with what's possible in the birthing room. You can talk to other people at the same stage in pregnancy and compare notes. Sometimes the variety of people and their different attitudes can give you some insight into your own experience and ideas. But a class can also expose you to the opinions and anxieties of others, which may not always help you feel better prepared. Finding a class that works for you may require a little thinking about your personality and your feelings about labor and birth. Are you aiming for childbirth without drugs? A class in natural childbirth may help you learn pain-management techniques and give you confidence. But if you're not sure what you want, you could feel pressured in the same class when the teacher stresses the importance of not getting an epidural. A class that talks about both options might be more useful. The perfect class may or may not be out there; you may have to put up with a little unwanted advice to learn what you need to know. If you know others who have taken birth classes recently, talking to them may give you an idea of each instructor's attitude and the tone of the classes.

You may also want to educate yourself about breastfeeding and newborn care.

→ See Breastfeeding Basics, page 282.
→ See Baby Care Basics, page 256.

> The classes force you to consider things you may not otherwise think about, plus it's a good forum for discussion. Feeling like I had some semblance of control was important to me during labor, so just knowing that what I was feeling was normal helped me a lot, if that makes any sense. And my labor was such that I did use every damn breathing technique we were taught! :) Hell, just being in a room with a bunch of other pregnant couples was a comfort to me.
> —anonymom

> It is true you can learn a lot from books, and classes can give you a lot of information that seems sort of useless. Having not given birth yet, it is hard for me to know for sure whether it will have been a good use of time, but I did feel like the opportunity to ask questions and discuss options in the class was really beneficial for me. Books don't usually answer back! But if you have someone else you can ask, then maybe a class is unnecessary.
> —anonymom

> We prepared with a Bradley-method class and it worked very well. I was able to relax between and during contractions because we had prepared for it; also we had practiced different laboring positions that helped a great deal. Both Bradley and prenatal yoga had encouraged strengthening exercises, like squatting and Kegels, and those were also helpful.
> —anonymom

> I'm preparing by avoiding thinking about it. I figure since billions of women have given birth, a class can't be that important.
> —anonymom

149

Definitely do classes!
No doubt they vary in value
according to your teacher but they're
very, very worthwhile. If nothing else, they
get you very familiar with the terminology
and the stages and details to expect. Nothing
anyone can say can prepare you for the actual
sensation of the pain, which is grotesquely
horrendous and can neither be anticipated
nor, thank God, really remembered, but
you'll at least know about it.
—anonymom

I read a great book
called *Birthing from Within*, as
well as Ina May Gaskin's books, so I knew
a lot of the breathing and visualization
techniques ahead of time. I also "practiced" for
labor by holding an ice cube on my wrist and
breathing/visualizing while my husband timed me
for a minute. I think anything you can pick up along
the way is helpful. I also did a lot of yoga and
meditation while I was pregnant, so I used
some of that focus in labor.
—anonymom

body prep

Some women feel better going into birth well groomed. Others don't care at all. It is true that you may not have much time after birth to deal with your cosmetic needs, so if you are upset by feeling unkempt, you might be better off taking care of some of this beforehand. Body preparation procedures like shaving and enemas used to be a standard part of birth prep in a hospital, but they are not often standard these days. You may be shaved before a C-section, and you can usually get an enema upon request (saves some from worrying about pooping on the table—still possible with an enema, but less likely).

what to pack

You may be in the hospital or birth center for 12—48 hours after the birth, or several days if you have a C-section. Obviously, the length of your stay has some bearing on how much you pack. Some people bring huge bags and try to cover every possible need; others feel good packing just the bare essentials. It's really up to you how far you want to plan ahead. You may have ample time to pack as labor slowly progresses at home. Here is a list of suggestions for various items you might want or need:

your stuff

- **Labor clothes unless you're fine in a hospital gown (or naked). Consider that clothes may get stained if you wear them during birth.**
- **Night clothes, robe, slippers, and underwear; you may bleed and sweat a lot, so consider bringing several sets.**
- **Maternity or very loose clothes to wear home—it's very unlikely you'll fit into your old clothes right away.** → See New Mom Fashion, page 186.
- **Comfortable support bra or nursing bra**
- **Toiletries (including lip balm to prevent dry, chapped lips during labor)**

baby stuff

- Infant car seat: required to take home baby → See Car Travel, page 359.

- Weather-appropriate clothing for your newborn (shirts that open from the front may be easier to get on and less irritating to a newly cut umbilical cord)

- Socks/booties/hat (some of which may be given to you at the hospital)

- Blankets (you will also get some from the hospital)

other stuff

- Insurance card and any hospital papers you have filled out → See Birth Certificate and Social Security Card, page 163.

- Birth plan, if you have one

- Any labor-support aids: props, massage oil, CDs, DVDs, focal-point item, favorite pillow, book or magazine for early labor, etc.

- Stuff for partner: change of clothes/shirt, toiletries, bathing suit if he or she will get in shower/tub with you.

- Camera, film, charged batteries, tapes, if you want to take pictures

- Any phone numbers of people you may want to call, prepaid phone card or calling card for long-distance calls using hospital phone (cell phones may not be allowed in hospital rooms)

- Snacks. You may be very, very hungry after the birth, and want a favorite food (or an alternative to hospital food). → See Restrictions on Food and Drink, page 127.

taxi!

Movies and TV shows love to show the pregnant woman and her anxious husband careening through traffic, arriving at the hospital in the nick of time. But first-time labor usually starts off pretty slowly, giving you room to consider the various transportation logistics and avoid traffic dramas. It's very rare for a woman to give birth in a car. When you talk to your doctor or midwife and/or doula about when to go into the hospital or birth center, consider transportation as well as how fast your labor is progressing. If it's rush hour, it may be a bad idea to wait until your labor is unbearable to get into the car—and it's not a good idea to drive yourself no matter how early in labor. You can relieve some commute stress by trying a rehearsal drive (this can be done when you go tour the facility). Ask in advance where you enter and where to park. If you plan to take a taxi or call a car service, keep phone numbers handy. (And if your water has already broken, a trash bag for the seat of the car will be appreciated!)

documenting
the birth

Photographs or videotapes of your labor, birth, and your newborn can be very powerful reminders of the experience and a way to share the moment with others in the future (including your baby, eventually). Hospitals, however, sometimes do not allow videotaping of the actual birth (the moment when the baby comes out). Some are more flexible than others when it comes to this policy. Also, if your birth partner will be doubling as birth documentarian, you may feel deprived of support during the intense phases of labor. The business of getting a great shot may distract from the immediacy of the experience on an emotional level. You can consider hiring a professional birth photographer. The pros are generally aware of staying in the sidelines and/or capturing the various moments with a particular style—they may also have good solutions for lighting problems that are common in birthing rooms. You may want to talk to whoever's doing the shooting about your preferences, so you won't end up with more or less detail than you're comfortable with.

We took photos before I started pushing and then right as my son was being cleaned off.... I love these because it was hard for me later to remember how he looked those first few moments.
—anonymom

I get ill when I hear myself during a contraction, but I am so impressed with me too! I was strong and I did a great job. It is awesome to see that.
—anonymom

Photos. Love them. Didn't want them, glad I have them.
—anonymom

It's a cliché, but after witnessing my wife's labor, I really did understand how much stronger women are than men. And when I saw my son's pinched face pop out, his mouth already twisted in a scream, I understood why we're wired to forget the first few years of life. But, of course, there's always a video camera to negate nature's decision to delete.
—anonydaddy

the birth environment

the setting

By far the majority of births in the United States (99 percent) happen in hospitals. Birth centers are becoming more popular—in 2004, there were 170 in the United States, up from 125 in 1984. Home births are less common, but have been proven a safe option for low-risk births. Occasionally home or birth-center births require a transfer to the hospital. Think about where you would like to give birth, then try to stay open to the alternatives. Each setting has its advantages.

hospital

Most ob-gyns now deliver exclusively in hospitals. A hospital birth provides access to a range of medical resources, such as anesthesiologists, neonatal specialists, and intensive care units.

STAFF: A lot of your contact with hospital staff will be with nurses. Depending on whether or not your doctor/midwife is present early on, you may also be examined by residents. You may meet more than a dozen nurses and half a dozen doctors in two days. As always, the quality of care depends on the caregiver. Some are great, some leave something to be desired.

PAIN RELIEF: A hospital birth will allow you the greatest access to pain-relief medicine. You may or may not have the ability to use other methods, depending on what else is going on (monitoring, etc.).

TOURING: Maternity wards and hospitals vary a lot. The best way to find out about a hospital is to go there. You can tour the hospital anytime during your pregnancy. Sometimes tours are formal and in groups (and need to be booked well in advance).

REGISTRATION: Preregistering at a hospital can spare you the annoyance of having to do it upon arrival. A preregistration package can be mailed to you or you may be able to pick it up during a tour.

INSURANCE: Insurance will cover hospital births—call your provider, however, to confirm that your particular plan covers your doctor or midwife *and* the hospital you intend to use.

ROOMS: Some hospital birthing rooms are comfortably designed, not unlike a hotel room (with a lot more beeping and blinking things). Others are in dire need of a makeover. Some rooms have showers, tubs, and/or reclining chairs; others are minimal. You can usually bring your own birthing ball or other

> Make friends with the nurses. They really are the first line and will be there during the birth. The better your relationship, the smoother things will go and the more questions you can ask over and over again. If you have never been in a hospital overnight before, it can seem a bit medical or overwhelming, so it is always important to keep asking questions to make sure all is okay.
> —anonymom

gear. Usually, delivery rooms are separate from recovery rooms, which are often shared. You may have the option to upgrade to a private recovery room if one is available, generally at your own expense. If you are interested in this option, talk to the hospital staff about their policy: You may be able to get on a waiting list as soon as you arrive at the hospital or you may have to wait until the baby's born. Shared recovery rooms run the gamut—both in terms of degree of privacy and quality of company (you never know who will be next to you).

Some policies you may want to ask about: "Rooming-in," which means that, barring any complications, the baby can stay with you from the moment of birth to when you leave the hospital; and "family-centered maternity care," which gives you the option of rooming-in or having the baby placed in the nursery (and brought to you for feedings).

LENGTH OF STAY: Insurance usually covers up to 48 hours for a vaginal birth, 3—5 days for a C-section. The length of your stay is generally calculated from the time the baby's born.

birth center

Birth centers are designed to provide women with a natural and homelike birth experience while providing access to more medical care than a home birth. Birth centers use fewer routine interventions and they usually have less medical equipment. Some centers are part of a hospital. Freestanding centers are affiliated with nearby hospitals, to which women are transferred in case of complications. So, a transfer can mean a quick wheel from one wing to another or a short ambulance ride. The average transfer rate is around 7—12 percent—most of these are not emergencies.

STAFF: Birth-center staff may include nurses, nurse-midwives, and nurse practitioners. Doctors may also be on staff or affiliated with the center. Midwives are usually in charge of births.

PAIN MANAGEMENT: Birth centers focus on nonmedical pain management, though some medication may be available. Epidurals often are not, so women who want one will have to be transferred.

TOURS: Birth centers often offer tours of their premises; if a center is part of a hospital, it may be a part of the hospital tour.

REGISTRATION: Since there aren't many birth centers, they are often quite popular. Centers may accept a limited number of births for any given time period. It might be necessary to register well in advance in order to plan your birth there.

INSURANCE: Birth centers usually take insurance, but you'll need to check with your carrier.

ROOMS: Rooms in birth centers are often described as more "homelike" than hospital rooms, though they may not be anything like your home. Labor, delivery, and recovery may all take place in the same room; rooming-in (having the baby with you from birth onward) is a common practice. Birth centers often have a number of birthing options, such as a whirlpool bath, shower, special chairs, and other equipment.

LENGTH OF STAY: Generally 6—24 hours after the birth. This can be an advantage or a disadvantage, depending on how you feel. Talk to your midwife about postpartum care and breastfeeding support; she may follow up with you at home.

home birth

Giving birth at home can add a dimension of freedom: You can snack and bathe, move around, light candles, go outside, etc. You can invite whomever you want. When the baby is born, you will already be at home—the transition to post-partum can be a smooth one. Another bonus: Midwives who perform home births are qualified to do prenatal care at home as well, which can make for very relaxed checkups.

The American College of Obstetricians and Gynecologists maintains that hospital births are the safest. But a 2005 North American study published in the *British Medical Journal* (and involving more than five thousand births) revealed that planned home births in "low risk" pregnancies, assisted by certified professional midwives, were just as safe as hospital births and much less likely to involve interventions. In this study, about 12 percent of the women who planned to give birth at home were moved to a hospital; the midwives estimated that 3.4 percent of the deliveries required "urgent" transfers. Though not a large percentage by any means, this does bring up the question of proximity to backup hospital care. If home birth is appealing to you, you will need to find a midwife who performs home births. She can advise you as to whether you are a good candidate. Consider the hospital backup plan (even visit the hospital) and prepare yourself emotionally for a rerouting if a complication arises.

All my friends asked weren't you worried? And of course I was, but I was also really confident in my midwife and in my body. I understand why it might not be for everyone, but my home birth was an amazing experience, and I'm really glad I did it.
—anonymom

> I had my daughter in a birthing tub. I have to say it was very good, although since that was my first child, I've nothing to compare it to. I am pregnant again (with a boy). I will opt for another water birth. It was natural and less "strict" but the pain of giving birth without medication doesn't let you think of much other than the pain!
> —anonymom

> I chose to do a water birth. The tub helped me so much; it helped to ease the pain of back labor as well as relax my body. It was such a wonderful experience, I recommend it to every woman. My husband was able to get in the tub with me so when our baby was delivered and placed on my chest, his was the first face our baby saw. It was a really amazing experience. My only wish was that I had gotten in earlier. Although after three hours we were very pruney!
> —anonymom

water birth

A water birth involves laboring and sometimes also delivering the baby in a tub of warm water. The idea behind a water birth is that moms and babies both feel a gentler transition. The baby goes from one warm, watery place to another. The mom's tissues and muscles are more elastic and relaxed, her circulation is flowing, and she may feel less stress due to the buoyancy provided by the water. Women who have experienced water births often describe them as very pleasant and pain relieving. Some studies indicate that with a water birth tears may be less severe and pain more manageable (epidurals are less likely). Although the research is very limited and there is little information about the risks of water birth—there's some controversy over whether the baby is more likely to become aspirated (breathe in fluid) in a water birth. Some studies show that a supervised water birth for a low-risk pregnancy is just as safe as a nonwater birth, and can be beneficial both in terms of reduced pain and interventions. One of the main obstacles to a water birth is finding a place to have one and someone experienced to assist. Some but not all birth centers offer the water birth option. Many water births are done at home in a special tub rented for the occasion.

the birth support team

Your doctor or midwife will be handling the birth of the baby. Unless you're at home, there will be nurses to monitor your physical health through the process. Anyone else you choose to have in the room during the birth is there to support you.

partners

Back in the day, births were women's business, attended by midwives and other women pulled from the ranks of the tribe. But as our society has become less tribally oriented, partners have become our major means of support. Including the partner in the birth room is a fairly recent phenomenon, after years of banning men from hospital deliveries. But at this point, partners can not only attend the birth but also get involved: coaching, cutting the cord, and even helping to deliver the baby.

Being at the birth is a way for partners to feel supportive and involved in the process and to share in the experience from the first minute. Many men emerge from the delivery room gushing with awe, amazement, and respect for their partners' strength. But being there can also bring up more complicated feelings. Even when partners educate themselves through classes, reading, and videos of birth, attending a birth for the first time can be really scary. While mothers have to go through the pain, partners have to see them suffer, and know there's little they can do to help. They may also have to witness some gory stuff. Some people can handle this better than others, but the general expectation (beyond the old gag about the dad passing out in the delivery room) is that partners will stay cool, no matter how they feel. Having someone there to provide backup support can be a huge help. This can be a professional (see "Professional Support: Birth Doulas," page 160), another family member, or a friend with whom both of you feel comfortable. The person can be in the room all the time or waiting for the partner to call and ask for help.

Talking before the birth about both of your expectations can help. Are you worried about acting crazy in front of your partner? Do you have concerns about how he or she might deal with the birth? Though it might be awkward to discuss this stuff beforehand (and truthfully, how you think you'll feel may be nothing like you actually do), it's a lot easier to talk about anxieties when you're not hooked up to machinery or groaning in pain. No matter how it goes for you, birth is pretty intense. You may not have the time or energy or clarity to talk to your partner the way you'd like to. In fact, you may be so overwhelmed that you act like a total freak. So you may want to prepare him for the possibility that you won't "be yourself." It can be a great relief to know going in that you're on the same page, or at least to know what the other page looks like.

If you decide that you don't want your partner at the birth, and you are both okay with that decision, it's totally appropriate to decide to choose another support person to help you through labor. Just because most partners attend the birth doesn't mean yours has to. Some people feel good about sharing this experience; others, for whatever reason, would rather keep things separate. You need to pick the support team that will help *you* feel the most confident. If that's not a partner, you may want to rely on someone else in your life.

> My husband was great; it's a good thing he is strong, because I really held onto him. I puked on him, too. That's real love.
> —anonymom

> When the Big Day came, I felt useful for the first and last parts, but not the middle. In the initial contractions, and the first few hours after arriving at the maternity ward, there's enough time between contractions to talk, to reassure, to calibrate. Then comes the transition phase, where I felt useless, toxic, even. Her pain exceeded any prior reference point—so much more than what she'd experienced or expected, she worried something was wrong (though all was fine). . . . You try switching pain-relief approaches from massage, to showering, to sitting on those rubber balls, but she's on to you, and gets really hostile for trying to deny or beguile her from her grief. This ninety minutes was the hardest part, obviously for her, but for me, too, because there was so much discomfort with so little seeming progress. Then, the nurse came in and, to our amazement, said she'd dilated four centimeters in a half hour, and was ready to have the baby "now." . . . I flatter myself that my excitement over seeing the baby's crown helped her ignore the pain in the last three minutes and push harder.
> —anonydaddy

Don't forget to consider the needs of your partner and make sure they have voiced them and you understand them. So much is justifiably focused on the mother that you might forget this.
—anonymom

Too many people were there. My midwife sent everyone home and my husband and I focused on each other. It worked.
—anonymom

My husband was great—he made all the nurses laugh and I brought lots of good music—bossa nova to help with the breathing and heavy Cuban salsa for the final push.
—anonymom

If I could do it again I would nix the husband. Here's why:

#1 He's a spaz. He can't hang with all that. Having to watch your wife deliver a baby is way stressful, gross, and frankly, he doesn't want to see "all that" and I didn't want him to either.

#2 He yelled at the doctor. Seriously, guys don't know anything about anything with this stuff. I told the doctor beforehand that I didn't want an epidural. Of course, she kept offering. When she would, he would freak out. He said I "caved" because she pressured me. I "caved" because I was entitled to change my mind on the spot not knowing a damn thing about what it would feel like to give birth.

#3 He pointed out at the delivery that the baby looked black. He was purple just because that's how it is, and he had some curly hair going on, but honestly . . . the doctor, nurses, and my family didn't think it was all that funny.
—anonymom

partner positioning

Some suggest that the sight of the formerly sex-specific vagina being repurposed as a birth canal can be damaging to a partner's libido. There are those who complain of graphic genital images haunting them after the birth, interfering with desire. Not everyone wants to see his baby burst forth into the world, possibly tearing apart his sexual playground in the process. If you suspect that the man in your life (though this could certainly be an issue for lesbian partners, too) may not be able to handle seeing you both ways, as it were, you may opt for him to stand close to your head, away from the hardcore birthing action. That way, he can squint at your contorted face and pretend you're having an orgasm instead of a baby. But do consider how this reflects on your partner's ability to see you both ways conceptually as well. You might be able to protect him from the crotchy conflict, but you can't protect him from the conflict at the heart of the matter: His lover has become the mother of his child.

other people

Some people love the idea of the birth room becoming a family reunion, surrounding themselves with everyone they love. Others can't bear the exposure or the distraction, and want a more intimate environment. Socializing can even inhibit the progress of labor. Hospitals generally limit the number of people present during a birth. Often two people is the maximum, but rules vary. Birth centers are usually more flexible. One of the benefits of a home birth is that you have total control over who's around.

Numbers aside, choosing the people who will witness this incredible event—and enormous challenge—is something to consider pretty seriously. You can't predict what will happen in the birthing room, and you don't know for sure

My husband and mother [were there] for my first birth along with my midwife. At the time, I thought my mom was great. She was supportive. She is a nurse, but didn't butt heads with the staff. She stroked my cheek. She held her grandson, and gave my husband small breaks. Afterward, though, it came out that her perception of the birth was much different. She had thought I had the worst birth ever. I didn't use drugs. I didn't need interventions. My son was born healthy. She really knocked down my self-confidence afterward (like months later when I heard how she felt). It created a rift with us for a while. I don't regret it, but wish it had been better for her. I still believe I had a good birth.

—anonymom

My husband was with me throughout. The midwife was there whenever we wanted her, as were the nurses. The midwife was wonderful—an incredible calming and reassuring presence. I remember her telling us "I'm here for you tonight. That's why I'm here." I felt great about all of them. They made it possible for me, for us, to have the birth we wanted.

—anonymom

I'll just never forget how calm and supportive the midwife was—she made me feel like it was all going to be perfectly fine, and it was. The loss of control and the pain of labor can be really scary, at least it was for me, so having that constant and calming reassurance was incredibly important.

—anonymom

how you'll feel. But you can start by choosing people you feel comfortable with, imagining some scenarios, and thinking about whether having these people around during whatever might transpire makes you feel better or worse. If someone you're considering is making the idea seem more stressful, maybe they're better off in the waiting room.

Of course, it's not always that simple. When someone wants to be there for your birth and you just don't feel great about it, you'll have to decide whether to hurt the person's feelings or compromise your own. You might end up feeling fine about the person's presence once you're in the thick of labor. Or not even notice they're there. Ideally, whoever's in the birthing room will be able to understand that your needs may change as your birth progresses and to adjust their behavior accordingly . . . even if that means adjusting themselves out of the room.

To that end, it's a good idea to set some ground rules with the people who will be with you at the birth. Are there things you'd like them to do? What do you definitely not want to happen? It's very important that your support team is willing to be flexible and to put your needs above their emotions and egos. You'll have a lot to worry about while you're having your baby; the less you have to worry about hurt feelings, the better.

professional support:
birth doulas

A birth doula, according to the Doulas of North America website, "is a person trained and experienced in childbirth who provides continuous physical, emotional and informational support to the mother before, during and just after childbirth." Our current medical model of care does not involve a healthcare provider's presence through most of the birth. Women who birth in hospitals often spend most of their labors without a knowledgeable person present to help them manage the experience. Having a doula can help pick up some of the slack. The birth doula (sometimes called labor doula or birthing/labor assistant) may be the only support person at the birth, or she may be in the room along with a partner and/or other family support people.

Some people worry about whether the presence of a doula will make a partner feel left out. Most partners who have had doulas at their baby's births find it a relief. Having someone dedicated to helping with pain management frees up a partner to provide other kinds of comfort. And having someone around who knows about childbirth can take the pressure off when questions or issues arise.

Doulas can help women birth without pain medication if desired, or help them understand any interventions they may encounter. There is mounting evidence that birthing with a doula can mean shorter labors, fewer complications and interventions, and possibly a more positive attitude about the birth experience. Cost is a major factor in the doula equation. Doulas are expensive and not covered by insurance. It's unfortunate that in our current medical model, we have to fork out our own cash for much-needed labor coaching and support.

Since the doula will be present at such an intense and vulnerable time, she should be chosen carefully. Interview the doula. Ask her how many births she has attended and how recently. Ask if she's worked at the hospital or center where you plan to deliver. Ask if she is certified with the Doulas of North America. Personality and sensibility are important, and sensitivity to your priorities is crucial. If you're thinking you may want an epidural, you will want to look for a doula who will be open to that rather than one holding fast to the cause of natural childbirth. If you're considering hiring a doula, ask for a number of references, including ones from women who have had a variety of types of births in order to find out how the doula handled those situations. A good doula understands the balance between pushing, cheering, and rolling with the punches. The doula is not there to make decisions for you; she's there to support you through your childbirth experience.

resources

Doulas of North America: DONA.org

after the birth

The final stage of labor involves birthing the placenta—this can take ten minutes to more than half an hour. Your caregiver may press on your abdomen or pull the umbilical cord to help ease the placenta out. Though the birth of the placenta is an important part of labor—getting the placenta out safely reduces the risk of any postpartum hemorrhaging—you may feel only mild contractions and have to push once or twice. Plus, your mind may be focused on the baby or the fact that the really hard part of your labor is finally over.

After it's out, your caregiver will inspect the placenta to make sure it is intact and then usually put it into a bucket of some kind. The placenta is quite large and bloody and covered with sinewy bluish or purple veins. Some find it to be a little gruesome and would rather not look at it. Others are curious to check out this significant organ that kept their baby alive for so long. In certain cultures the placenta is revered as a great symbol of the cycle of life and may be ceremoniously buried or consumed (it's said to offer a lot of useful nutrients). Once the placenta has been delivered, your doctor or midwife will examine you to see if you need stitches (if you've torn or had an episiotomy, you'll need to be sewn up). Often the area is numbed so the stitches don't hurt too much.

> I'd asked the nurses not to offer me the chance to cut the umbilical cord. I consider this a well-intentioned but ultimately condescending gesture for dads, a terribly important job that everyone watches that proves only how unessential dads are—kind of like letting little kids press the elevator button. The nurses pushed the scissors at me once, then twice. Like a Victorian drawing room guest, I accepted only after the third offer. I turned to the camera, snipped the shears, and just at that moment, the bairn frog-kicked right over the umbilical cord. I damn near cut her big toe off. I'd have a restraining order on me now if I'd returned our daughter to her mother nine-toed after ninety seconds in my care. So get someone to hold the feet if you're cutting the cord.
> —anonydaddy

postbirth protocol

Here's a rundown of standard procedures you're likely to encounter in the hospital after your baby's birth. Some of these apply to birth-center births as well. If these practices are not part of your immediate postbirth experience, you may need to discuss them at your first pediatrician visit.

It may be possible in some situations to modify or even decline these routine procedures, but the rules vary. Some are mandated by law in certain states. In other cases, your options may depend on the flexibility of the place or person you're dealing with. If you are interested in forgoing any of these procedures, it's a good idea to research the rules as well as the potential ramifications of opting out or postponing.

cord blood banking

Cord blood is a rich source of stem cells, and an industry has grown to give parents who can afford it the opportunity to store their newborns' cord blood for potential later use. If a situation comes up where the child or a relative with a matching blood type needs a transplant, cord blood can be a safer and easier option than bone marrow. The March of Dimes estimates that parents who do not have a prior history of genetic disorders or cancers that could be treated with stem cells have about a 1 in 20,000 chance of being able to use the blood they've stored. Cord-blood banking is not cheap; there is usually a substantial initial fee and a yearly maintenance cost. It is also possible to donate cord blood to a public bank for the use of others, although certain tests and restrictions apply.

resources
A Parent's Guide to Cord Blood Banks:
parentsguidecordblood.com

> Ask each cord blood-banking company as many questions as you can think of. What happens to the cord blood if they close down, or how many families have chosen them to date, and how many people have actually used the cord blood to date … these questions can help you get a realistic idea of what is going on.
> —anonymom

UMBILICAL CORD: The umbilical cord is cut immediately after birth in most hospital births. If you want to wait longer—some say this is beneficial to babies; others say it may lead to more jaundice—speak to your provider to see whether she is amenable. The cord may be cut by the provider or by your partner (if everyone involved thinks that's a good idea).

CLEANING: Your baby will probably be removed quite soon after birth to be cleaned off and wrapped up unless you specify otherwise. Newborns need to be kept warm. Hospitals generally wrap up babies in blankets to accomplish this. Another option is keeping the baby against the warmth of the mother's (or another's) body, often with blankets on top. If you do not want your baby to be bathed (this will obviously remove the birth gunk but can also lower a baby's body temperature and take time away from you), be sure the staff knows that. Baths are routine in many hospitals.

APGAR TESTING: The Apgar test (named after Virginia Apgar, the pediatrician who designed it) is performed 1 minute and 5 minutes after birth. The test assesses the baby's skin color, muscle tone, heart rate, breathing, and reflexes. Each is scored from 0 to 2, and the numbers are added up to form a total. A lower score means it's more likely a baby will need additional care or observation after birth.

MEASUREMENTS: Your baby will be weighed and measured after birth, usually immediately.

FOOTPRINTS: Footprinting of infants is done for identification purposes, although they are not always legible enough to read clearly. The AAP and ACOG both no longer universally recommend footprinting because so few of the footprints studied were legible. The practice continues in many hospitals, perhaps more as a tradition and to provide parents with keepsakes.

ID BRACELET: In hospitals, mothers and babies are fitted with matching ID bracelets. The bracelets are checked when the mother/baby pair is discharged (and possibly at other times during the hospital stay). As a further precaution, some hospitals have begun to use electronic bracelets that set off alarms if babies are removed.

VITAMIN K SHOT: Vitamin K shots have been given to U.S. newborns since the early 1960s. About 1 in 10,000 babies has a vitamin K deficiency, which can prevent blood clotting and cause major problems in the rare newborn it affects. There's some controversy about a link between vitamin K and increased risk of childhood leukemia but no studies have found a conclusive connection.

EYE OINTMENT OR DROPS: Babies are routinely given antibiotic eyedrops or ointment shortly after birth. This is considered controversial by some because the antibiotics protect babies from getting eye infections from gonorrhea/chlamydia bacteria, and most mothers do not have these diseases. However, the eyedrop treatment has evolved as a public health measure to protect the few babies at risk. One concern is that the eyedrops blur the baby's vision during the period immediately after birth, when newborns are otherwise more likely to make eye contact with parents. If you want, you can ask nurses to postpone the eyedrops until you have had a few minutes or more to look into each other's eyes. Depending on how cooperative your nurse is, you may get some time before the ointment is applied. However, the antibiotics are often required by state law.

SCREENING TESTS: In the United States, all newborn babies are screened for various disorders while in the hospital, using blood taken by pricking the baby's heel. Requirements for tests vary by state. Parents may opt to test for additional disorders as well. For information on newborn screening including which tests your state requires, and how to arrange for additional testing if desired, ask your OB or pediatrician before the birth, or look up your state with the National Newborn Screening and Genetics Resource Center (genes-r-us.uthscsa.edu).

HEPATITIS B SHOT: Some hospitals give hepatitis B shots to all newborns unless the parents opt not to do so. If you are sure that you and your family are hepatitis B—free, your baby may not need this vaccination at this time. This is a good thing to discuss with your pediatrician when you meet with her before the birth.

PHYSICAL EXAMINATION: Your newborn will be examined by a pediatrician within the first day of life. If the pediatrician of your choice does not work at the hospital where your baby is born, you will either be assigned a pediatrician from the hospital or given a list of affiliated doctors to choose from. You will have your first visit with your child's regular doctor within a week.

birth certificate and social security card

Registering the birth (getting a birth certificate) is a process that can be started at the hospital or birth center—you fill out a form, sign it, and then it's sent to the county offices to be processed. You can apply for your baby's Social Security card at the same time, which is pretty convenient and can save a lot of hassle at a Social Security office later on. You'll need to have picked out the name. If married parents have different last names, you may need to bring your marriage certificate.

If the father is not going to be involved (or you are not sure whether he is), you can talk to a lawyer to see what your options are regarding the father space; you can also leave the father space blank. Birth certificates can be changed later on, if necessary. If you have a home birth, your midwife should be able to walk you through the birth certificate process—you can also check with your State Office of Vital Records for information.

resources
Social Security online: ssa.gov/reach.htm

meet your newborn

newborn appearance
Some common physical traits of newborn babies (all are temporary).

DARKER SKIN TONE
Skin may be purple or red; hands and feet may be bluish.

SWOLLEN GENITALS AND NIPPLES
Related to the mother's hormones. Girls may also have some vaginal discharge.

MILIA
Tiny white spots on face; also see "Baby Acne," page 256.

ERYTHEMA TOXICUM
A common red rash that looks like flea bites.

SQUISHED FACIAL FEATURES
Eyes may be smaller or shut.

VERNIX
This oily, white slime protects the skin in utero and may be present at birth.

MOLDING
An elongated head (from squeezing through the birth canal).

STORK BITES
Small red/pink patches, mostly on upper lip, near eyes, and on back of the neck.

LANUGO
A downy fuzz that may be more prominent in premature babies.

The first time I saw my son after birth, I have to admit . . . he looked nothing like I thought he would! I was actually thinking, "Are you sure that's my baby??"
—anonymom

She looked like nobody in the family! She looked like an old man. It was shocking and I felt fear that I couldn't love her! That passed quickly.
—anonymom

I said, Hello, there you are. You're a boy. It was amazing to see him, after feeling him for so many months. He looked right at me. He was big, with big eyes, and very cute, but gooey.
—anonymom

Don't expect the Gerber baby to come out of your vagina—newbies don't always look so hot!
—anonymom

He was so perfect, beautiful and blond! I am part Asian and dark haired. I was surprised that the other genes kicked in.
—anonymom

bonding on command

In *Parent-Infant Bonding,* first published in 1976, pediatricians Marshall Klaus and John Kennell described a "sensitive period" right after birth when the mother and baby have a natural window for bonding: "We believe that there is strong evidence that at least 30—60 minutes of early contact in privacy should be provided for every parent and infant to enhance the bonding experience."

The results of their work, along with the efforts of La Leche League and childbirth activists, led to the practice of putting mother and baby together immediately, or soon, after birth, so that this important bonding could take place.

The emphasis on postbirth contact came as a reaction to the status quo at the time, which was to separate mother and baby immediately. To put an end to this practice, the results of bonding studies were shouted from the rooftops and the moments after birth were exalted as a "crucial time" that could have permanent repercussions for the mother-baby relationship.

On a chemical level, there's lots going on in the hour after birth; even with the fuzziest newborn eyesight, the baby often has the ability to find the nipple, which leads to colostrum letdown, which leads to uterine contractions, which help shrink the uterus. In this way, bonding is a basic physiological set of reactions. But bonding is often described as a loving "dance," with baby and mother locked into each other's every move, every touch. Some mothers feel this right off the bat. But for others, dancing (even conceptually) is out of the question. Babies may be whisked off to the NICU immediately after birth. C-sections take time to complete. The lingering pain or shock of labor can blow all other

> When they brought my son to the room to stay with us, he was asleep; I immediately noticed one ear was stuck to his head and didn't yet know that this was merely due to the fact that infant ears are so soft. Instead of kissing him or something, I pointed at him from three feet away and said, "Is there something wrong with his ear?"
> —anonymom

Should a mother otherwise committed to care-giving miss this rendezvous with her infant, and begin to commune the next day, there are no measurable ill effects—provided someone else keeps her warm and safe in the interim. . . . Bonding right after birth is by no means essential for the development of love. It can, however, facilitate the process.

—Sarah Hrdy, *Mother Nature*

> Although I found him gorgeous, I don't think I bonded with him for a few months. The older he got, the more I fell in love with him.
> —anonymom

> A few hours after the birth of my son, I had a strange and unexpected feeling of detachment and boredom. I thought that would be the moment to bond to the max with the little one. Instead, I felt the need to do something completely different. So I ducked into a little room and watched fifteen minutes of *Curb your Enthusiasm.* Having done that, I came back to my new life with baby and everything was great.
> —anonymom

165

feelings out of the water. The presence of others can obscure any opportunity for private emotions. The sight of the baby may well freak people out before it fills them with love. Do these scenarios lead to less-bonded babies? According to studies, it doesn't seem like it. The long-lasting effects of initial bonding have recently been questioned. While immediate postbirth bonding may help foster connection between mothers and infants, it seems that it's a bonus, not a necessity. → See Bonding Pressure, page 198.

> It wasn't what I thought it would be like at all. I felt cheated out of a birth experience (labor, pushing, vaginal birth, baby placed on your chest . . . bonding . . .). I felt no connection to him at all. It wasn't "the most amazing experience of my life." I really didn't have a birth plan or a set idea in my head. But this sure wasn't it!
>
> —anonymom

> This will sound awful, but I was so disappointed when I first saw her. Not because she wasn't amazing—she was. I was disappointed to know that the pregnancy was over. I wasn't going to get that attention anymore, and I wasn't going to be "glowing." She was so beautiful, though, all alienlike.
>
> —anonymom

> It changed my brain. It made me a mother. That pain was indescribable! I feel proud of my births! I did it.
>
> —anonymom

emotional aftermath

Some people seem to be mainlining adrenaline and pure joy for days after their babies are born. Others are content and serene. The highs of birth, however, can be accompanied or followed by some less glorious feelings. Sometimes these are a direct result of things not going according to plan (a rather common occurrence). But sometimes it's just the enormity and intensity of birth that can overwhelm you. These feelings are a normal part of the process and don't mean you're not thrilled about your new baby. → Postbirth feelings can feed into postpartum ones. See Emotional Landscape of Parenthood, page 188, for more.

> I must say that the minute I gave birth, I was absolutely overcome with happiness that I wasn't pregnant anymore. I know a lot of people love being pregnant but I was not one of them.
>
> —anonymom

> I just kept saying to myself, I can't believe they let me just leave the hospital with this little person. Shouldn't there be a class? Certification? Something official?
>
> —anonymom

> The best part is when you are still in the hospital being cared for and medicated—the flowers, the calls from friends and family, it's just a love fest.
>
> —anonymom

dealing with disappointment

Even if you weren't aware that you had any fantasies or expectations to begin with, you may feel let down, sad, angry, or just vaguely unfulfilled after giving birth. Coming to terms with your disappointment can be difficult in the face of something as wonderful as a new baby. But when so much of the prep women do for childbirth focuses on pumping themselves up for a positive experience, it makes coming off a less positive one that much harder. Birth is a complicated process. Remember how little control we have over much of it. Your birth experience might have made a deep emotional impact. But your feelings about the birth will probably diminish, and your feelings about your baby will almost definitely grow.

167

posttraumatic feelings

It's common to have some posttraumatic feelings after birth. These usually subside after a while. Sometimes parents find that telling and retelling the story helps normalize the experience (or lets the reactions of others confirm that it was indeed completely hellish). If feelings about the birth are still freaking you out well after your postpartum bleeding has stopped, you may be dealing with posttraumatic stress disorder. Recent studies show this affects somewhere between 2 and 5 percent of women after birth. Counseling is usually recommended.

postpartum support

After the birth, a new mom might feel like old news. All eyes are on the baby. Her trusty doctor wants nothing to do with her until the 6-week visit. Even her own mother, if she's around, is probably more focused on the adorable newborn than on her grown daughter, plastered to the bed in the background. But mothers need mothering, too, and so do fathers. Everyone's postpartum needs are different, but most people could use some kind of help. Unfortunately, some parents have a hard time getting the support they need after their babies are born.

handling hostess stress

Sometimes it's hard to not "host" even when the most generous people come over to help out. Here are some ways to help make visits as stress-free as possible:

- Put a clear time limit up front to avoid extended stays.
- Don't feel obliged to let anyone hold the baby unless you want them to.
- Don't feel compelled to schedule visits before you're ready.
- Don't dress for visitors. Some even suggest staying in your pjs.
- Keep refreshments to the bare minimum.

why help may be hard to come by

- We don't always live near our families, so it's not easy for them to come help.
- Our culture values independence and expects people to be able to go it alone.
- People are afraid to interrupt the intimacy of the early days of parenthood.
- There's a fantasy that motherhood should be instinctual, so help shouldn't be necessary.
- People may just not know what to do!

how to get the help you need (or really, really want)

The first step to good postpartum support is to feel okay about asking for it. Wanting or needing assistance is a normal part of new parenthood (whether that means a shoulder to cry on, someone to hold the baby, or someone to get you a glass of water). If you're feeling like help would be good for you, listen to yourself.

When people ask what they can do to help out, don't say no without thinking about it. Though it can sometimes seem a real hassle to make lists of chores for your loved ones (or even paid help), people won't be able to tell from your strained smile that you're really in desperate need of trash bags but can't get up the nerve to ask.

Even if you've got hands-on help up the wazoo—the house gets cleaned, someone's on night duty, and the freezer's full of casseroles—you may still feel like you're missing something. The kind of support that goes beyond "chores" can be hard to pinpoint, but here are lots of less tangible kinds of support that all parents need to make a healthy transition.

New parents need support to . . .

- Go through a range of emotions without feeling "wrong."

- Talk about their birth experience as much or as little as they want.

- Tell people to go away when being a host is adding stress.

- Talk to other new parents about the details of baby care, and parent reality: sleep, feeding, depression, what kind of nipple to buy and where. Sometimes we just need to just see other new parents *being* new parents to help us feel less like aliens. → See Emotional Landscape of Parenthood, page 188.

division of labor

Delegating isn't always easy. Mothers, especially, can wind up feeling like they're responsible for all the little (and big) details of new parent life. Just to clear up any confusion, we've provided a list of tasks that can be accomplished by someone else, and a couple you'll probably have to handle on your own.

what others *can do*

- Buy diapers, buy wipes, change diapers, throw away diapers, buy any other baby-care items, bathe baby, clean bathtub, tend to baby's cord, dress baby, undress baby, do laundry, burp baby, rock baby, take baby for a walk, hold baby, feed baby a bottle, wear baby in a sling or front carrier, rent a breast pump, buy breast pads, buy nipple ointment, sterilize pump or bottle parts, do any or all bottle feeding, make pediatrician appointments, go to pediatrician appointments, read up on baby care, locate resources for feeding and sleep help, start a child-care search, buy food, order food, cook food, clean up the kitchen, deal with social arrangements, make coffee, make sure there is coffee, make sure there is milk, make sure there is whatever else anyone needs in the house, do the dishes, write thank-you notes or e-mails, change sheets, do laundry . . .

> The first day that it was just me and the baby, I called a girlfriend begging her to come over so that I could eat and do something without having to constantly hold a baby, but my friend had plans, and I kind of freaked out. I got to where I was just begging for someone to help me, but also telling myself that this is what I'm supposed to learn to do by myself.
> —anonymom

what others *can't do*

- Give birth, breastfeed.

the support team

The ideal postnatal support people will be sensitive to your need for autonomy and privacy while taking care of the things you ask them to do. If you're not comfortable with the person being around, it's not really a supportive situation.

BABY NURSE: A baby nurse is usually an experienced nanny with expertise in newborn care (not a registered nurse). She may come during days or nights or may live in for some or all of the newborn period. At night she will get up and feed the baby a bottle or bring the baby to the mother for breastfeeding and then settle him down again. She may be helpful in setting up something resembling a regular feeding and sleeping routine. Baby nurses are completely devoted to baby care and often do not handle any household duties. They generally need meals provided. Since baby nurses have tons of experience with newborns, they often have a "magic touch." One drawback is that unless they are also great teachers, parents can feel helpless and hopeless when that magic touch has to leave. It's important that you communicate your priorities to a baby nurse when you're considering hiring her, and again when she comes in to work. Although many baby nurses support breastfeeding, they are not usually experts. Baby nurses often want to make themselves useful, which may mean offering bottles, which may not be the best thing for the breastfeeding pair in the long run.

→ See Getting Off to a Good Start, page 282.
→ See Caregivers and Your Milk, page 309.

> I had my mom with me for six weeks, my sister [who] lived down the street, my pesky mother-in-law hovering around whenever I'd let her in the door, and my absent-minded husband who became a master of eye-rolling every time I asked for a glass of water. . . . Lots of help. Too much help. . . .
> **—anonymom**

> I have hired a twenty-four-hour baby nurse but am leaning toward unhiring her because I'm concerned that the kind of postpartum care I'm looking for is not the kind she's used to providing. For example, I don't want to give bottles at all if possible in the very beginning, so it's not like I'd be saving sleep by having her feed the baby at night. We also plan to sleep with the baby near us, while she'd have to be in another room. I know she's fairly probreastfeeding but I do think she mostly works with women who want to give bottles (pumped or formula) and I don't want to have to push against someone else's beliefs about babies if that someone is supposed to be working for me. However, doing it alone seems quite scary.
> **—anonymom**

POSTPARTUM DOULA: Unlike a baby nurse, a doula (a word derived from the Greek "female slave") is there to take care of *you* so that you can learn how to take care of your baby. What exactly she does to help varies from family to family and from doula to doula. Many are fonts of advice and information about baby care. But doulas are generally dedicated to helping parents get comfortable with baby care themselves instead of just taking the baby off the parents' hands. Most doulas know a lot about breastfeeding, and all will support it. They may also supply other kinds of emotional and logistical support, perhaps meal preparation, massage, or helping with housework. Doulas may work days, nights, or both. They can come as often and for as long as you arrange it, though there may be a minimum number of hours. Doulas tend to be pretty expensive and are really varied in their expertise (as well as personality).

If you are shopping for a doula, look for someone who feels like a good match for your temperament and seems to share your values. Though doulas are trained to listen rather than preach a particular parenting strategy, you still want someone who'll be reassuring to you and your way of doing things. It's important that the doula is someone with whom you feel you can communicate. Doulas are not medically trained or qualified therapists but they tend to know quite a bit about a new mother's physical and emotional situation. So the right doula can be a great resource for getting the kind of medical or psychological support you may need.

NEW MOM GROUPS: You can find groups through pre- or postnatal exercise groups, midwives, hospitals, pediatricians, playground conversation, the Internet, or new mom friends. They may be focused directly on new moms, breastfeeding, or newborn care. They may also be called playgroups, though in the first few months, it's not really the babies who are doing the playing. Groups can also form less formally among friends (or friends of friends) who have babies around the same time. If you're feeling enterprising and can't find an established group in your neighborhood, you can try starting one of your own by approaching other moms, putting up flyers, etc.

HOUSEHOLD HELP: It's great if you can pay someone to help you clean house, do laundry, cook, or manage any of the other tasks that are piling up in your life, but if you can't, there may be other people in your life who can help out. When people offer to help, and you can't think of a job for them, consider asking them to make dinner or help you keep your house from becoming a total pigsty. It might not be what they had in mind, but if they want to help . . .

> I was not prepared at all to care for my baby, but I had a lot of support from female family members. I opted not to take newborn classes because I wanted my own experience, but having "experienced mothers" around gave me more confidence.
> —anonymom

> I sort of wish we had a bit more assistance the first few weeks, just so we could be better rested . . . my husband took a week off of work, and then I was by myself with the baby, which was completely terrifying at first—it was like having some sort of strange foreign exchange student that I was completely responsible for!
> —anonymom

> It was so hard to have my in-laws come stay with us for a week after the birth of our son. I would suggest getting into your own routine and then allowing houseguests. We got far too much "motherly" advice and I felt banished to my bed every waking hour.
> —anonymom

GRANDPARENTS: Grandparents are often so excited about the new baby that they can become your new partners in baby obsessing. In some communities, the grandmothers and aunts play a huge role in caring for the mother and/or the new baby. On the other hand, if your parents are not particularly interested in (or capable of) much baby care, or need a lot of help themselves, you may become more taxed than assisted by their presence. We've talked to so many parents who were entirely surprised by how they responded to their parents or in-laws during the newborn period. So, try to keep the possibilities as open as you can, while you figure out what you need and want. → See Family, page 218.

FRIENDS: Friends who understand a bit about the whole drama of a new-born will probably respect your need for groceries, errands to be run, short visits, and privacy. They will also forgive you for any self/baby-obsessed behavior. → See Friends, page 223.

INTERNET SUPPORT GROUPS: Internet sites can be very valuable resources for new moms for exchanging advice and worries and for alleviating loneliness or that feeling of being the *only one* who has a hard time with x, y, or z. Websites can help you find people to meet offline, too.

resources

After the Baby's Birth: A Complete Guide for Postpartum Women by Robin Lim

Mothering the New Mother: Women's Feelings and Needs After Childbirth, a Support and Resource Guide (Revised and Updated 2nd Edition) by Sally Placksin

Postpartum Survival Guide by Ann Dunnewold, Ph.D., and Diane G. Sanford, Ph.D.

The Post-Pregnancy Handbook: The Only Book That Tells What the First Year After Childbirth Is Really All About—Physically, Emotionally, Sexually by Sylvia Brown with Mary Dowd Struck, R.N., M.S., C.N.M.

> My mom stopped by a few times. Other than that, I thought I was Superwoman and could do it all. I was sorely mistaken....
> —anonymom

> I decided not to find someone else to watch him in the early months because I want to be with him all the time and it is really not easy to find someone, and when the need is not exactly pressing, you can delay and delay. In a way it is like a job where you have a hard time getting help when you create a system where you believe you are the only one who can figure it out.
> —anonymom

The best thing I did, for my second baby, was buy myself two new pretty pairs of pjs (I got the kind that has a tank underneath and a button-up cardigan on top) and then kept them on for the whole first week. It helped remind me, and *everyone else,* that I was recovering. When friends stopped by, I felt dressed enough, and then they didn't stay too long. It also helped me with the mental/emotional transition. Then, when I was ready, I got dressed and started the new life with baby.

—anonymom

We never allowed more than one or two visitors at a time; asked them to bring food rather than gifts (they all brought gifts); did not wake the baby for anyone (even my mother); they could watch him sleeping or hang out and wait till he woke up.

—anonymom

The most difficult thing was juggling all of our friends and family who wanted to see the baby—my husband and I needed alone time with our daughter and with each other. . . . It was hard not to hurt people's feelings, but also to stand up for what we needed as a family.

—anonymom

I loved having visitors for the first two weeks. It was nice to hand him off to people so I did not have to hold him all the time. Then the constant entertaining hit me and I did not have visitors for the next two weeks.

—anonymom

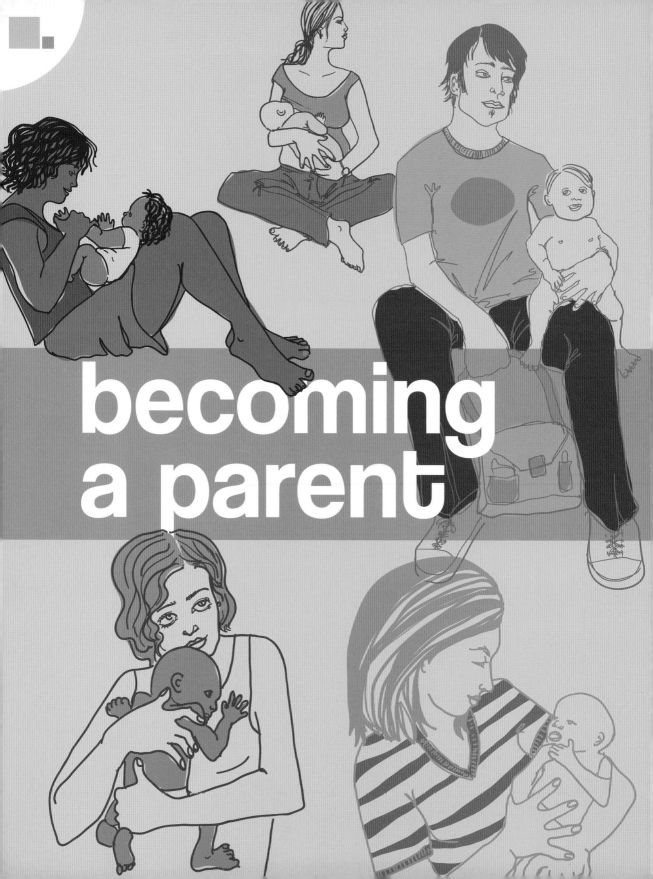

becoming
a parent

It's not like the fact that parenthood changes your life is some big secret. We were told our lives would be more meaningful. We were told our lives would be over. We tried to ignore the cliché warnings—still, they were disturbing. It was scary to imagine the end of life as we knew it. It was depressing to think that the previous life had no real meaning. After thirty-odd years of defining ourselves according to what we did or made or felt, we were suddenly a little unsure of who we'd become. And after nine months of being the center of attention, we were suddenly shoved aside as the whole world wrapped itself around this small creature who'd come to stay. We were more exhausted and emotional than ever, but our feelings seemed strangely irrelevant. Adjusting to the demands of a baby and recovering from birth were plenty of work. Adjusting to the changes in ourselves was something else entirely.

Roles shifted. Priorities realigned. Relationships changed. We fought with our partners less, and then more, and then the same amount . . . just about different things. Both of us went through whole weather patterns of emotions and perceptions, wondering, "When will things ever get back to normal?" The answer, for better or for worse, is probably never. Don't panic: Becoming a parent will almost definitely alter your life to the core, but we can pretty confidently say that the way it is now is not the way it will stay. Eventually, you'll get into a groove. It might happen before the stitches heal, or it might take months. But it will happen, and when it does, the prebaby you and the postbaby you will start to feel a lot more aligned. For us, it wasn't always seamless: We still missed lazy Sundays with the paper, but we could see how that feeling translated to a baby sleeping peacefully on our chests. We haven't solved a crossword puzzle since, but we do enjoy a not-unrelated sense of satisfaction when the nap battle is finally won. There are parts of ourselves that make more sense now that we're parents. And there are parts that don't fit quite so easily but still feel like a crucial part of who we are. When you have a baby, you evolve in a world of ways. Try not to be afraid of what you're turning into. You'll still be you . . . only different. This section will look at how parenthood changes your body, brain, and life.

the postbaby body

healing

We were expecting labor to be a nightmare. The healing phase hit us like a left hook. Though having the baby *out* was certainly a relief, we found the days after birth to be surprisingly difficult: lots of responsibility, little sleep, lots of pain, and little preparation. Yes, we'd heard about the hemorrhoids. But no one had mentioned the major constipation and gas. (Those intestinal issues loom almost as large in our memories as the pain of birth itself.) And we would have liked to know that while we would enjoy 9 months without periods, we would be wearing maxipads(!) for over a month straight afterward. The pain was definitely tempered by the joy of our new babies. And the adrenaline didn't hurt, either. We do have friends who healed almost painlessly, and many more who didn't think it was nearly as bad as we did. Still, we make a point now of warning people, perhaps more than necessary, that the first days or weeks postpartum might be pretty rough. We felt like it would have been a lot easier for us if we had known what was coming.

when to call

Call your doctor whenever you want! Just because women are not scheduled for a postpartum checkup for 6 weeks doesn't mean concerns don't arise. It can be hard to distinguish between "normal" postpartum healing and things that require medical attention. Call your ob-gyn, midwife, or family doctor with any and all questions you have, even if you just want some reassurance. Here are some symptoms you shouldn't ignore:

DEFINITELY CALL YOUR PRACTITIONER IF . . .

- Your bleeding is extremely heavy (more than one pad an hour).
- You have bright red bleeding more than 5–7 days postpartum.
- You're bleeding heavily again after bleeding has been tapering off.
- Your cramps are very strong and painful after more than a week.
- Your bleeding smells bad (not just like menstrual blood).
- You're passing large clots (bigger than around a golf ball).
- You're having pain or burning when urinating.
- You've got a red, painful area on your breast.
- You've got swelling or pain in your leg.
- You've got a fever above 100 degrees after the first-day postpartum.
- You're feeling faint or dizzy.
- You're nauseous or vomiting.

→ See C-Section Recovery, page 181.

Everyone talks about how labor is so hard—labor (and I didn't have an epidural and it lasted 36 hours) was a piece of cake compared with what came after. I had a couple of pretty decent "rips" and what felt like bruising to the general area. And due to the fact that the placenta wouldn't come out on its own, I lost a lot of blood (I was temporarily very anemic). That combined with the incredible nipple pain that I was experiencing at the beginning of breastfeeding and the fact that I was afraid of going to the bathroom made me distracted from appreciating this cute little baby! I wasn't prepared for that.

—anonymom

Oh my God. I couldn't sit for ten days, which made nursing painful, and I even took that stupid plastic donut in a taxi with me when I went to the doctor so I could sit on it.

—anonymom

The smell of my sweat for the first few days was unbelievable. It was unlike any body odor I had ever encountered. More like something you'd find in a zoo.

—anonymom

I guess I should have prepared myself better for postpartum as opposed to labor in the last few weeks of pregnancy. Not that labor and delivery is not an important part of pregnancy and motherhood, but in all honesty, my body was better prepared for labor than it was for motherhood, and yet I was convinced it was the other way around.

—anonymom

The most painful thing about the entire pregnancy (apart from the actual labor) was managing the ass, frankly. I remember having to cut my walks into tiny segments so that I could rest my cheeks. The scraping against those lunar pebbles also chafed my skin so that it felt like the kind of blisters you get with new shoes. I never used paper to dry myself. Now, I start with paper but I still have to wash myself after every no. 2, the Indian way with a bucket. They say it's more hygienic anyway. The hemorrhoids haven't disappeared, and I don't imagine they ever will (unless you go for surgery, which isn't a very appealing thought—not quite yet, anyway). After about 10 weeks, they stopped hurting because they popped back in again without manual assistance.

—anonymom

It felt like a bar of steel holding the area between the anus and the vagina together, as if that whole area had been casted, molded. Papier-mâché! I felt very uncomfortable about the idea of going to the bathroom, but because it was hard and the skin tense, it also made it very difficult physically. I used herbal therapy—Saint-John's-wort worked as an anti-inflammatory cream—and compresses of witchhazel.

—anonymom

I wish people had been honest with me. I can't complain, I had an easy pregnancy and labor. But I had a tough time after. Nobody told me that breastfeeding could be hard, impossible. Nobody told me that a baby with jaundice could go back to the hospital. After that happened to me, other moms I know said it happened to them. Strangely, they never told me. When I asked them why, they said they did not want to scare me. I wish they had just told me the truth. So now I tell the truth to my pregnant friends. Yes, labor and delivery is painful. Yes, they will make you feel guilty if you don't breastfeed. No, breastfeeding is not easy and maybe you won't be able to even if you want to with all your heart. Don't get me wrong. Having a baby is the most wonderful thing that happened to me. I just wished I had known the truth so I wouldn't have been depressed and crying for the first two weeks thinking I was the only one going through all of this.

—anonymom

bodily byproducts of birth

BLOODSHOT EYES, "BLACK" EYES: Intense pushing can burst tiny capillaries (veins) in the eyes, causing black or bloodshot eyes. They are not dangerous or painful although they may look dramatic. They usually go away in a few days, but sometimes last longer.

DRUG HANGOVERS: Headaches, nausea, skin rashes, constipation, itching, aches and pains, and/or tingling or numbness in legs can follow epidurals, narcotics, and other drugs used in labor. *Wait for the drugs to leave your system. Treat constipation and headaches. Tell your doctor about any lingering effects.*

BACKACHE, PELVIC ACHE: Might be from labor-related muscle strain or from being in awkward positions while anesthetized. *Rest. Do some light exercise. Work on posture. Don't strain. Once the stomach gets stronger, there will be less pressure on the back.*

GAS AND BLOATING: Gas can be very painful or mild and is often the result of slow digestion or air trapped in the abdomen during surgery. *Introduce solids gradually. Talk to your doctor about suppositories, enemas, over-the-counter medication (containing simethicone), or Vicodin and Percocet (though these can cause constipation). Chamomile tea can help, too.*

CONSTIPATION: Anesthesia, pain relievers, iron supplements, and C-section can all slow digestion. Sore perineum, stitches, hemorrhoids, tender and weakened pelvic floor muscles = fear of a bowel movement. *Drink water. Increase fiber. Move around. Be brave: Stitches were made to withstand pressure. Enemas, stool softeners, or glycerin suppositories can help.*

SWEATING. HOT FLASHES. LOTS OF PEEING. All the water your body stored during pregnancy is suddenly free to flow . . . and it does. Whatever doesn't come out via your kidneys comes out as sweat. This drenching detox can happen any time of day. It can start 24 hours to a week after labor, and often ends within a month. *Drink water. Avoid caffeine. Call your doctor if you have a fever.*

BLEEDING:
→ See Bleeding, page 180.

PAIN FROM EPIDURAL NEEDLE: The back can be sore around needle insertion areas. *Mention any lingering epidural issues to your doctor.*

CONTRACTIONS AND CRAMPS:
→ See Involution, page 180.

URINARY PROBLEMS, URINARY TRACT INFECTION, INCONTINENCE: Postpartum incontinence is very common and is caused by weakened pelvic-floor muscles. *Do Kegels. Talk to your doctor about a urinary tract infection (antibiotics may be prescribed). Unsweetened cranberry juice can help. Keep clean.*

CROTCH PAIN: Bruises, scrapes, rawness, cuts, and tears equal soreness, burning, and stinging pain for days or weeks. Stitches may pull on sore tissues and cause itching. *Ice area, try compresses, use witch-hazel pads.* → See Keeping It Clean, page 180.

HEMORRHOIDS: Varicose veins in the rectal area may pop out from the stress of labor. They're not dangerous but can cause pain and may bleed. They usually recede over time. *Soothe with witch-hazel pads, hot and/or cold compresses. Try sitting on a donut-shaped pillow. Kegels may help. Your doctor can recommend a medicated cream. Don't avoid bowel movements. Hemorrhoids can be removed with surgery if necessary.*

No one ever told me that when I came home from the hospital (and this is after what was considered a good vaginal birth) that I would be having contractions every time I breastfed (with resultant gushes of blood); that I would suffer major and totally upsetting constipation (and resultant enema from husband on the floor of my in-laws' bathroom); that I would sweat through two sheets a night no matter the bedroom temperature; that going to the bathroom—just to pee—would be a three-act drama including a water spray bottle for the cleaning, maxiMAXIpads for the blood, and witch hazel for the 'roids!; that my breasts would be so rock hard that I would develop sudden fevers of 101 for the first—count 'em—three weeks (I had mastitis); and that my pelvis and back hurt so much that sitting hurt like hell. But as soon as the birth is over, it's like . . . you're over! Even the ob-gyn was like, See ya in six weeks.
—anonymom

SORE TAILBONE: Birth can injure (and in rare cases break) the tailbone. *Try a donut-shaped pillow; ask doctor about pain relief options.*

bleeding

All remaining lochia (tissues, blood, etc.) needs to come out of the uterus after the baby is born. At first, bleeding is heavy, soaking about five pads in 24 hours. Clots (up to the size of a golf ball) and mucus are common in the early weeks. Eventually, this blood will turn brownish, then pink, then a yellowish color. Bleeding should stop entirely within about 4—6 weeks. Bleeding can be heavier with a C-section, twins, a very large baby, fibroids, or placental problems. Unusually heavy bleeding or large clots can be an indication of delayed postpartum hemorrhage, an emergency situation. Call your doctor or go to the ER if you experience heavy bleeding and feel faint. → See When to Call, page 176.

what to try

- Use maxipads (do not use tampons for 6 weeks).
- Consider disposable underwear.

involution

After the birth, the uterus needs to shrink from the size of a watermelon to the size of a pear. This process is called involution, and it happens quickly to discourage hemorrhage or infection. In total this takes about 4—6 weeks, but a lot of the heavy-duty shrinking and tightening take place in the days following birth. Most new moms are very surprised to find that these contractions can be strong, and sometimes painful (some say they're like bad menstrual cramps). Breastfeeding actually helps speed up this process, since the hormone oxytocin, released during feedings, also makes the uterus contract. Very noticeable contractions are common while nursing in the first few days. These fade as time goes on.

what to try

- Go to the bathroom frequently to take pressure off the area.
- When a contraction comes on, breathe deeply and massage your lower belly.
- Lie down on your side or stomach and press pillows against your abdomen.
- Use hot compresses.
- Doctors sometimes prescribe painkillers for the first couple of days postpartum.

keeping it clean

Visits to the bathroom involve some pretty fancy cleaning maneuvers in the first few weeks. Gentle cleaning can help prevent infection and speed up the healing process:

- Change pads frequently.
- Wash hands before wiping (front to back).
- Rinse with a perineum bottle (a squirt bottle supplied by the hospital or midwife), a cup, or from cupped handfuls in the shower.
- Avoid rough toilet paper (try medicated and/or unscented wipes).
- Try squirting cool water over the perineum while urinating to help with any stinging.
- Try compresses: cold, hot, cold followed by hot, or soaked with witch hazel.
- Take a warm bath or soak in a sitz bath (a small plastic basin that fits onto your toilet seat).
- Place a witch-hazel pad over your maxipad.

c-section recovery

C-section healing is affected by lots of things: the circumstances of the surgery, the length of labor beforehand, and whether other procedures (episiotomy, forceps, vacuum) were used. Recovery from a scheduled C-section is usually quicker than from an emergency one, partly because unanticipated C-sections are often preceded by long labors. Some women experience pain for a couple of weeks postpartum, while others feel the effects of surgery for months. Either way, it can be very frustrating and exhausting to deal with postoperative recovery, general postpartum recovery, and a bouncing new baby all at once. Here are some common concerns and ways to deal with them:

MOVING AROUND: Post-op moms often say that for a couple of weeks, any movement—picking up the baby, brushing teeth, sneezing—reminds them that they've had an operation. The abdominal muscles, central as they are, are used for most physical activities. Therefore, women are encouraged to take it easy: Get help around the house and refrain from picking up anything heavier than the baby. However, some activity is important for postoperative circulation, respiration, and digestion. Immediately after surgery, doctors and nurses often ask moms to wiggle their toes and fingers. Short, gentle walks are encouraged soon thereafter. Driving is not recommended until the incision has healed because of the risk of sudden movements.

THE INCISION: After 2—3 days, the incision becomes tight and sealed. The scar soon heals from red to pink and then fades to a lighter line. The incision might itch as it heals. After about a week, it's safe to gently apply some vitamin E oil or calendula cream to soothe itching. If bacteria has been introduced during surgery, an infection can emerge weeks after birth. This requires medical attention (antibiotics are usually prescribed).

call the doctor if

- Your stitches come undone.
- Your incision gets red, swollen, and hurts under the surface.
- You notice pus.
- You have a fever.

> I had a C-section after seventeen hours of induced labor proved unsuccessful. I had a complication—I lost half of my blood volume—so I was really anemic, pale, and a tad extra tired for a while until my body recovered. And I was not ready for the whole postpartum neverending period thing that seems to go on forever. Yuckola. It was my first experience ever wearing a pad, and I made my husband go buy them from the store—I think he bought every possible make and model!
> —anonymom

> Try not to joke with anyone the first few days—it just hurts your stomach way too much. Oh, and coughing and sneezing go right along with it. Holding a pillow to your stomach helps a tiny bit.
> —anonymom

breastfeeding after a c-section

Giving birth by C-section doesn't directly interfere with your ability to breastfeed, but recovery and hospital issues can make it harder in the beginning. Here's what you can do to make breastfeeding easier if you have a Cesarean birth:

MAKE IT CLEAR THAT YOU WANT TO BREASTFEED. Communicating your priorities beforehand is extra-important when recovering from a C-section—both because hospital policies may not be ideal for breastfeeding and because you may be out of it during your recovery. Let your doctor and nurses know to bring the baby to you for feedings and that no bottles or pacifiers should be given in the nursery.

BE CONFIDENT ABOUT YOUR ABILITY TO BREASTFEED. Unexpected C-sections can be demoralizing for mothers who were emotionally invested in the idea of a vaginal birth. But breastfeeding can work just fine after a C-section.

GET CLOSE TO YOUR BABY AS SOON AS POSSIBLE. Getting to know the feel and smell of your skin will encourage your baby to breastfeed.

DON'T BE AFRAID TO NURSE UNDER LOCAL ANESTHESIA OR PAIN MEDICATION. You can nurse your baby whenever you're both ready, ideally right away—even before your local anesthetic has worn off. This can help you both get a taste of breastfeeding before the pain of surgery kicks in. Medication can help speed your recovery. Speak to your doctor about choosing a good pain reliever that won't cause problems for your baby. In general, pain is more likely to be an issue for breastfeeding than pain medication, so there's no reason to deprive yourself of relief.

GET HELP WITH POSITIONING. Side-lying and clutch-hold positions tend to be more comfortable for C-section moms. At first, you can even nurse flat on your back if you need to. Try to get assistance from the nursing staff or a knowledgeable breastfeeding support person about the best ways to hold a baby after a C-section. Have a partner or another helper watch the positioning and latch suggestions so you can get help at home, too.

→ See Getting Off to a Good Start, page 282, for general advice about getting nursing going.

> My C-section became infected and opened a bit. Nurses had to come to my house twice a day for two weeks to clean and pack the wound with gauze for healing. It was a serious and emotional time. Things slowly got better but recovering from the C-section prohibited me from breastfeeding very long. I just couldn't handle both at the same time.
> **—anonymom**

> Due to the Cesarean, I wasn't lactating immediately and felt like I'd been hit by a truck for two days. It took at least four days to start feeling even fractionally a mom. Luckily, my husband stayed with me most of the time in the hospital for a week and this really made for an excellent beginning as he learned how to do things at the same time as I did (when to feed, how to do the diaper, the bath). He actually did this stuff before me due to the Cesarean. It really made him understand how important he is and how being a parent is learned rather than totally innate.
> **—anonymom**

body image

A postbirth body may seem strange and unfamiliar. The surface wounds usually heal pretty quickly, but your feelings about your body might be going through changes for a lot longer. Though most everyone is happy to get that watermelon out from under their rib cage, there are lots of reasons women miss their pregnant bodies: the attention, the feeling of fullness and usefulness, the glow, the relief from worrying about a flat stomach. The loss of "specialness" a woman often feels after giving birth can add to the prevailing pressure—to become thin and sexy as soon as possible, so she can get back into the limelight as a sexually attractive woman. But giving birth and nurturing a baby can introduce a positive image of a body with a purpose beyond looking attractive. This can give women a new-found confidence.

body parts

HAIR: Many women notice their hair falling out in alarming quantities in the months following birth. This is caused by the same phenomenon that makes hair extra-thick during pregnancy. All the hairs that remained in a growth phase throughout pregnancy enter a falling-out phase about 2—5 months postpartum. This is technically called postpartum alopecia. Though hair is usually lost over the whole scalp, it may or may not be noticeable. Hair loss is not permanent, but it can take up to 18 months for hair to return to normal thickness. While it's growing back, you may notice little tufts at your hairline. These will eventually blend into your hair; cutting bangs or layers can ease the transition. If hair loss is accompanied by sudden fatigue, forgetfulness, dry skin, and cold, check with a doctor to rule out thyroid issues, which sometimes occur postpartum.

BELLY: You may have heard that you'd be wearing maternity clothes home from the hospital. But you may not have anticipated being asked "When's your baby due?" on your first solo trip out of the house after birth. Postpartum bellies do look surprisingly pregnant. It takes up to 8 weeks for the uterus to reach nonpregnant proportions, and the padding around it can take much longer. The ligaments, which play an important supporting role for the organs in your abdomen, can take up to 6 months to realign. There's often some surplus skin in the midsection even after the weight is lost. Looser or differently aligned skin may also cause your belly button to change size or shape. Some women's torsos shrink up seamlessly, while others are left with a lot of squish and sag. The amount of slack in the skin depends on the muscles and fat beneath, as well as skin type, age, history, and heredity.

I felt like I instantly morphed from mystical vessel to functional animal, and was left in the corner nursing my wounds (and my newborn).
—anonymom

Before having a baby I concentrated on things like were my feet too big, did I look fat, was my nose big, really stupid stuff. After witnessing my amazing body give birth to a baby, then produce milk to feed her, and heal itself, I began to see that my body was fantastic—big feet and all!
—anonymom

The third or fourth month after the baby is born, your hair starts falling out! I never heard that. It was disgusting. But the main problem for me was I made this huge effort to leave my baby so I could get my hair highlighted at great expense. All the highlighted blond hair fell right out and the hair growth was all dark. No, this is not at *all* earth shattering! But it was a DRAG and expensive and avoidable!
—anonymom

Around the time when the "happy hormones" leave, you look down in the shower and see all this hair floating down the drain. It left me feeling quite sad, I remember.
—anonymom

183

> Within the first
> few days, my boobs
> became rocks and I looked like
> a porn star even with my "after
> baby" body. I just kept looking in
> the mirror at myself thinking,
> "Wow . . . I'm huge!"
> —anonymom

BOOBS: Saggy boobs are caused by two things: gravity and the swelling of pregnancy. Your boobs will expand (and shrink, leaving extra skin) whether you breastfeed or not. If you nurse, your breasts will probably be enlarged while you're feeding frequently. A mother's cup size often peaks in the month or so postpartum. If you're not nursing, you'll probably go through a period of painfully engorged breasts, followed by some degree of deflation. Some women feel depressed about their breasts after they've weaned, or after birth if they don't breastfeed. Many moms are surprised to find that the change is less radical than lore had led them to believe.

SEX ORGANS: As pornography has gotten more mainstream, the idealized body has forged a new frontier: the crotch. The ideal vagina, in keeping with the ideal of femininity in general, is supposedly one that looks pristine and youthful, not one that shows signs of use. Vaginal births, while they generally don't result in gaping holes between the legs, may result in a little wear, tear, and stretching. This can make the labia larger. Women have lately taken to getting plastic surgery to make their labia more uniform and girlish looking. We thought it was a given that all vaginas were supposed to be unique, but apparently, not everyone agrees. → See Vagina Anxiety, page 211.

SKIN: Dry and/or oily skin, dandruff, and breakouts are common for many postpartum moms. Most of the time these issues resolve on their own, but a dermatologist may be able to suggest skin-care regimens if the situation is really bugging you. If you have any moles that have changed during pregnancy, check them out with your dermatologist. Stretch marks, whether they popped up during pregnancy or after the baby's birth, are probably the most common postpartum skin complaint. There are various treatments available, but their effectiveness is questionable.

WEIGHT LOSS: There is no magic formula for postpartum weight loss. Some women don't put on much extra pregnancy weight. Some lose what they gain within weeks and without effort. Many others find themselves carrying pregnancy weight for 9 months or more, no matter what they do. There are so many factors entering the postpartum weight situation. The way you put on and take off weight, postpregnancy and otherwise, is hugely affected by your genes, as well as what you put into and do with your body. If you want to diet, many doctors and nutritionists emphasize going slowly and giving yourself time to lose the weight. Make nutrition the top priority; eat when you are hungry and avoid junk foods.

> I suppose
> my breasts now
> are a tad of a
> disappointment;
> just as I never knew
> how big they could
> get, I'm surprised at
> how saggy they can get
> after only one child!
> It's amazing looking at
> them and seeing all of
> the wrinkles and
> old-lady lines on
> them when I hoist
> them up.
> —anonymom

breastfeeding and dieting

Many women feel hungrier when breastfeeding than they did during pregnancy, or for that matter, at any point in their entire lives. Some women find that they are able to eat much more than usual and still maintain (or even lose) weight. Others feel as if their bodies are clinging onto extra pounds and only start dropping them once they wean. Breastfeeding mothers burn a lot of calories making milk, though weight loss does not necessarily correspond. It's not clear why some breastfeeding women lose weight and others hang onto it. Most doctors do not recommend substantially restricting calorie, carb, or fat intake while breastfeeding. In fact, many recommend 500 extra calories a day. In addition to depleting good nutrients and energy, here are a few problematic things that can happen to a breastfeeding mother if she goes on an extremely restrictive diet:

- Rapid weight loss (more than a pound a week) may decrease milk supply.

- Toxins, such as environmental contaminants, PCBs, and pesticides, are stored in body fat. Rapid weight loss can release these toxins into the bloodstream, which may lead to higher toxin levels in the breast milk.

- Low-carb diets can cause ketosis. This happens when the body burns fat instead of glucose, causing toxic, acidic ketones to build up in the bloodstream. It is unknown if ketones pose a risk to the breastfed baby, but even the major carb-diet gurus recommend that breastfeeding moms keep up their carb intake.

exercise

A new mother's body is still doing a lot of transforming: Stomach muscles are out of place, ligaments and joints are still loose, and there may be stitches, sores, bruises, or backaches. Hormonal changes and sleep deprivation have a huge impact on energy levels.

The American College of Obstetricians and Gynecologists says it's okay to exercise as soon after birth as you want, as long as you feel up to it, though too much too soon is never recommended. C-section moms should wait 6 weeks. Sometimes just caring for a baby can be enough physical work for women to feel the benefits of a bona fide workout. Many moms find that gentle exercise helps the healing process, boosts energy, and encourages gradual weight loss.

Postpartum moms have a few spots that may be in need of special treatment and/or workouts: the pelvic floor and the abdominal or core muscles. There are stretching and tightening exercises you can do to strengthen these muscles (see "Kegels," page 58). Also, if you are, to borrow a Zen expression, "mindful" of your body while you tend to your baby, you can actually strengthen muscles and avoid strains or aches. When you pick up the baby, bend your knees to protect your back. When you nurse, sit up straight. Don't sit the baby on one hip all day; switch positions.

BREASTFEEDING AND EXERCISE: It's totally fine for a nursing mom to do moderate exercise. Because working out with milk-heavy boobs can lead to some soreness and leaking, you may want to feed first and get a good sports bra. Some moms just don't have the urge to exercise while breastfeeding. This may or may not be related to hormone levels or the fact that making milk is already burning a lot of calories.

> It's taken me nine months to "lose" the weight but my bod looks nothing like it did before (not that it was ever great...)—things shift, droop, soften.
> —**anonymom**

Of course, we all hear about models and actresses who get their figures back within weeks of giving birth. What the press does not reveal is the cost required—not only in financial terms (personal trainers, dietitians, and figure-sculpting equipment, even surgery) but also in terms of the potential future health problems resulting from dieting and exercising too soon after childbirth.

—Sylvia Brown,
The Post-Pregnancy Handbook

> I loved being pregnant. I felt great and thought my body and belly *rocked*. It's the aftermath that sucked.... The last thing you want (or need) to do is worry about being fat—yet it seems people feel the need to comment just how "great" So-and-so looks after just having given birth. It's an unwritten contest to see how long it takes women to "regain their figure." UGH.
>
> —anonymom

hot mom = not mom

Shaping up has always been a concern for new mothers, but now they're expected to do it with lightning speed. Celebrity moms appear svelte and smiling just days after giving birth. Due to exercise? Diets? Genes? Surgery? Just plain luck? Who knows. And pity the poor high-profile mom who's caught on camera with a little residual flab showing. Will she *ever* lose the weight?? Is something *wrong*?? It's hard not to have unrealistic expectations when the fantasy of snapping back like elastic-girl is everywhere.

Beauty, in modern-day America, means perfection, and perfection means showing as little impact of time and experience on your physical self as possible. Of course carrying and birthing a baby changes your body. Yet women who want to be seen as beautiful are expected to erase any evidence of babies (just as they're expected to erase the signs of too much sun, or just too much time on the planet). It sucks that on top of the real work of being a mom, we're all supposed to be worrying about stuffing ourselves into jeans or obsessing over stretch marks or wondering whether the fact that we've had kids makes our labia unappealing. How are we supposed to feel good about our bodies when all the "hot moms" we see look like they're not moms at all?

new mom fashion

The immediate postpartum period is rarely a shining style moment. Due to leftover belly girth, maternity wear is often the best option in the first weeks. (If you happen to be breastfeeding in hot weather, you may not be wearing a shirt much anyway.) Fashion entrepreneurs have come up with a new concept called transitionwear to assist new moms with their postpartum fashion crises, and spend a little money in the process. As far as we can tell, this is usually really stretchy clothing, sometimes with a little belly camouflage.

Your look will likely go through some changes along with your lifestyle. Women sometimes struggle with the idea that they're *supposed* to change their image when they have babies, not just because of practical considerations, but because they're concerned about what's "proper" for a mother who's no longer on the market for a mate. (See "Where's

image consciousness gone wild

Rumor has it that some massively image-conscious moms schedule C-sections a few weeks before their due dates to avoid putting on those last few pounds and give themselves time to take off weight before their first public appearance. Some may even postdate their baby's births to make their physiques seem even more miraculous. It's hard to say whether this rumor is based in reality or postpartum envy, but either way, it's a disturbing idea.

> When I was three months postpartum, I encountered a mom with a baby the same age. I immediately started blabbing about how crazy it was, how little time there was for my own stuff, how despite warnings, I could never have imagined how overwhelmed I'd feel. "I know!!" she said. "I've even resorted to waxing my own eyebrows." I was stunned. In the entire period since my son's birth, I had not once consciously considered having eyebrows, much less grooming them. But she did teach me something: No matter what the baseline, motherhood takes everyone down a few notches (at least for a while).
>
> —Rebecca

the Mystique?," page 212.) On the other hand, grooming is one of the few wholly sanctioned "me time" activities for new mothers (which may have more to do with being palatable than being pampered). But many moms find themselves skirting a delicate balance between slovenliness and self-indulgence. Too little grooming, and they obviously don't care about their partners. Too much, and they obviously don't care about their children. Of course, everyone's threshold varies; one person's daily routine is another one's disarray.

A few stereotypical postpartum fashion solutions:

Throw in the towel immediately . . . or eventually (perhaps after some futile attempts at regaining clothing composure early on). Succumb wholly to the practical: comfortable shoes, yoga pants, disposable T-shirts. Figure you'll pick up the ball again when your kids are old enough. Or maybe you won't.

Plunge further into your hippie leanings, transforming from flower child to earth mama. Wrap yourself in long loose skirts and tunics, celebrating your body's changing curves. Make your baby sling the cornerstone of your wardrobe. Ignore the oppressive voice of mainstream fashion, so irrelevant to nature.

Stage a full-fledged war against "looking like a mom." Never leave the house without a blow-dry and fresh manicure. Visit your bikini waxer before your 6-week OB appointment. Wear heels to the playground. Dress for a hot night out, every day. Go to Paris to observe French chic mommies and emulate their technique.

baby body image

The idea that mothers love their babies no matter what they look like is part of the vernacular: *"A face only a mother could love."* But it's not necessarily true that how a baby looks doesn't affect a mom's feelings. Almost all babies share proportions that we find aesthetically pleasing. In fact, babies' cuteness is thought to be a major reason we put up with their general pain-in-the-ass-ness, which makes being cute an asset from an evolutionary perspective. But just as there are ideals for adults, there are ideals for babies, and not all babies look like the ideal. There are some studies showing that babies who are less attractive get less attention. Since attractiveness is so subjective, it's hard to know what this means. Parents of babies who are different looking may have to readjust their own expectations about what a baby "should" look like, as well as learn to manage the responses of others. People seem to exercise the same freedom of expression about babies' bodies as they do about pregnant ones. Parents often find themselves feeling defensive about comments on their babies' weight or appearance. "She's a big girl" can feel like a thinly veiled "She's *too* big." It's trite but it's true: All babies are unique and should be considered on their own terms.

the postbaby brain

emotional landscape of parenthood

Most of the time we hear about stark poles of postbaby emotions—utter bliss and utter despair. If you're not euphoric, you must have postpartum depression. But in real life, the postpartum psychological terrain is a lot more varied. Feelings are complex and messy and contradictory. It's totally normal to feel ecstatic and lonely. Elated and anxious. Overflowing with gratitude and seething with resentment. It's even normal not to feel much of anything at all, like you're on autopilot.

Here are just some of the emotions you might go through (within the course of a year or a day):

Spaced Lonely Bored Angry Serene Confused Worried

Confident Dazed Euphoric Depressed Shocked

Anxious Happy Spent Unstable Blissed Out Sad Proud

> I hate to say this, but newborns are boring; why does nobody tell you that it's boring until they are like six months old?
>
> —anonymom

> I was euphoric for the first week. . . . The next week or two it hit me, though. Sleep deprivation set in and I felt awful. I started worrying that I really didn't love her because I had lost the euphoria.
>
> —anonymom

> I was lonely, sleep-deprived, and anxious about everything. The pounds melted away because it seemed like every time I sat down to a meal, my daughter started to cry. I also resented my husband because his life seemed to be just slightly different while mine had turned upside down. Oh, and also, he planned a barbecue *at our house* the day after our daughter had her first night of not sleeping, when she was five days old. I had a breakdown in the bathroom, wailing, "WHY WON'T YOU SLEEP? PLEASE SLEEP!" My husband blissfully slept through the whole thing.
>
> —anonymom

It seemed like a dream, like I was caring for someone else's baby. When were they coming to pick her up??
—anonymom

I had a few roller-coaster days. Mostly my feelings were more easily hurt, particularly by my spouse.
—anonymom

I had some postpartum issues where I felt unstable and superemotional, I would cry over anything (good and bad). I felt as though a lot of friends and family offered to be there for me and then they weren't—now, in retrospect, I realize I didn't ASK for help/support.
—anonymom

I couldn't believe that I was a mother. How can you adjust to such a life-altering change so quickly? One minute, you are a couple, and in the next minute you are a family. It was just shocking.
—anonymom

For the first few days it felt just magical, then it got confusing.
—anonymom

I felt incredibly capable and confident—some crazy protective instinct took over and for a while it seemed I could survive on very little food and very, very little sleep. I think I barely even looked up from the baby for weeks. But the confidence (or whatever instinctual insanity it was) had a dark side: I felt a strong hostility to the outside world (damn phone), and a primal urge to sort of *envelop* my baby and retreat.
—anonymom

I was exhausted, depressed, and somewhat scared of what I had gotten myself into.
—anonymom

I didn't feel like I had anything left in me to deal with the everyday. I wouldn't have eaten had someone not put food in front of me.
—anonymom

I cried to my husband and said, "Why would nature make the first few weeks so hard as to make you resent your baby?" It just didn't make sense to me, and I thrive on being able to make sense out of any situation (even, and especially, the hard ones).
—anonymom

In hindsight I realize I was just sort of out of it. The amazing thing was that the adrenaline rush that happened immediately postpartum lasted for two weeks.
—anonymom

I struggled with the fact that I had a boy and my heart was set on a girl. I felt ashamed of being disappointed.
—anonymom

189

the continuum of depression

You can feel depressed without having postpartum depression. You can have thoughts about something awful happening to your baby, even about doing it yourself, without being at risk of harming her. Every smidgeon of negative emotion that enters a new mom's mind is not a sign of a clinical disorder. It's a matter of degree, and of how those feelings are processed. In a recent study at the Mayo Clinic, 89 percent of mothers and fathers reported having intrusive, upsetting thoughts about their baby being harmed: suffocating, drowning, being kidnapped, etc. "For most parents, this is just mental noise," said Jonathan Abramowitz, psychologist and director of the OCD/Anxiety Disorders Program at the Mayo Clinic. "They dismiss it and move on." But when those thoughts are constant or insistent—you cannot make them go away or find a way to put them in perspective— you may be grappling with something more serious.

Postpartum care is very limited and rarely includes any real psychological assessment. So it may be largely up to you to decide whether or not you are worried about the way you feel. Unfortunately, depressed moms often feel hopeless, like help won't do them any good. A partner can be crucial in getting her the support she needs. Postpartum depression and anxiety are serious problems that require treatment. If you take action, things can get better! Support groups, therapy, and medication are just a few of the options that have been shown to help. → See Emotional Resource Rescue, page 204.

I think I was depressed until my son was over a year old. I stopped working to stay at home with him, and I was bored out of my skull, as well as frustrated that I couldn't do anything other than care for him. I didn't get treatment, so it's no wonder I was depressed during my second pregnancy, too. I got treatment following my second child's birth. I kinda like being a mom now.

—anonymom

Almost everyone has some sort of depression after having the baby. (I said almost, I know not everyone does.) With all the feedings, changings, lack of sleep, missing the time you used to have with your husband, missing the time you used to have for yourself, and the lack of time for normal everyday things like eating and showering— you do get a little down.

Everyone expects new moms to be full of joy (which we are) but not to be full of anxiety, experience waves of sadness, and feelings of deep inadequacy to the core of our being. After becoming a mother, I finally understood all those stories you hear about mothers going on family vacations and disappearing; or even the mothers who totally lose it and harm their babies. Even if I knew I would never, could never do these things, I understood them for the first time.

—anonymom

For me, I can remember a point where I had horrible thoughts. I just couldn't take it anymore and I wanted to throw my son against the wall. Of course, I would *never ever* hurt my son, but ... sometimes those thoughts come across your mind. It's normal, though, as long as you don't act on your thoughts. I'm here to say that it does get better and there is a light at the end of the tunnel. If you feel that way, please get help. You can talk to your doctor, ob-gyn, midwife, or counselor—or even other moms. Also, if at all possible, when you feel that way, at that very moment try to switch the baby responsibilities to someone else. Even if your husband is sleeping and has work the next day, just wake him up and tell him he needs to take the baby, even if it's for fifteen minutes while you take a shower, a walk, or a short nap.

—anonymom

signs to look out for

- Bad feelings that are continually present and don't respond to improvements in your situation (more sleep, more help, etc.)
- Thoughts or feelings that make it hard for you to take care of yourself or your baby
- Persistent obsessive thoughts (often involving hurting the baby and/or yourself)
- Panic attacks
- Feeling like nothing can improve the situation
- Refusing sleep/food
- Having no positive feelings for the baby at all

I felt depressed, overwhelmed, anxious (mostly about the future, and I mean WAY into the future like twenty years!), detached from my baby, which was scary. But I didn't feel suicidal nor did I ever have thoughts of hurting the baby. I did have thoughts of him being thrown against a wall or tossed over a bridge . . . not by me but just the action. That was scary. I didn't know where that was coming from.
—anonymom

[I wish I had known] that the postpartum would hit me that hard and it was *normal*. Even after the doctor told me it was normal and put me on Paxil, I still just wanted it to go away as fast as it could. It was a whole new emotion/feeling for me. I've never had PMS, never had bad periods, never had a roller coaster of emotions during my cycle. I had a very easy pregnancy, no emotional highs and lows then either. So when this hit, it was completely foreign to me.
—anonymom

baby blues

"Baby blues" is the official name for the whacked-out state most moms find themselves in for some portion of the first week or so postpartum. Even amid overwhelming joy, and irrespective of other factors, almost all women experience some emotional mayhem early on. About 80 percent of new moms feel a form of the "baby blues." This is largely attributed to a huge plummet in estrogen and progesterone. Some people think that this phenomenon is related to other kinds of posttraumatic responses, and is as much about what a mom has been through as her chemistry. It's easy to imagine stuff that might contribute to these intense emotions, like, oh, for example, the labor and delivery you went through. Or your new overwhelming responsibilities. Or utter exhaustion. Don't judge yourself, your marriage, or anything else in your life too harshly for the first couple of weeks. To us, this time felt less like the blues (which imply a kind of quiet, even romantic, soulfully depressed state) and more like cacophony . . . highly experimental free jazz maybe?

I came home from the hospital two days later in a state of alternating hysteria and catatonia. I knew about postpartum depression, but this? Killer waves of incompetence crashing through my body and making me too frantic to even understand what was happening to me? . . . I had pictured the initial entry into newborn Hell as Dead Woman Walking, on Seconal or something, like Neely in *Valley of the Dolls.* That turned out to be excessively optimistic.

—Susan Squire, from "Maternal Bitch" in *The Bitch in the House*

> It was my first week back from maternity leave and I was eating with a bunch of coworkers. Someone asked me what it's like being a mom and I said something like, "It's great. I love him so much, he's amazing. It's so awesome but sometimes I'm like 'You're such an asshole!' " This did not go over well. There were two loud gasps, one guy (with three kids) laughed. I had to backpedal . . . "I mean of course I love him, it's just at 2, 3, 4, 5 A.M. when he just won't lie down and sleep! . . ." Later one of the women said she was "sure that other mothers felt this way, they just didn't say anything about it."
> —anonymom

the code of silence

You're in line at the drugstore with your screaming infant and a basket of products you're hoping will get her to stop screaming. Your bleary eyes catch a magazine photo of a gorgeous, glowing mother cradling her gorgeous, glowing baby. We all know by now that these impossibly perfect images are the products of marketing and spin. Yet many moms on the street seem to project the same kind of magical maternal bliss.

Joy and excitement are a big part of most new parents' experiences, but they're not all of everyone's. If bad feelings were allowed to be a normal part of the postpartum experience (because *they are*), women would be a lot less freaked out about having them. But trying to connect to others and express less-than-gleeful feelings is not always easy. People might pretend they don't know what you're talking about. Or bristle at the negativity. Or give you an earful of "the bright side." Sometimes it takes some exploratory socializing to find out who you can blab to. If you're having a tough time finding moms who are willing to admit that they ever feel anything other than joy, check out some of the memoirs we list at the end of this chapter.
→ See Postpartum Support, page 168.

> Reality bites sometimes, so let's not pretend that it doesn't simply because our children are so amazing and so precious and grow up so fast. Today's mothers and mothers-to-be need and deserve some doses of reality. If not, they are being done a great disservice by the media and by healthcare professionals, and I believe they are, in fact, being set up for a much greater fall when they struggle and stumble along the way.
> —anonymom

> I know one rebel mom who made it a habit to say "I'm sooo sorry" whenever she saw a mother with a newborn. It's a little hardcore, for sure. (Plenty of people moved their strollers rapidly in the opposite direction.) But she did it because she knew that when she was a new mom, she could have used a little less congratulating and a little more sympathy. It's damn hard work!
> —anonymom

> I feel like no one ever talks about how miserable it can be. I mean, it seems everyone makes it out to be, "It's hard but it's all worth it." That's true, but they gloss over the fact that it can be *so miserable* at times. There were times I was regretting the decision to have a baby. Then I'd become racked with guilt for feeling that way. I thought there would be ups and downs, but I was just in the "down" for a while (not depressed, just not enjoying it). Again, the guilt for feeling that way . . . even my own sisters never divulged the misery. Maybe it was just me, but I doubt it.
> —anonymom

According to Postpartum Support International, here are the official symptoms of the four postpartum psychiatric mood disorders:

postpartum depression and/or anxiety

- Occurs in 15 to 20 percent of mothers
- Onset is usually gradual, but it can be rapid and begin any time in the first year

symptoms

- Excessive worry or anxiety
- Irritability or short temper
- Feeling overwhelmed, difficulty making decisions
- Sad mood, feelings of guilt, phobias
- Hopelessness
- Sleep problems (often the woman cannot sleep or sleeps too much), fatigue
- Physical symptoms or complaints without apparent physical cause
- Discomfort around the baby or a lack of feeling toward the baby
- Loss of focus and concentration (may miss appointments, for example)
- Loss of interest or pleasure, decreased libido
- Changes in appetite; significant weight loss or gain

obsessive-compulsive disorder

- Three to 5 percent of new mothers develop obsessive symptoms

symptoms

- Intrusive, repetitive, and persistent thoughts or mental pictures
- Thoughts often are about hurting or killing the baby
- Tremendous sense of horror and disgust about these thoughts (ego-alien)
- Thoughts accompanied by behaviors to reduce the anxiety (for example, hiding knives)
- Counting, checking, cleaning, or other repetitive behaviors

dads and depression

Since hormones are only one of a number of possible causes for PPD, we should not be surprised to discover that dads are affected, too. In fact, male cases are becoming more common as we learn more about the illness. And fathers are just as likely to feel guilty and ashamed of depression as women are. They may feel that it's hard to ask for help: "What do I have to complain about? I don't even have to do the hard work!" Plus, men are supposed to be tough. But it's vital to address depression. Thinking through the sadness can help you find a way to resolve it whether with your partner, other dads, in support groups, or therapy. Time will help. But untreated depression can spiral out of control, so it's not a good thing to ignore.

I wanted everything to be completely scrubbed clean in a full-on, psychedelic "out damn spot" kind of way. Since I was basically chained to the couch for weeks, I couldn't really act on the impulse, which made it excruciating at times. I would stare at the dust bunnies across the room as I nursed. At night I lay awake for hours mentally painting over a small circle of unpainted plaster on our bedroom ceiling. Eventually it went away (the patch is still there).
—Ceridwen

postpartum panic disorder

- Occurs in about 10 percent of postpartum women

symptoms

- Episodes of extreme anxiety
- Shortness of breath, chest pain, sensations of choking or smothering, dizziness
- Hot or cold flashes, trembling, palpitations, numbness, or tingling sensations
- Restlessness, agitation, or irritability
- During an attack the woman may fear that she is going crazy, dying, or losing control
- Panic attack may wake her up
- Often no identifiable trigger for panic
- Excessive worry or fears (including fear of more panic attacks)

postpartum psychosis

- Occurs in one or two per thousand
- Onset usually 2 to 3 days postpartum
- This disorder has a 5 percent suicide and 4 percent infanticide rate.

symptoms

- Visual or auditory hallucinations
- Delusional thinking (for example, about infant's death, denial of birth, or need to kill baby)
- Delirium and/or mania

resources

Beyond the Blues: A Guide to Understanding and Treating Prenatal and Postpartum Depression by Shoshana S. Bennett, Ph.D., Pec Indman

The Mother-to-Mother Postpartum Depression Support Book by Sandra Poulin

The Postpartum Husband: Practical Solutions for Living with Postpartum Depression by Karen R. Kleiman, M.S.W.

This Isn't What I Expected: Overcoming Postpartum Depression by Karen R. Kleiman, M.S.W., and Valerie Raskin, M.D.

The Center for Postpartum Health: postpartumhealth.com

Depression After Delivery: depressionafterdelivery.com

Postpartum Progress Website: postpartumprogress.typepad.com

Postpartum Support International: postpartum.net

does ppd have an evolutionary function?

THE MODERN SCIENCE INTERFERENCE THEORY New mothers are meant to be close to their babies. If modern medical birth creates distance, moms can feel disconnected and depressed.

THE INEXPRESSIBLE HOSTILITY THEORY The protective impulse a mother feels for her baby can involve strong feelings of aggression and hostility to the outside world. This may be a leftover hormonal response from the days of serious predators. These days the threats may be less tangible, but moms can still feel defensive. And that aggression, if not expressed, can be turned inward as depression.

THE CRY FOR HELP THEORY PPD is a subconscious way of saying "I NEED MORE SUPPORT."

→ See Thinking About Parenthood resources, page 374.

behind the scenes: why do i feel this way?

HORMONES: At the end of pregnancy, progesterone and estrogen are at thirty to fifty times normal levels. Three days after the birth, they drop close to zero. Progesterone and estrogen can act as antidepressants, so the rapid decline can cause dramatic emotional changes. The breastfeeding hormones prolactin and oxytocin, increased after birth, can have relaxing and bonding effects. The balance of hormones is different for each woman and affects women's moods in radically different ways. Hormones can be a cause of postpartum mood disturbances, or can just change the way a woman processes an already stressful situation, positively or negatively.

→ For more on breastfeeding hormones, see pages 217 and 316.

EXHAUSTION: If one bad night's sleep can change the whole way you look at the world, imagine what seventy-three bad nights can do. Fatigue is considered a major contributing factor (maybe even a cause) of PPD, as well as depression in general. Lack of sleep can make you more susceptible to illness, which can push exhaustion to a whole new level. Having to take care of your baby at the expense of taking care of yourself can lead to intense stress, anger, and resentment (not to mention an unshakable head cold). → See Sleep Deprivation, page 341.

THE BACK STORY: How did you get here? Maybe it took three difficult years, four specialists, endless acupuncture sessions, and oceans of positive thinking. Maybe it was a surprise after a one-night stand. Maybe you spent ages trying to adopt, or got a call the week after you filled out your applications and brought a new baby home that afternoon. Maybe one of you wanted it more than the other, and the other one was willing (or not) to go along for the ride. If this baby was a mammoth effort, you may be extra-exhausted by the work it took just to get you to this point. And you may feel added pressure to be nothing but happy, despite the letdown that often comes after such incredible efforts. Unplanned pregnancies can affect your feelings, too, as can difficult ones, previous miscarriages, or any big challenge that happens on the way to having a baby. The effect can go either way, and may not be what you expect.

i want my life back!

Few people are surprised by the idea of their lives being transformed by babies. But many are shocked by the magnitude. You may realize, for example, that you'll be giving up sleep, or working late, or all-night parties, or haute cuisine. You may not

> I felt like I had been run over by a giant truck. It was simultaneously very challenging, rewarding, relationship affirming, and emotionally charged. Oh—and did I mention exhausting? It was exhausting. The first day that my husband went back to work and left me home with the baby, I was in tears thinking that I could never do it by myself. Now, six months later, I'm in tears thinking about going back to work on Monday.
> —anonymom

> You just don't understand what sleep deprivation can do to a person until you experience it. Add postpartum mood swings, a screaming baby, and a sore body (including blistered, bleeding nipples) and you wonder why more moms don't sew themselves shut after birth.
> —anonymom

> It's always time for something...a nap, a bottle, a meal, a bath, a new diaper....
> —anonymom

> I miss staying late at work when I suddenly have a good idea.
> —anonymom

195

> When you're breastfeeding and the baby has just fallen asleep and the doorbell rings and it's the burrito you ordered (because you haven't eaten all day) and you look across the room to your wallet on the counter and you're like, how am I going to get the burrito?, that is the kind of "hard" I don't think you can prepare for.
> —anonymom

realize that you will, at first, be so tied to the couch that you will not even be able to get up to reach the case of spring water you thoughtfully purchased while still pregnant (much less have a relaxing bath with the lovely postpartum care package you received as a gift). Even when you're told to indulge and take some time for yourself, you may be reminded that *"a happy mom means a happy baby."* Even "me time" is baby time when you're a new mother.

And then there's the permanence, the thud of real-ization that, if you're lucky, you'll have this kid for the rest of your life. This is not a trip or an adventure from which you return to your old life with cool pictures, feeling wiser or more fulfilled. You may (eventually) be able to spend a weekend away from your baby, but you can never spend a weekend away from being a parent. Sometimes we need some time to mourn the loss of the old life—a life that was just yours to enjoy and screw up exactly as you saw fit. Shock, anger, denial, and all the other fun emotions associated with grief are a normal part of growing into your new healthy parent self.

> I can't help but to feel terrible guilt if I go shopping or other things without my baby. I feel like my time is better spent with my son, instead of at the mall, or the supermarket, or the nail salon. By the way, I've only indulged in these luxuries once since he was born. See, I feel guilty even admitting I got a pedicure.
> —anonymom

> I keep reading about how I can have a couple glasses of wine every now and then while breastfeeding. But it's not just wanting to drink more than "the occasional glass of wine," it's about missing the pure joy of making a whole string of perfectly irresponsible decisions . . . to have those extra few martinis, to dance at that bar even though there is no dance floor, to smoke a cigarette even though you quit, to ramble on about all these things you probably will never do. That is what I miss.
> —anonymom

> I miss sleeping until whatever time I wanted. I miss having the option to sleep or not. I also miss little things like going places without having to get ready for two hours. Not that I don't want to go places with my son, but it's very discouraging having to pack so much stuff just to go to Target. Or for an afternoon walk.
> —anonymom

> I can't even imagine how I'm going to get back to my creative work. I don't even have time to set up my paints, forget about painting.
> —anonymom

but enough about me . . .

Letting go of your prebaby identity can also be a relief. A baby can inspire some positive changes, like quitting smoking or other self-destructive behaviors. It's amazing how much more appealing a brisk walk in the park is when you don't have a hangover. The lifestyle makeover vibe isn't limited to the physical. Babies can also boost self-esteem or at least shut out self-loathing: Moms and dads who spent hours obsessing about the minutiae of me, me, me—be it status or wrinkles—may find that once they're parents, they just don't care about that stuff anymore. Maybe it's the sheer busywork of baby life that distracts from any unproductive navel-gazing or masochistic interior monologues. Sometimes it's the profound reshuffling of priorities that eliminates the narcissistic clutter: In the face of tangible worries about your baby's well-being, those obsessive rumblings may seem less important. This is certainly not a universal experience (some of us can always find time for self-scrutiny). And new parental obsessions and anxieties can quickly fill the place of old nonparental ones. But in the meantime this refocusing can be a welcome fringe benefit of the Mommy/Daddy metamorphosis.

It completely changes your perspective. And certainly takes the focus off yourself, which I'm really grateful for. . . . I'm so tired of thinking about myself. I'm kinda sick of myself.

—Brad Pitt on *Today*, July 14, 2006

the time warp

Time with a new baby can move s-l-o-w-l-y. You feed the baby. You change the diaper. You look through a picture book. Twice. You take a tour around the room, the house, the block. And by some miracle, only 15 minutes have passed. For many people, the slowing down of time can be a pleasant break from the rushy-rushy adult world. People describe a peacefulness, and revel in the chance to observe and experience things that they'd otherwise be missing. Not everyone gets so Zen about it, of course. Some are just bored out of their minds. The flip side of the slow-motion effect is the crazy fast-forward feeling, when parents turn around to find that their babies don't seem so much like babies anymore. Ergo, they're growing up. Ergo, you're growing older . . . and confronting your mortality. This can stir up all manner of feelings.

197

parenting outside the norm

A child's view of what's normal is defined by what happens in her own home. But the cultural standard of "normal" varies tremendously. Families who don't meet other people's expectations of normal may face assumptions about how their differences—things like religion, age, gender, gender preference, physical ability, race, etc.—might reflect on their parenting. If difference is something you've been dealing with all your life, you've probably developed tools to handle people who judge you. But prejudices can be especially resonant for new parents, who often feel insecure about their new roles (whether or not their families fit the mainstream profile). Even confident parents can feel frustrated and undermined when they have to fight other people's perceptions on top of the work of just being a parent. No one knows better than you what it's like to be a parent in your situation, but finding others who can relate to your experience can be helpful.

→ For resources for specific parenting situations, see page 374.

difficult/high-need/demanding/ "hurting"/hard babies

However you want to describe it, some babies are way, way harder to handle than others. And those babies are difficult for a zillion reasons, only some of which can be diagnosed. Constant crying, extreme lack of sleep, health worries, knowing your baby's in pain and not being able to do anything about it . . . parents of high-need babies can find themselves grappling with a messy mix of expectations and envy on top of a lot more work than the average parent. The easier a baby is, the easier it is for you to enjoy your time with him. It should be obvious, but we sometimes have to remind ourselves that the opposite is true, too. → See Colic, page 258; Preterm Babies, page 269.

bonding pressure

People talk about bonding like a romance novel fantasy, in which parent and baby's first lingering eye contact sparks the sound of a thousand imaginary violins. If this happens to you, by all means enjoy the music. But bonding is not really about feeling fireworks. It's about building a relationship. Sometimes this happens instantly; sometimes it takes time: days, weeks, months. On the most basic anthropological level, bonding is about feeling enough connection to keep you from leaving your baby in a bush. If you're feeding, caring for, and holding your new baby—whether or not you're feeling warm and fuzzy while doing it—you're bonded enough for now.

It was love at first sight, but then it was harder, maybe right around the second month. I felt really rundown then; maybe the adrenaline wore off, maybe the sleep deprivation started taking its toll, but suddenly I really wished I had constant help and wanted to hand over the baby all the time, and sometimes just felt very disconnected from him.

—anonymom

After two days in the hospital, I came home with my baby and the strangest process of bonding between us started happening. It's hard to explain without sounding extremely corny, but the bottom line is I thought I was her. I remember lying on the bed with her beside me and my husband would come in to stroke my head and I thought to myself that he must be more careful because my skull would break. I lay in a heap, curled up, and looked at the world as if for the first time—bewildered, exhausted, and utterly new to the world.

—anonymom

the extreme vulnerability of a newborn baby (in specific)

Unlike other species (like, say, gazelles, who are literally born running), a human baby needs an enormous amount of care and protection. This can instill a sense of strength, competence, and awe at your protective abilities. But newborn parents sometimes find themselves near obsessed with all the ways their baby could be hurt over the course of an average day. Suddenly everything is a potential danger. A dad we know took down all hanging pictures, just in case one fell. People can't sleep because they're too busy checking to be sure their babies are breathing. When parents get used to being parents and babies get a little sturdier, this particular kind of obsessing tends to lighten up.

the existential vulnerability of the human condition (in general)

As much as we desperately want to protect our children, at the end of the day, we're all vulnerable to the unknown. Having a baby can give you new empathy about the horrors of war, natural disasters, disease . . . any tragedy you can imagine. And imagine you may. It can be hard to watch sad stories about adults—never mind children—without thinking about how devastated the parents of the victim must be. This can be a bit debilitating when it comes to watching the evening news.

> I love being a mom, but nothing can prepare you for all the worst-case scenarios that pop into your head at every stage of your baby's life.
> —anonymom

> I think on the fourth day I burst into tears imagining terrible things happening to her. I thought I was bound to accidentally hurt her at some point and couldn't bear it. She felt—and was—so vulnerable. It blew my mind.
> —anonymom

> When my baby was a newborn I was constantly afraid I would smush him or drop him or who knows what. It was such a relief when he got bigger and stronger! Or maybe I just got used to it!! Those first few weeks though, yikes!
> —anonymom

> Any films with babies or children either fill me with anger and disgust at the cloying talk or start me sobbing at the awful things that befall them.
> —anonydaddy

> She's six weeks old and I am obsessed with death and dying. I'm afraid my husband will drop her, or she will gag on a velour hooded onesie, or just die of SIDS. I leave her in her room and I manage to sleep but every time I pick up the paper, I feel like all I read are baby tragedy stories and I start to cry. I feel so happy to be in love, and so frightened.
> —anonymom

> I now see pictures of moms and their babies in war zones or impoverished areas and think, "You know what? That woman loves her baby as much as I love my baby. And she wants for her baby the same things that I want for mine." And my heart just breaks for her.
> —anonymom

> I can't even watch commercials for sad things about kids anymore. In fact, I can hardly watch sad movies anymore whatsoever. Or watch the news. Or read the newspaper. When horrible things happen to grown men, I think about their mothers.
> —anonymom

199

> I just knew I was scarring this perfect little being for life with bad energy vibes.
> —anonymom

> I can't afford the best schools, the special camps, the lessons... that's where the anxiety comes from. What you hope is that what you can't give in money, you can make up for in other ways.
> —anonydaddy

> I always thought I'd be a laid-back mom but now that I'm here, I'm amazed at how many thoughts are darting through my mind. Did I leave enough milk with the babysitter? Did he wake up so many times because I am not sending a clear and confident message about sleep time? Should I be more alert in the morning to get him off to a good start? Now I feel like I am actually an uptight person and there's nothing I can do about it.
> —anonymom

this will go on your permanent record

First-time parents often worry that whatever they do will leave an indelible impression. You may think you're stressing the baby out with your anxiety, bumming her out with your negativity, or just generally ruining the kid with every misstep. The advice industry feeds this idea by constantly harping on the notion of setting up bad habits, leaving little wiggle room for flexibility and flux. Despite our cultural obsession with the spongelike minds of babies, "infant determinism" may be overrated. According to medical researcher John Bruer, what happens in the first three years does not do irreparable harm except in the most extreme cases (and sometimes, not even then). You're going to be in this baby's life for a long time. If you don't hold her exactly right for a couple of weeks, you'll have ample opportunity to make it up to her.

Bruer quotes Steve Petersen, a neuroscientist at Washington University in St. Louis, as saying that neurological development so badly wants to happen that his only advice to parents would be "Don't raise your children in a closet, starve them, or hit them in the head with a frying pan." Petersen was, of course, being flip. But the general conclusion of researchers seems to be that we human beings enjoy a fairly significant margin of error in our first few years of life.
—Malcolm Gladwell, "Baby Steps," *The New Yorker*, January 10, 2000

the anxiety trap?

In her book *A Potent Spell: Mother Love and the Power of Fear,* author/psychotherapist Janna Malamud Smith suggests that our society actually cultivates mothers' anxiety. Anxiety serves a purpose, she says, making mothers focus all their energies on worrying about their children instead of advocating for universal healthcare or otherwise making a nuisance of themselves. In other words, anxiety preserves the status quo. And when mothers bear so much of the burden of responsibility for their kids' welfare, they also bear the biggest burden if their children get sick or hurt or die. So they're trapped into obsessive vigilance—for fear of the ultimate punishment. Where does the basic desire to protect our children end, and the culturally induced paranoia begin? It's hard to say. We can't necessarily avoid the worries, but being aware of the forces at work may help to put them in perspective.

> I find that my main stay-awake anxieties have to do with cash money! We work so hard, and try to be with our baby as much as we can and have hardly any time for anything else (this has been a huge strain on our marriage). I feel robbed and angry about it.
> —anonymom

People who become parents via adoption or surrogacy experience many of the same emotions as birth parents: joy at the baby's arrival, disbelief that they have suddenly become parents, fear that they won't be able to bond enough, fear that they won't know how to comfort the baby when it cries. But becoming a parent without the pregnancy can give these emotions a different tenor. There are also many adjustments unique to these experiences. The range of emotions is as diverse as the families involved: The feelings of a gay couple adopting a third-world orphan may have little in common with those of the grandmother who takes custody of her teenage daughter's baby or the couple that struggles with infertility before using a donor egg and a surrogate.

The road to the baby has a lot to do with it. After months or years of pitching themselves to agencies and birth mothers, parents may feel pressure to live up to the ideals of perfection they've put forth (which can slam especially hard against the reality of constant feedings and sleepless nights). The negative feelings that come up can be difficult to acknowledge with the long-awaited baby finally in arms, but these feelings are normal for all new parents. The particular challenges of nonbiological parents are being increasingly recognized and discussed. Speaking with others in similar situations, and explaining the difficulties and joys to friends and family members can do a lot to alleviate the pressure. → **See Adoption and Surrogacy resources, page 374.**

beyond good and evil

Our culture has well-defined ideas about motherhood and fatherhood. And you may be bringing some ideals of your own to the parenting party. You may see yourself as the laid-back mom, the rock-'n'-roll mom, or the jet-set career mom; you might want to be an ecoanarchist treehouse dad or a super-chill-money-is-not-important dad. You both may want to be the kind of eternally glamorous parents who simply *do not change* after the baby's arrival. Or energetic, youthful parents who will easily connect with their teens. The trouble, as usual, is where fantasy meets reality. Chill Dad may start to think that being broke is not that chill. Rock Mom may find that she's not as comfy as she thought with strapping her baby into that rickety tour van. The glamour parents may find they actually prefer staying home in spit-stained sweatpants. The parents we become may bear zero resemblance to the parents we imagined we'd be.

These fantasies may come from real values or important priorities; they can also come from insecurity or a resistance to growth and change. Raising kids is hard enough without worrying about fitting into a fantasy. In order to inhabit our new parental roles, the ghosts of the perfect (or perfectly imperfect) mommy and daddy need to be exorcised. Each time an image of what you *should* be feeling comes into conflict with what you *are* feeling, step back and try to recognize whether you're grappling with the problem at hand or just some mythological idea of what a parent should be.

the good mother: selflessness and sacrifice

Since mothers are the ones who can carry, birth, and breast-feed babies, it is sometimes assumed that it's a woman's nature to give, give, give. And that all our giving should flow from us "naturally" without complaints. Through the pain of childbirth. Through the angst of colic. Through the scabby nipples and swollen, streaked-balloon breasts. A good mother will give her life for her baby—literally, of course, but figuratively, too—her career, her body, her identity. But the perfect all-sacrificing mom is a fantasy. If you feel conflicted about your choices or sacrifices, you are no less maternal than someone who makes them with ease or even pleasure.

→ For more on work and sacrifice, see The Balancing Act, page 226.

bad mom

If the good mom hovers like a deity, the bad mom is more of a dark cloud, crystallizing into finger-wagging warnings and rapping us on the hand whenever we cross the imaginary line. Even when we call ourselves "bad moms" as a joke, it begs the question What is a bad mom? The bottom of the barrel is clear: baby-killers, dangerous drug addicts, people who leave their kids alone in a car for an hour in a heat wave. How about a mom who parks her kid in front of the TV? A mom who would rather be getting a pedicure than playing This Little Piggy? Someone who drinks a little while pregnant? While breast-feeding? Someone who doesn't try to breastfeed at all? Anyone who doesn't do everything exactly in the optimal interests of her child? In that case, aren't we all bad moms?

the good daddy: provider anxiety

For all of our progress, there is still a lingering sense in our culture that a man is not a "success" if he can't provide his family with the best of everything. (In same-sex partnerships, one partner may adopt the provider role and feel the same pressures.) A dad may not be expected to change diapers, but he's still expected to pay the bills. After all, the mother is carrying the baby; shouldn't he at least be able to carry the rent? It's apparent from the first time

> I now know that I can't be the perfect mother and don't want my son to think I can be. I have lightened up, laughed more, and humbled myself so my child will be able to see my faults and continue to love me unconditionally as I love him. I wish I knew that at the beginning of becoming a parent. Have had to endure some emotional ups and downs to get to this point but it has given me more perseverance and hope.
> —anonymom

the good-enough mother

The "good enough mother" is a fancy psychoanalytic concept (developed by British psychiatrist D. W. Winnecott), but simply put, the "good-enough mother" is someone who can strike a healthy balance between her needs and the needs of her infant. Though she starts off with "an almost complete adaptation to her infant's needs," she gradually eases up and "adapts less and less completely." More generally, Winnecott talks about how kids need to feel that they have gotten love and attention from their parents without feeling that they're destroying them in the process. And moms need to feel like it's okay to care about themselves . . . so that they aren't, in fact, destroyed in the process!

he tells friends about the baby and is met with semijokes like "You better get a second job." While it may be fine for a single man, or even a couple in love, to live in a tiny space with no real savings, is it okay for a family? As one new dad said to us, "Bringing a child into a world filled with war and misery is one thing, but bringing that child into a studio apartment is another." The solution to financial problems is not always clear or easy, but it is clear that unrealistic ideals don't help. Like the idea of the perfect mother, the perfect father (who bears the burden of his family's finances unfailingly and unquestioningly) is a fantasy that can undermine a father's confidence about his real-life role as a parent.

death of a maiden: **older** parenthood

Women in their late thirties and their forties are "in their prime" . . . until they get pregnant. Then the language gets a little less optimistic. *Advanced maternal age. Elderly primigravida. High-risk pregnancy.* The large majority of thirty-five-plus women who get pregnant have healthy pregnancies and healthy babies. Still, it can be a struggle to shrug off the assumption that you've got more to worry about. And difficult, sometimes, to contend with assumptions about older parents. People might imply or joke that you'll be too tired to run after toddlers, or that you'll be less in touch with "the kids" later on. Or more grimly, that if you have your children when you're older, you'll be dead before they have children of their own. But who knows? People live to be a hundred; people die young unexpectedly. And age is only one factor in staying on top of what your kids are up to. Being a young parent is no guarantee that you'll be more connected than someone older. As older parenthood gets more common (the number of parents in their thirties and forties has been steadily climbing), these stereotypes may start to feel much less relevant. Age may feel like an advantage, making parents more stable, more focused, more confident. Feeling that you are ready to move on to the next phase can make some of the sacrifices of early parenthood relatively easy.

But since older parents may have a more solid (or stubborn) sense of who they are, having to adjust to a new life and identity can be tough. People who are more set in their ways may feel they have more to lose when their lives change. It can also be hard to separate the effects of having a baby from the effects of just getting older. Parenthood can be an easy scapegoat for a sagging physique and a sagging social life. If you are an older parent surrounded by mostly younger ones, you may feel out of place or isolated. There are support groups especially designed to combat this. But you may also find that once you're out there in the reality of parenthood, age isn't much of a factor at all.

➜ For resources, see Older Parenthood, page 375.

> I'm thirty-three. This is my first and most likely only pregnancy. I absolutely think that my age and the fact that this is a once-in-a-lifetime experience for me is making me appreciate even the difficult stuff.
> —anonymom

> Age definitely was a factor in my approach. I wanted to do everything as well as I could. I researched everything thoroughly, and I did not take the word of my practitioners at face value. I don't think I would have been as proactive when I was younger.
> —anonymom

> We're a relatively old couple (me thirty-nine, Mom thirty-four) and Mom was a caffeinated smoker who'd been on the Pill since the Reagan Administration. We were keen to conceive. We figured the upside from waiting longer to get married—more secure in choice of partner and in finances—would be balanced by a long winding road to pregnancy.
> —anonydaddy

It made me crazy when I went into the doctors' office and they reassured me that I wasn't "too old" at "thirty-one." I guess they are so used to people being worried about the age thing that they just assumed I'd be worried, too. . . . The only thing this "reassuring" comment did was make me feel really, really old!

—anonymom

It is such a drag that our bodies are in prime shape for babies when young though our minds are only ready (for baby, and for partner in many cases) way later on. In some ways I think I'd be a great mom to a teenager right now but what if I had conceived with my high school boyfriend? I mean, he's nice and all, but my God . . . and what about the life I've been able to live without worrying over child care, plus demand feeding and immunization schedules? I am so much happier to be grinding sweet potatoes and scanning for choke hazards now after having lived many lives.

—anonymom

I feel like I was 100 percent ready for this kid and I thank god because this is not a *small thing* and if I hadn't have been ready (i.e., younger), this would be twelve million times harder than it already is!

—anonymom

emotional resource rescue

Reading a passage in a book that touches on your own experience can do a lot to keep you from feeling like a lunatic, or at least remind you that there are others out there who are just as crazy as you. Plus, the authors can be so damn funny, they make it hard not to laugh at their sorry situations—and maybe your own.

PERSONAL STORIES

Any issue of *Brain, Child* magazine (brainchild.com)

Anything by Erma Bombeck: old school, hilarious, and still relevant: "I lost everything in the postnatal depression."

The Bitch in the House: 26 Women Tell the Truth About Sex, Solitude, Work, Motherhood, and Marriage by Cathi Hanauer (editor): anthology of essays and stories by women who have different (i.e., real) ideas about what it means to be a woman, wife, mother, nonmother . . .

Child of Mine: Original Essays on Becoming a Mother edited by Christina Baker Kline: includes writing from Allegra Goodman, Naomi Wolf, Meg Wolitzer, and others.

Down Came the Rain by Brooke Shields: Celebrity mom comes forward with the story of her postpartum depression.

Getting a Life by Helen Simpson: subtly hilarious stories about parents of young children and the (often disturbing) thoughts that occupy their minds.

Inconsolable by Marrit Ingman: a beautifully written, candid, and fast-paced portrait of utter baby chaos by an Austin mom raising a painfully allergic and colicky baby and nearly losing everything (her mind, her marriage, etc.).

A Life's Work by Rachel Cusk: a brilliant book by a novelist who really captures every contradictory moment of new parenthood. The chapter on Ferberizing is pure poetry.

The Mother Knot by Jane Lazarre: a searingly honest account of the reality of new motherhood in the 1970s. Apparently, not much has changed. Totally nails the feelings of alienation and isolation, identity and creativity conflicts.

Mother Shock: Loving Every (Other) Minute of It by Andrea Buchanan: A new mom muses (amusingly) on the good and bad parts of her experience. There's a great chapter on quitting breastfeeding.

Operating Instructions: A Journal of My Son's First Year by Anne Lamott: A classic, this story of a single woman who is both a new mother and recovering addict is reassuring, inspiring, and funny.

Rise Up Singing: Black Women Writers on Motherhood by Cecelie Berry: essays, stories, poetry by many great writers (Maya Angelou, Alice Walker, etc.) on motherhood—sad, funny, historical, celebratory, smart.

SUPPORT/GUIDANCE FOR PARENTS

Becoming the Parent You Want to Be: A Sourcebook of Strategies for the First Five Years by Laura Davis and Janis Keyser: an extremely open-minded workbook and guide to the day-to-day decisions of parenthood.

Everyday Blessings: The Inner Work of Mindful Parenting by Jon Kabat-Zinn and Myla Kabat-Zinn: a Zen-based parenting book.

Parenting From the Inside Out by Daniel Siegel and Mary Hartzell: discusses how parents' personal history affects their parenting.

MORE RESOURCES ABOUT THE STATE OF MODERN MOTHER/PARENTHOOD

The Mommy Myth: The Idealization of Motherhood and How It Has Undermined All Women by Susan J. Douglas and Meredith W. Michaels: an in-depth analysis and outrage over celebrity images of motherhood. Big on breaking down impossible standards.

The Mother Trip: Hip Mama's Guide to Staying Sane in the Chaos of Motherhood by Ariel Gore: a combo memoir/guide/call-to-arms by mommy/revolutionary Ariel Gore, founder of *Hip Mama* magazine.

Perfect Madness: Motherhood in the Age of Anxiety by Judith Warner: a look at our culture's obsession with perfection and how it particularly oppresses mothers.

Of Woman Born: Motherhood as Experience and Institution by Adrienne Rich: oft-quoted poet and feminist's classic treatise on the complicated feelings of motherhood.

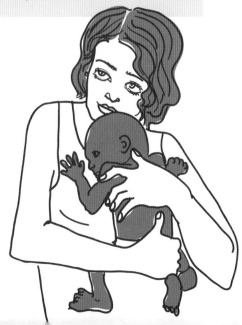

the postbaby life

parents and partners

In this chapter we sometimes refer specifically to relationships between lovers or married people, but a partner can be anyone you share the work of parenthood with—both the child care and the ultimate responsibility.

conflicts

All the intensity, newness, vulnerability, and sheer logistical problem-solving that come with having a baby can put any relationship in the salad spinner. Depending on what your relationship was like prebaby, these stresses can feel like minor tremors or major blows.

Here are some fun things coparents might go through:

NEW BABY FIGHTS: Imagine you and your partner are in a rental car driving through the countryside of a foreign country. Night has fallen, neither of you speaks the language, and the hotel is nowhere to be found. Your maps and guidebooks seemed so comforting a little while ago but now nothing matches up with what you're seeing out the windshield. Things are getting grim. At first you may be civil and optimistic with each other: "Maybe this way," one of you will say, or "Hmm, what about that road?" But the more dead ends you hit and wrong turns you make, the more the insults start to fly. "Maybe that way" becomes a sarcastic "Smart move" soon enough. "Let's try this road" becomes "Why don't we just drive around in circles all night?" And the insults only grow deeper and deeper, the main task no longer finding the hotel but finding the right words to describe just how hopeless, incompetent, and fundamentally wrong the other person is. All your partner's flaws come rushing to the surface and suddenly, as you make yet another fruitless turn on to an even darker street, you see nothing but weakness (or bossiness) and bumbling (or arrogance) sitting on the other side of the emergency brake. Of course you'll eventually find the hotel. But in the meantime some terrible things, maybe some things it will be hard to unsay, have been said.

This is what having a newborn in the house can do to a couple. Since you're both lost, confused, and looking for answers, you can't turn to each other . . . so instead you turn on each other. We've heard stories of couples digging into each other with the meanest, most hurtful comments they could muster over whether to install blackout blinds or how to attach baby mittens to a onesie. At first the fights may seem impulsive and irrational. But they can continue and deepen, latching on to preexisting issues. It can be hard to remember that sleep deprivation, a colicky baby, or just general insecurity may be the real problem.

LEARNING TO NEGOTIATE: What do you do when a choice comes up and the two of you have different ideas about what to do? You negotiate a path

New mothers often find themselves barking things like "Be careful!" when their partners pick up, change, or rock the baby. Is this because moms are more anxious? Are dads less so? Why does this happen? Meredith Fein Lichtenberg, doula and all-around expert on the postpartum experience, had this to say on the subject:

> "All new parents feel some anxiety and doubt and it's easy for the new mom (who usually spends more time with the baby at first) to be the one to express it—not because she is a woman or because she is more anxious, but because she is literally with the baby more, or because we live in a society where women tend to be more likely than men to express their negative feelings. Whatever the reason, if the mom says something expressing anxiety or caution—even if it's what both parents naturally feel—it's easy for the dad to grab the opposite role to create balance. Then he makes some laid-back response: 'It's all going to be okay!' and, at worst, she thinks he just doesn't appreciate the gravity of the situation. In reality they are saying the very same thing:

> "HER: *Be Careful! (meaning—this baby is Awfully Important to me!)*

> "HIM: *Don't worry—it's no big deal. (Meaning, I know! This baby is awfully important to me, too! I can't even bear to think of something going wrong.)*

> "What a shame that they often think that they disagree!

> "So what can you do? Humor is really helpful for this kind of thing. If you hear yourself telling your partner to do something completely obvious, a light remark or joke, 'Oh, I'm turning into my mother!' or 'Gosh, who on earth said that?!' can help deflect the moment. If you can get time alone with your partner later, it might be helpful to candidly say, 'I hear I'm saying all these cautious things and I just want you to know, I don't really mean to imply that you don't know what you're doing—I'm just saying it because I'm nervous and I want everything to go okay.' And if you can't bring yourself to say any of these things? Try leaving the room. If you don't watch your partner with the baby, you will not have to resist the temptation to correct his every move. It might be best for all three of you!"

that *both of you* can live with, just like you did with all those choices you came across before you had a baby—like what movie to see, or where to go on vacation, or how to handle a family drama. This can happen any number of ways. It may be that the person who's least attached (or the one who just can't stand the fight) just gives in. But if one parent becomes too dominant a voice in each decision, the other may begin to drift a little, or feel insecure about his or her own parenting abilities. And in order for both partners to feel connected to child raising, both voices must be heard. Maybe you'll take turns, or figure out which areas matter most to each of you and take the lead on those. Or maybe you'll figure out a middle path. Each couple has their own style of negotiating, though it may not always be the most productive one. Parenthood is an ideal time to work on yours, because the forks in the road will just keep on coming.

what's the problem?

According to researchers Jay Belsky and John Kelly, whose book, *The Transition to Parenthood,* is based on interviews with 250 couples, new parents usually fight over one of five things:

- division of labor
- money
- their relationship
- career and work
- social life

JEALOUSY AND COMPETITION: Competition between parents can take many forms. It can be so obvious that it's almost embarrassing, or so subtle, neither parent even notices it's there. Here are some things that can trigger jealousy:

- She gets to be so much closer with the baby.
- He's got it so easy.
- I wish I got to go out and be in the world, go out for drinks, feel important.
- I wish I could stay home with the baby (and nap).
- I used to be the center of attention.
- She used to look at me that way . . .
- I wish the baby would look at me like that.
- S/he gets to have all the fun with the baby while I have to do all the work.

As your child's needs change over the years, so will the time you spend meeting them. But babies do get different things from each parent, so there will probably be times when one or the other is preferred for a particular kind of company or comfort. It's easy to end up feeling like the other partner is the "fun one" or the "nurturing one" or any other pigeonholing description. But, as you get used to being a family, you will each find your own ways of soothing, nurturing, and loving your baby, as well as getting him to laugh hysterically.

(SUR)VIVE LA DIFFERENCE: Chances are that at some point you may have different ideas about how to raise your kid. Even when you and your partner are on the same page about particular routines or strategies, each person will probably have his or her own way of going about things. Keep in mind that while babies enjoy consistency, the important thing is that he knows what to expect from each person, not that every person in his life acts the same way. The baby benefits from a variety of experiences and influences; different kinds of parenting energy and techniques are a good thing.

OUT OF SYNC: Your own feelings of ambivalence or frustration or vulnerability can be hard enough to reckon with, so when you detect them in your partner, they may cause panic. What if he/she freaks out? Will I have to carry the burden of this new life all alone? We'll both be terrible parents. We'll end up hating each other. What if we've made a huge mistake???!!! If one partner was always lobbying for a baby while the

> It's so incredibly hard not to be jealous sometimes of just how much more *voluntary* fatherhood seems. Yeah I know there is an incredibly close bond between mother and baby and if push came to shove I don't think I'd trade it, but sometimes I really wish I could get as separate as he can. If I get out of my mother head for a couple of hours, it's an event.
> —anonymom

> Emotionally, it wreaks havoc on a marriage, especially the first couple of months—as the mother you are always doing more, I don't care *how* liberated your husband is—breastfeeding is something only you can do and at times you are just tired and in need of a stiff drink.
> —anonymom

> I don't mean this to sound bad, but I just think the first year of your baby's life is profoundly different for father and mother . . . they relate differently.
> —anonymom

other hesitated, blame games can pop up when things get rough. "This is what you wanted, isn't it?!" may be the spoken or unspoken sentiment underlying a stressed-out fight over a broken car seat or a screaming baby. You may both miss your old lives, but with different intensity—or at different times. It's not easy to see your partner going through periods of doubt or aggravation. And it's definitely harder to feel connected when your emotional lives are not synchronized. But this does not spell disaster, it just spells humanity.

SHARE THE BURDEN: A parent may want more help but find that no one else knows the crucial information: the pediatrician's name, the diaper size, or what website to consult when the baby breaks out in a rash. This happens a lot with moms, but there is no inherent reason for a mom to be the maestro of all the little details of child life. Relinquishing control (which is what delegating is all about) may not come easy, but it can keep a balance in the relationship.

EVOLVE TOGETHER . . . AND APART: Since you'll both be having moments of newfound confidence and total cluelessness, you may need to develop some skills in being both supportive *and* vulnerable at the same time. Part of this is accepting each other's inse-curities as a normal part of the process. Another is respecting that partners change at different rates and in different ways.

> I became less patient because I put all my energy into the babies. Much snappier, bitchy, difficult. But then again I think in some way our relationship got deeper, we admired each other's capabilities as parents, we depended on each other more.
> —anonymom

baby breakups

There are many reasons a couple might break up soon before or after the arrival of a baby. Sometimes the split isn't directly related (but since the baby is bound to have an impact on the relationship, it may be a factor). The stress of the pregnancy or the new baby can be too much for the relationship to bear. Though the baby may be the trigger, it's not usually the real cause. A new baby can bring other problems to light, whether they're individual issues or things that have been brewing between partners. Whatever the motivation, a breakup with a new baby on the way or in the house can be pretty trau-matic, piling big changes onto big changes. Aside from the emotional issues, there are logistical concerns to be worked out: What will the relationship between your ex and your child be like? It is generally advised to set up official custody arrangements, even if you are remaining friendly. The way these issues play out can bring up a whole new set of emotional concerns. Counsel-ing can help provide an outlet for the added stress that may arise, as well as help you make a plan you can both live with.

single parenthood: going it alone

The most recent census data counts ten million single mothers and two million single fathers in the United States. Some people raise children alone by choice; others become single by circumstance. Some are single indefinitely; others, intermittently. Though there's a big difference between taking on parenthood alone from the start and raising kids with a partner who isn't around, many of the fundamental issues are the same. However you get there, going it alone is a lot of work. It means one person has to do more than one person's job. Single parents are usually working parents, unless they're getting money through other means. For many single parents, finding a reliable support system, including child care and emotional support, is crucial. The "village" model works for a lot of single parents, who share responsibilities with other parents or people in the community when help is needed. But some really thrive on feeling independent, managing the needs of a whole family and household on their own.

If looking for a partner is on your agenda, the all-encompassing demands of a new baby can add anxiety to that situation. Most people, whether they have partners or not, find it difficult to balance their personal lives with their parenting lives in the early months (or even years). Although you may not want to ignore the urge to get out and look, it's important to cut yourself some slack during this intense period. It will almost definitely be easier to find time for yourself (and maybe someone else) as your baby grows up.

Although single parenthood is pretty commonplace these days, parents may still find themselves dealing with judgment, directly or couched in sympathy. Negativity about single parents usually comes from a place of ignorance—if you're feeling judged, seek out other single parents, who may have a perspective closer to your own, or at least be able to relate. → For resources, see page 374.

sex

Talking to new parents about sex can sometimes be very uncomfortable. They tend to lower their voices to whispers (as if their love life is a world-shattering conspiracy) or launch into loud, self-lacerating comedy routines. The tone may vary, but the warning doesn't: "You'll never have sex again." It's easy to understand why sex is unappealing right after birth. It's not quite as easy to understand why your sex life hasn't snapped back into shape six months or a year later. There are lots of things that come into play. Some are obvious, such as sleep deprivation and the constant threat of interruption. Others are more subtle, such as the need to rethink your ideas about sex and your body.

Here are some of the many factors:

no time, no sleep, no clue

Stress, exhaustion, fights, and full-on freak-outs don't leave much space for seduction. New parents often spend the better part of the first year staggering around in a sleep-deprived haze, trying to fit the components of their nonbaby lives into a few fleeting moments. Scheduling a shower can be hard enough, let alone getting in the mood for sex. There's a reason sleep deprivation is used for torture, not pleasure. And that joke about new parents fantasizing about sleep more than sex? Needs are needs.

> Given the choice between intimacy and sleep for the first six months, I would always opt for sleep. It took a couple of breakdowns and the possibility of divorce before we finally talked things out and really reconnected. It is so easy to let the baby take over and let the marriage fall by the wayside.
> —anonymom

> I hear of the hormone levels being all wacky, but personally I just feel it has to do primarily with lack of sleep. When you're the only one who gets up with the baby because you have what he needs, it takes a toll on you, and all you want to do when you have a chance is *relax*! Having sex takes a lot of extra energy!
> —anonymom

what's the deal with 6 weeks?

Six weeks postpartum, most moms are given their doctor's go-ahead for sexual activity. What this means is that it's no longer dangerous to have sex. It doesn't mean that by this time you should want to have sex, or particularly enjoy it if you do have it. Many people, maybe even most, take a lot longer than six weeks to even think about sex, much less have sex.

> We don't have sex that much. When we do, it's great, but the frequency has definitely taken a hit. But, of course, we'll never truly know if it was the baby or not. Couples without children slow down, too. Sometimes, I worry about it, though. One person told me the main thing was not to let the child come between my wife and me. I didn't know what he meant at the time, but I do now, and he was right. The marriage, or partnership, must be the primary relationship in the house, at least from the adult perspective.
> —anonydaddy

> Sex after we've had the baby has improved in some ways and gotten worse in others. My wife sees herself as a mother, so her ability to let go, to be sexual in certain ways, has changed, so her desires in terms of specific activities and behavior during sex has changed. In other words, she used to give me blow jobs pretty regularly and now she doesn't. Ever. Unless it is my birthday. And even then, they seem like a chore to her. In general, sex seems to be a little less passionate and a little more efficient than before. Of course, for the first few months, we were just nervous the baby was going to cry and we were going to have to stop, so it was hard for either of us to concentrate or get in the mood. The good news is that I think her body changed physically from having a baby and she definitely feels more physical pleasure from intercourse than she did before she had the kid and that's nothing but good good goodness.
> —anonydaddy

vagina anxiety

There's a lot of hype about what happens to a woman's vagina after childbirth. The mythology of the stretched-out, gaping, flappy vagina is mean-spirited and false, yet remains a source of utter terror to many. The vagina was meant for birth as well as sex; that's why it's so flexible! Yes, babies and aging can lead to less muscle tone in that area (Kegels *do* help), but the idea that birth will leave you with an orifice the size of a beer can is just plain crazy. → See Kegels, page 58.

baby love

Though not everyone is attracted to babies in general, most people are very attracted—in a sensual, even "animal" way—to their own babies. Studies have shown that a mother can instantly recognize her own baby's scent and is magnetically drawn to it. We tend to almost involuntarily kiss our babies every few minutes (or even seconds) when we hold them. They are "delicious," "scrumptious," we want to "eat them up." Moms and dads often rhapsodize over favorite baby body parts: the

> It's somewhat horrifying to admit, but the very first thing I said when my baby was born was not "Is he okay?" but "Did I tear?"
> —anonymom

> I was always cradling, holding, kissing him, smelling him; I was basically a step away from licking him (like a cat). It probably all sounds kind of gross, but I really had little choice in the matter: He was just so soft and divine and *new*. By comparison my husband seemed very, hmm, scratchy and old? The situation was kind of a mess (I felt guilty, husband felt rejected). As the intense physical aspects of newborn motherhood eased up, our sex life started to improve. I also had to make a conscious effort to remember how to feel sexual, not just sensual.
> **—anonymom**

nape of the neck, the curl of the upper lip, the tiny round shoulders. And the urgency of a baby's need can remind parents of more mature expressions of longing—sating the desire of a hungry baby echoes (or maybe even defines?) the basic desire/satisfaction loop of human sexuality. Listen to the language of lust if you need proof: "Baby, I got what you need," "I'm hungry for your love." All this kissing and tasting and smelling and needing are the kinds of uninhibited sensual behavior we more often associate with another kind of love.

So what does this mean for your sex life? If one partner (often the mother in the early months) is more involved with the baby, the other partner can become jealous. Watching the woman you love cooing and yearning for someone else—even if it is your own tiny, helpless, and adorable infant—can be hard to take. If both parents are equally hands-on, resentment may play less of a role, but all that sensual baby love can divert physical, loving attention away from each other. However this affects a relationship, it's worth remembering that, for better or worse, baby love almost always gets less encompassing as time goes on.

where's the mystique?

Women often feel they need more than healing time to relearn their bodies as a source of sexual pleasure. Just as it's difficult to suddenly inhabit a public and nurturing body during pregnancy, it can be equally hard to regain

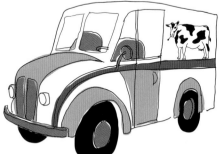

your private, sexual body after childbirth. Husbands or lovers may need some transition time, too. Partners who get involved with OB appointments, birth prep, and birth itself have certainly seen enough to demolish any mysteries about their significant others' nethers.

Unfortunately, our culture doesn't tend to "celebrate" the maternal body as a font of sexuality. The madonna/whore complex (mom=purity and love, whore=sex and desire) has been around forever, and it doesn't seem to be going anywhere anytime soon. There's a not-so-subtle message out there that motherhood and sexuality don't mix. Some people imply

the maternal body vs. the sexual body

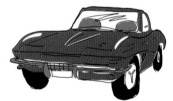

there's an evolutionary motive: Women can be sexual only when young and ripe, because that's when they're fertile. Once they've gotten their babies, they don't have the biological imperative to express (or elicit) desire. Conveniently, this theory also holds that men are designed to be sexual for a long time and across all phases of life. A related myth suggests that women (especially moms and older women) prefer the cuddle to the orgasm; that they are more "sensual" than "sexual." But these myths are exactly that: myths. In reality, all people—men and women—are capable of healthy sexuality throughout their lives, but it helps if they're not stifled by false ideas about what is or isn't appropriate.

We also hear lots of tales of boring "married sex." It can be easy for newly married parents to imagine a grim future. Once people become parents, the story goes, priorities change, and passionless sex is inevitable. While this is certainly a depressing stereotype, it taps into some really tough (or maybe tender) truths. As parents, we often start to value different qualities in ourselves and our partners: qualities like capability, responsibility, a "good influence." These qualities don't really compute with the characteristics we tend to associate with good sex: bad, loose, carefree. At the very least, sex requires letting go. As a new parent, that's often really tricky, since you're so keyed into being on guard and on call at all times. Instead of partners in romance, you are now partners in responsibility. Getting loose enough to enjoy sex is sometimes so much of an effort, it no longer feels . . . loose. Of course, all parents experience varying levels of stress about this. It can ease up as you ease into parenting, or deepen with each new added responsibility and/or kid.

breastfeeding and sex

Though many couples view breastfeeding as an obvious physical obstacle to getting on with their sex lives, the bigger picture of baby care (and all it involves for both partners) may sometimes be the real culprit.

The repurposing of the boob from a source of erotic pleasure to a source of food can cause some confusion. This is especially true in cases where the mother's partner is a "boob guy" (or girl). Partners may feel they have been usurped in their role as the sole beneficiary of the breasts. Mothers may

the pros and cons of service sex

What if your partner wants to do it and you don't? Differences in desire are a fact of life in relationships, especially in times of stress (new parenthood definitely qualifies). There's a huge amount of pressure on new moms to not forget their husbands' needs while tending to their newborns. Since so many studies seem to indicate a good sex life leads to a long and healthy marriage, women are often encouraged to have sex whether they want to or not. It's amazing how little is mentioned of the mother's sexual and emotional needs. Mothers can end up feeling like sex is something else they have to give . . . "for the good of the family." But doing it when you don't want to can create resentment, and make you feel detached. Ideally, the focus should be on finding your own urge for sex rather than only satisfying your partner's.

the milf phenomenon

The lovely term "MILF" stands for "Mom I'd Like to F*ck." The idea of a mom who is also supersexy can be a relief from the dowdy suburban stereotype. Finally, mothers are allowed to be desirable. Sounds progressive. Problem is that the MILF, as depicted on various websites and in movies, looks more like a porn star than a real-world mother. Her stomach is superflat. She wears slutty, tight clothes and flirts with young boys. Hmmm. It's nice that moms can be seen as sexual, but why can't we be sexy when we look like ourselves and not like blow-up dolls?

→ See Hot Mom = Not Mom, page 186.

> I had a lack of interest, but I'm not sure if that can be attributed to the physical demands of breastfeeding or just the overall exhaustion from having a new baby.
> —anonymom

> No libido at all while nursing. It's hard to want more physical contact when you already get all you can handle all day.
> —anonymom

> Tender? Yes.
> Overused? Yes. For the first six months I found it really hard to offer my body up to both the men in my life. Now, at nine months, I feel more independent of my baby and the sex life is back on track (still breastfeeding all the time, however). The problem now . . . my boobs are seriously on the droop. They are swinging low. It's really kind of upsetting. They have already deflated to a little smaller than prepregnancy and they are sort of flat against my chest.
> —anonymom

> I can't feel into it if my body is ready to nurse. I can't be thinking fun kinky thoughts when this happens. Totally kills the mood.
> —anonymom

miss the old days when the boobs were for foreplay instead of reminders of the baby. Boobs may leak during sex, which can be awkward (and messy, if you care). Sulking and/or hostility from partners can add a dimension of guilt and resentment. At the end of a long, hard day of giving, a nursing mother can feel like her partner is just another needy mouth to feed.

On the other hand, enhanced boobage can boost sexual confidence. Breast implants, after all, do bear a striking resemblance to milk-filled boobs. In fact, there's a whole world of websites depicting breasts squirting milk (in a manner vaguely reminiscent of other bodily expulsions). Some consider this a fetish, but it can also be viewed as a sheer celebration of the lactating breast. There's no reason breast milk shouldn't be incorporated into a couple's sex life, if it works for both of you.

Breastfeeding hormones can interfere with sex, too; the same substances that suppress ovulation can also suppress lubrication and desire. But there are some potential hormonal perks for breastfeeding moms. The hormones involved in milk delivery not only elevate feelings of tranquillity and bonding but also can actually help get you "in the mood." Regular bursts of oxytocin (the "love hormone") while breastfeeding can juice up sexual pleasure all around. Some nursing moms feel their orgasms much more intensely due to increased oxytocin levels.

→ For more on sexual feelings and associations with breastfeeding, see Is Breastfeeding Sexual? page 316.

> My husband loved the big boobs and was very sad to see them become little nuggets of nothing when we weaned!
> —anonymom

> It makes me feel sexy to have such voluptuous breasts! My husband loves it even more. He actually finds the milk sexy. . . . I worry that I will leak.
> —anonymom

> Ever since I was pregnant, I haven't really liked the new look my breasts took on. My partner says he thinks they're beautiful and sexy. While I was worried he'd no longer see them as sexy but as a tool, it's me who ended up seeing them as a tool, rather than sexy.
> —anonymom

> I didn't want my husband touching me. My boobs would leak and it would just get messy and remind me that the baby is in the next room.
> —anonymom

> I feel like the sexual feelings I once felt about my breasts are gone. I used to feel like that's what made me a woman; now I just feel like they're feeding tools only. It's very hard to get in the mood.
> —anonymom

> I think that my husband was rather jealous about it. I think he felt left out of the bonding that was taking place at that time between me and the baby.
> —anonymom

COSTUMES AND SCENERY: New parents are often urged to call on the familiar trappings of romance. Some say candlelight. Others say garters. But the gist is the same: Set the stage and the sex will follow. Milk-stained clothes and a living room littered with the detritus of infancy are not generally considered erotic. Whether the simple act of changing the lighting or your outfit can segue you into romance is another question. Some people go for traditionally sexy garb and situations. Others find them phony. If you've never been into stockings and high heels before, you might not be into them now, either. Even if you're a longtime fan of lingerie, trying to force yourself back into old ensembles when you're not feeling it (or when they don't fit!) might just make you feel even less enthusiastic. So, if the idea of dressing up or staging a romantic scene appeals to you, by all means try it. Maybe you will be transformed like an X-rated Cinderella . . . maybe you'll just feel like a pumpkin in a garter belt.

AFFIRMATIONS: You are more than a parent. You are a beautiful, intelligent, witty, engaging, multifaceted individual. We count on our partners to provide all these strokes and more. But this stuff often gets lost when you're both obsessed with babies and sleep and freaking out over new identity issues. Remind yourself that your interests extend beyond feeding and excrement by venturing outside of your immediate family environment. When you feel the urge to emerge, try to use your body in ways that make you feel good, whether it's working out, dancing, or yard work. Seek out people and situations that make you feel smart, funny, interesting, charming, and hot. Flirt. Go to museums and look at art . . . and cute art students. Go to Home Depot to get supplies for your project . . . and get a glimpse of hot carpenters. If possible, without a crying baby.

EXPECTATIONS: Will sex ever be "like it used to be"? Plenty of couples get right back in the groove without much ado. Lots of others find themselves exploring new sexual identities and frontiers after birth. Sometimes this takes a while. Give yourself time to make the adjustment. Obsessing too much can interfere with any efforts to resurrect your former lust—with the sexuality that may be yet to evolve.

when sex **isn't** the problem

Sex, at least the good kind, is an outgrowth of love and intimacy. No amount of jump-starting or ego boosting is going to make you feel like having sex with someone you're feeling bad about. Sometimes addressing underlying problems will help the sex part fall into place.

→ See Parents and Partners, page 206.

SCHEDULING: Building baby-free time into your schedule can make sex an easier proposition. Some people structure the day around this, feeding the baby and putting her to bed early enough to allow for evenings alone as a couple. Or there's the "date night" option, where someone else takes care of the baby so Mom and Dad can take care of each other. Scheduling date nights can be a great thing to do. But if couple time is limited, there's a lot of pressure to use it to its fullest. This can sometimes backfire; we've both wasted some date nights exploring our potential for unfettered fighting. The "sex appointment" can also be a turnoff since we like to think that sex is lustful and spontaneous. Sometimes the best option is to see date night as a time to get connected just by doing things together rather than expecting to have a mind-blowing romantic encounter every time. A low-pressure evening out may make you more likely to seize the moment next time the baby conks out for an unexpected bonus nap.

INTEGRATION: The toy-stacking, bib-snapping reality of parenting may not seem so sexy. But that's not to say that family time needs to be entirely stripped of adult fun. Some parents try to integrate their sexuality into their new lives, instead of switching it on and off as they move in and out of "parent mode." This doesn't mean exposing your kids to inappropriate acts or language. Or using your breast milk in sex play (but hey, if it works for you, go for it). It's talking about grown-up stuff at the dinner table rather than making the baby the only subject of conversation. It's having a flirty sense of humor, or remembering that you don't have to wait until your baby's asleep to even touch each other. It's embracing parenthood as a part of who you are rather than just a role you play, and seeing that you can be a romantic partner and a caring parent at the same time.

JUST DO IT: It's as true in the postpartum bedroom as in the high school physics classroom: Objects in motion tend to stay in motion. Objects at rest tend to stay at rest. The longer you go without having sex, the harder it is to get it going. After a long break (weeks? months? years?), making sex happen can seem like a huge, monstrous, insurmountable effort. It's a little like going to the beach. Getting there is such a drag—the schlep, the traffic, the slimy sunscreen—you're tempted to skip it. But when you get there, you remember how much you *love* the beach! In fact, you wonder why you don't go to the beach more often. It's the same with sex when it's been a while. The more you do it, the more you want it. But first you've got to break the ice, or at the very least, be open to the idea. If you want to have sex but feel disconnected from your desire, you can try going through the motions for a while and letting your body's response take over. This is different from faking it; it's more like rolling a stalled car downhill and popping the clutch to help the machinery kick into gear. Sometimes keeping a whiff of sex in the air (by being physi-

> Body, looks, and sexuality were *not* a problem during my pregnancy. I felt sexy and my husband and I continued to have fantastic sex, *but now* as a mother I am sorry to say I have *no* desire and when I do have the itch to get busy, there is a very small window that both my husband and I have to be on board at the same time.
>
> —anonymom

cally close, flirting, talking about sex, etc.) can make it all seem more feasible. Sometimes it just takes a leap of faith. You liked sex once. Maybe you still do. There's only one way to find out.

postpartum fertility

Women who are not breastfeeding may see the return of their menstrual cycle as soon as the first month postpartum. Since lactating usually suppresses menstruation, breastfeeding moms may have weeks, months, or occasionally years before their period returns. Many factors influence this time frame, including how much breastfeeding is going on and the mother's own hormones and rhythms. Many moms find that menstruation returns when breastfeeding decreases a little. This can occur when supplements, pacifiers, or solids are introduced or when there are longer stretches between feedings. Others find they need to wean entirely before getting their period. A breastfeeding mother may experience an irregular cycle.

Breastfeeding suppresses fertility, but it doesn't always prevent conception. And it's not always clear how fertile you are while breastfeeding, so if you don't want to get pregnant, you'll need to stay on top of your birth control situation. You can consider using condoms, a diaphragm, a cervical cap, or an IUD, all of which are safe for breastfeeding. Natural family planning, vasectomy, or tubal ligation are other options. Nonbreastfeeding moms can use the Pill or other hormonal methods without extra precaution (breastfeeding moms, see below).

NATURE'S BIRTH CONTROL? Breastfeeding mothers can try the old-school method of letting nature do the child spacing. The technical term for this is Lactational Amenorrhea Method, or LAM. It theoretically offers about 98 percent protection from pregnancy for the first six months, but we personally know more than one person who's gotten pregnant while using it. (Of course, we can't vouch for how strictly they were following the guidelines.) But if it's important for you to avoid pregnancy, other methods may be in order.

LAM can be used only when

- **Breastfeeding is 100 percent exclusive (no supplements).**
- **There have been no periods postpartum (any bleeding is a sign of fertility).**
- **Feedings are frequent: The baby goes for no more than four hours between daytime feedings, and no more than six hours between nighttime feedings.**

BREASTFEEDING AND HORMONAL BIRTH CONTROL: Both progesterone and estrogen have been approved by the AAP for breastfeeding women. As far as we know, they do not hurt babies, though anecdotal evidence suggests that hormones can make a baby fussier. It's also possible that very young babies (under six weeks) may not be able to process the hormones easily. Hormones, especially estrogen, can also affect supply. You should talk to your doctor about which kind to take, making sure to consider the following:

- **Progestin-only birth control is the preferred choice for breastfeeding moms.**
- **Estrogen-containing contraceptives should be avoided for the first six months or until solids have been well established.**
- **Always go for the lowest dose possible.**
- **If supply or baby's weight gain seems to suffer, discontinue.**
- **Hormones can have side effects, such as headaches and nausea.**

it takes a village (but maybe not the one you're living in)

family

The modern family can include single parents, unpartnered coparents, adoptive parents, biological parents, step-people, friends, donor dads, surrogates, baby daddies, two moms, two dads, significant others, ex—significant others, grandparents with significant others, and probably a lot of other possibilities we're forgetting. The idea of family can be flexible, but the reality is solid: "Family" is who the baby learns to trust and count on regularly. They may or may not share genes.

having a family/becoming a family

When you become a parent, you very literally define your own family and your own jurisdiction. As you move forward, you have the opportunity to think about what parts of your family history you want to carry on and what parts you want to change. Having a baby can turn you toward tradition or it can cement your distance from it. If you want to raise your kids exactly as your parents raised you, you might not feel the need to stake out your own turf. But if you have some new ideas about how you'd like to do things, you may have to establish your new role as the parent of your child rather than the child of your parents.

Our experiences—as children of divorce, children of marriage, oldest kid, youngest kid, "problem" kid, whatever—not only shape who we are but what kind of parents we want to be. Most people have strong feelings about how they were raised and want to either emulate or totally renounce their parents' approaches. Many people follow their own parents' model by default, if not by plan. A feeling that something was wrong in your childhood—abuse, intense overinvolvement, lack of affection or structure, to give just a few examples—may push you to try to provide your child with a different experience. The popular psychology concept of the "inner child" has helped reinforce this idea. People who feel hurt by their parents' choices may try to heal those wounds through the choices they make for their own children. ➜ See Parents and Partners, page 206.

Maybe the simplest way to deal with the nomenclature of newfangled family life is to take a cue from the Spanish and add a con (for with) to relationships to incorporate just about anyone. Or it may be useful to nationalize *machetunim*, the catch-all Yiddish word for in-laws and other relatives.

—Bob Morris,
New York Times

> I have forgiven my parents for what I deemed my imperfect childhood. My father finally sees me as a grown woman and my mother has the utmost respect for me as a woman. Finally.
> —anonymom

> I am even closer to my mom because on the days that I feel like I could lose it at any minute, I call and talk to her and I know she has been there. I respect my parents more, too, knowing the feelings they had for me and my siblings as children.
> —anonymom

> I have learned so much about my own childhood by watching my parents with my baby. Not all of it's good. In fact, there have been some pretty disturbing revelations. If I were in therapy, I would be having a field day with this material.
> —anonymom

parents as grandparents

When parents become grandparents, a lot of things change. Their babies have babies. They may feel proud of you for carrying on the lineage and grateful for the chance to enjoy maximum love with minimum responsibility. They may feel the need to show you how it's done. They may just feel old and want to distance themselves from the elderly granny category. They may be reminded of how stressful parenting was for them, for their career, or their marriage. When you have a child, you can gain new understanding about what your parents went through—maybe that emotional breakdown in the station wagon that "scarred you for life" was entirely justified after all. But you may also feel revulsion: Am I turning into my mother? (Or father?)

Most likely, there will be some times when you feel like you wish your baby's grandparents were more helpful, or less nosy, or more interested, or less dogmatic. Most people have a few things they wish were different about their parents. Some of these may extend to the grandparent arena, too. All the stuff that made your relationship with your parents complicated beforehand will still be around afterward. And that stuff can reverberate when you see them playing with, disciplining, or otherwise influencing your new baby. But no matter how involved your parents are in your baby's life, they aren't his parents. So they won't have the same effect on him as they had on you.

> My mom refers to the days and nights she has my son as her time with him. Being Korean American, we see family as circular, not linear. My mom and my son speak Korean to each other, she cooks him gourmet Korean meals, and takes him to lunch to meet her friends and play with their grandchildren.
> —anonymom

Well, there's certainly no more doubt about the source of my food issues. Since day one, my mother has obsessed about every single drop of milk or spoon of cereal that has gone into my baby's mouth. Recently she suggested I put my six-month-old on a diet!
—anonymom

My mom makes comments like "We just threw you in the back of the van" or "The baby will sleep if she's on her stomach" or "Your obsession with potential allergies is like a new kind of eating disorder." She wants me to see that being a mom doesn't have to be so stressful. But in her day she didn't have all the safety recommendations and studies we have now. When she threw her kid in the back of the van, she wasn't actively rejecting safety guidelines, not to mention breaking the *law;* she was just doing what she thought was good. . . . I am just trying to do the same thing. (Un)fortunately now there is a lot more info out there about what's good and safe for babies, which is all hard to shrug off.
—anonymom

When my wife and I were contemplating having a baby, I asked my father how he and my mother came to the decision. His reply was "What decision?" He didn't mean I was an accident so much that couples of his generation didn't agonize over the question. They just had the kids. It's what you did. At the time, I envied the clarity, but now I'm grateful for all the hemming and hawing. When I look at my son, I see somebody with a lot of thought put into him. He was years in the making.
—anonydaddy

generational **divide**

Parents can be an incredible resource for parenting advice. After all, they've done it themselves. They may know tricks or be able to offer some big-picture perspective. But they may also have done a little rewriting of history over the years and forgotten what really happened when they were in the thick of new parenthood (selective amnesia being one of our best human defense mechanisms). When they tell you that they just put you in your crib and you slept through the night right off the bat, they may not be remembering the whole story (the part about you crying for several hours, or the part where someone went in and comforted you to sleep). They may know little to nothing about the whole newfangled parenting universe, and they may not have a whole lot of

respect for it, either. They may stubbornly stand by no longer fashionable ideas. They may be skeptical of trends—having seen a few come and go in their time. Going with your new program may mean accepting that the way they raised you was wrong, which makes it harder to get behind all this so-called progress: *"You turned out fine!"* True enough, hopefully. But that doesn't change the fact that you may want to do things differently. A couple of things that can help ease your parents into your approach: Reassure them about the things you loved about how you were raised. And try not to rub the latest research in their faces if it makes them feel bad. After all, your big ideas may well be proven wrong by the next generation.

in-laws

Much of the way we feel about parents can apply to in-laws. But there's also the added issue of the difference between their family culture and your own. It can be fascinating and/or terrifying to watch your in-laws with your baby and get a glimpse of how your partner was raised.

Some people are surprised to find their in-laws easier to deal with on baby matters than their own parents. It may be easier to assert your authority with someone who never held much authority over you in the first place. A little polite distance can keep things from getting too complicated. But distance can mean weirdness, too, especially during more vulnerable moments. Even if your backgrounds are similar, all families have their own ways of dealing with situations. Relationships that are touchy or difficult can get more so when differences in child-rearing values are expressed (just as with your own parents).

aunts and uncles

Siblings may embrace the new role of aunt or uncle with ease, or they may feel awkward, jealous, competitive, or just plain removed. The role is entirely personal and can be heavily determined by cultural expectations, individual inclinations, and proximity.

Siblings without kid experience may have absolutely no idea how to deal with the situation. Those who are most definitely not into the breeding thing (at this point, anyway) may be a little freaked out by your new baby-centered lifestyle. It's important to respect your differences, if this is the case. These feelings may change as time goes on.

family expectations

When a family member doesn't seem particularly interested in your baby, it can hurt. But sometimes a relative does not feel connected because there just haven't been that many opportunities for bonding. If you feel comfortable with it, you can ask the person whether he or she is up for hanging out with your baby alone for a while, even if that just means watching him while you make dinner or take a shower. If one family member is with your baby a lot, the others may feel left out. The ensuing drama can make holidays and birthdays extra-tense, and make extra work for you in negotiating and placating. Your child's relationships with his family will evolve over time. Babies are a particular taste, and as yours grows into a toddler and then a kid, there will be new ways to connect. Of course, there may be people in your family who just aren't interested no matter how old your kid is. If you're feeling the lack of extended family love, you may be able to create your own kind of family from friends you can count on.

missing parents

When one or both of your parents is not around to be a part of your new life, it can bring up strong feelings of loss and sadness—both about not being able to share your new baby with your absent parent and about not being able to reconnect to your own early childhood. Feelings of grief and anger can also come up for people who have estranged or otherwise absentee parents, parents with mental illness, or who just feel very distant (physically/emotionally) from their families. If you were adopted, you may feel the lack of your biological parents in your life in a whole new way. What traits will emerge from your side of the family? What skills? What diseases? Coming to terms with these missing pieces of your family may seem harder now that you're starting one of your own. But a new family can also feel like a new beginning.

asserting your autonomy

Your family may have strong feelings about your parenting choices. There may be traditions they want upheld or things they wholly disapprove of. Names and ceremonies are common issues, but opinions can be pretty far-reaching: what you'll do about work, child care, where the baby will sleep. . . . You'll have to decide how much of a role you want your family to play in your parenting. Since you're starting a family of your own, you may need to filter out other influences in order to really hone in on your own ideas.

What happens when a family member does something with your baby that you're not crazy about? What's worth fighting over? In the beginning, it can be hard to tell. Everything seems crucial when you don't have a frame of reference. And older relatives (especially those who at least semi-successfully raised you or your partner) can wield serious authority. Despite your lack of logged hours as a parent, this is, in fact, your baby. The buck stops with you, whether or not you have a clue about what you're doing. Still, you may not want to point out every single infraction. Even though you read that TV can cause ADD, one afternoon a week with talk shows blaring in the background is unlikely to addle your baby's brain. You can opt to provide your relatives with a printout of the AAP report on kids and TV, or you can shrug it off. Either way, it probably won't make one bit of difference to your baby. Unless there's something seriously screwed up going on (as in abuse), the issue is less about how other family members will influence your baby than how they make you feel. When your rules are being disregarded, it doesn't do a lot for your trust. But then constant needling on your part can make your family feel hurt . . . not to mention feel less like spending time with your baby. The situation can get more complicated when you're relying on them for child care.

It may take a while to learn what's worth ruffling feathers over and what isn't, and there may be some hurt feelings in the process. Letting people know what is important to you up front can help stave off future conflicts. Framing things in the context of your own wishes rather than what's "better for the baby" can help people feel more like cooperating and less like they're being attacked. But do realize that your baby is just as likely to be gaining rather than losing out from variation in experience. And remember:

> Make sure your family knows that you are the boss. The mother and baby are the only things that matter for several weeks. It doesn't matter if the mother-in-law hasn't had a chance to hold the baby yet today or if your husband thinks you should all try to have new family pictures taken. JUST SAY NOOOOOO!
> —anonymom

> My mother and I have had huge arguments and it's been nice to establish myself as my own woman and to have my own style of being a wife and mother.
> —anonymom

> To me the word "parent" connotes responsibility, as opposed to "mother," which requires only love, and I honestly didn't feel like a "parent" until my daughter was about five months old, just a few weeks ago. We were visiting my parents, and my dad was telling my mom not to let random people hold my baby. I spoke up to say that I would decide who would hold her and who would not on an individual basis! I was not questioned or challenged by either of them, and this was when it really hit home with me that I was the person most responsible for this little person.
> —anonymom

Everyone has the same interests at heart here, although they may not have the same exact idea of how to accomplish things. This person loves your baby, too.

friends

OLD FRIENDS, NEW BABIES: Friends with babies can do a lot to smooth the transition to parenthood. They can commiserate, or lend you clothes and equipment, or at least know what you're talking about when you ask whether the cheese is pasteurized. It can be a great relief to socialize with someone who knows the ropes and is accustomed to having conversations in thirty-second chunks. But it can also be a little sad to lose the intensity of those pre-baby friendships—when what used to be a cocktail party full of smart, interesting people in meaningful conversations morphs into a roomful of hunch-backs chasing crawling targets (possibly chatting incoherently about the one piece of culture they've been able to digest in months . . . but more likely mumbling about something related to food, sleep, or other bodily functions).

And then there's the bigger stuff, like clashing ideas about raising kids. Ideally, you'll be able to respect each other's takes on things and ways of handling situations. But that doesn't always come naturally. You may get a lot of "The newborn phase is the easy part!" or "Babies find bright colors overstimulating" or other equally questionable proclamations. "This is how it is" usually means "This is how it was for us." As always, a spoonful of salt should be taken with advice, especially advice you don't care for. And a truckload of understanding will help you forgive your friends for giving it to you (and maybe keep you from giving similarly inconsiderate advice to them). Whether or not you use pain relief in childbirth or how you trick out the nursery probably won't make much of a difference in your friend-ships. But parenting choices can reveal fundamental con-flicts that may not have been clear before you had kids. Many friendships survive—or even thrive on—debates and differences. But friends have broken up over less. As time goes on, and you both get more confident about your parent-ing, differences may not matter as much.

BABY-FREE FRIENDS: Your friends without babies may have valid anxieties about what will happen to you now that you're becoming a parent. Will you be boring? Will you be unable to carry on a dialogue without discussing or attending to the needs of your infant? How will you ever have time for their nonparent problems? Having a baby changes your focus (sometimes even before conception). And early parent-hood is often a total-immersion experience. Your friends might accuse you of being "preoccupied" with the minutiae

> I have a friend who I think is a terrific mother. The best part? She never pushes *anything* on *anyone*. How does she manage to refrain? I don't know. I sometimes find myself doing the things that irritate me the most. I.e., just wait until teething, just wait until the baby's born . . . but she never does. And she always has the best way to put advice when it's asked for. A little smile, a shrug, and then . . . her best guess for an answer. I love her for it.
> —anonymom

it's not you, **it's me**

Hanging out with friends should be a positive experience. If you walk away from someone—more than once—feeling bad about yourself, think about whether this friendship is working for you. Keep in mind that it might not be what your friend is giving you that's causing your bad feelings, though . . . sometimes talking to or seeing other parents can inspire our own insecurities to come to the surface. Think about what might be provoking your response (see if you can pinpoint the moment when things turned) and you might be able to tell whether your friend upset you, or you upset yourself.

of pregnancy or baby life, or "obsessed" with mother/fatherhood when you feel like you're just trying to do what it takes. You can try to explain to your friends just how hard, or fun, or miserable or meaningful it all is. But you can also forget the speeches and try to meet your friends on more common ground. They, in turn, need to accept that your life will revolve around your new baby, at least for a while. It can be hard to reassure your friends that you'll be back when you're so swamped in new parenthood that you don't feel so sure of that yourself. But eventually most people's interests will expand to include things that do not involve babies. If you do remain entirely baby-centric, you'll probably find that your friendships adjust accordingly.

A new baby can heighten anxiety for and increase pressure on friends who are ambivalent or not in the right situation to have babies themselves. Friends who have decided not to have kids may question their choices or feel surer than ever when they see what you're going through. Being conscious of what you say to your friends in the first place can keep bad feelings at bay. For example, saying "Having a baby is the most important and wonderful thing you can do . . . I just feel like my life didn't really begin until I was blessed with my little miracle!" might make someone who hasn't had a baby feel as if her life is meaningless, or at least like you see it that way. Being sensitive to other people's circumstances will go a long way in maintaining connections with people who are in different situations from you.

> A good amount of my single friends are not such good friends anymore. They can't relate. . . . They have *no* idea what my life is about. . . . In a lot of other ways it strengthened my relationships with people. I suppose I saw less of childless friends and more of people with children, which is good and bad.
>
> —anonymom

What about friends who are actively trying to have kids and are dealing with infertility or loss? It's hard to know how to act around someone who's longing for something you've got. Issues of guilt and jealousy can be difficult to talk about at a time when joy seems like the only acceptable emotion to voice. Talking about this stuff is never easy. You may just want to avoid raising the issue. But your friend who is trying to conceive (or mourning a loss) might appreciate the support of your awareness, and feel relieved if she's given permission to feel a bit of inevitable pain in the face of your happiness. It's obviously a bad idea to gloat about your baby, but painting a false picture of parental misery may be transparent and insulting. Talking about the weird stuff you both

> Friends . . . I am seeing them a bit more through the prism of how much they are understanding of how a baby changes your life. For example, I took the baby to Boston with me and tried to see a friend on her lunch hour as we were a ten-minute cab ride from her. She had the lunch hour free, but wanted us to come to her rather than the other way around. She just didn't see how it would have been so much easier for her to "hop in a cab" than for me and baby to "hop in a cab" (more like bundle baby all the way up, take the car seat, stroller and base, reinstall car-seat base in a cab [pack up stroller], maybe or maybe not distract/calm crying baby, get in the cab, tell cabbie where to go in an unfamiliar city, take baby, car-seat base, and stroller out of cab, find exactly where I'm going, find elevator . . . get to destination, baby may be hungry or need a change right away, etc. . . . But she didn't offer to make it easier on me). And technically she has no obligation. So, I was like, don't worry about it . . . and we just missed out on seeing each other. Oh well.
>
> —anonymom

224

feel can alleviate tension and remind you of what connected you in the first place. It can help to acknowledge the loss of the friendship as it was. It's important to enter into conversations with an open mind and the understanding that you both may have some less-than-happy things to say. You may have to let your friendship fade into the background while your friend takes on her own challenges, or comes to terms with her situation. If you do feel like your friend would rather not be in touch right now, try not to take it to heart. If there's a way you can let her know you care about her without pressuring her, great. You may even want to tell her directly that you're letting her take the lead. Otherwise, it will hopefully just be a matter of time before you're able to reconnect.

MAKING NEW FRIENDS: Other new parents are an invaluable resource when you have a new baby. If you don't have a prefab new parent posse, seeking out new parent friends may involve a little effort. Being able to talk to other new parents is so important, but how do you do it when you don't know any? → See The Support Team, page 170.

Online parenting networks can really help you feel like you're not alone. But they won't get you out of the house and into the world, which is crucial. Find something you enjoy—or can at least manage—doing with your baby (or with other pregnant people, if you haven't had your baby yet) and try it out for a while: regular walks, baby and me classes, or whatever else seems mildly appealing. Try not to put a huge amount of pressure on any one situation, however. The idea is to expose yourself to a wider range of people and find some you enjoy talking to, not to evaluate the potential of every mom you see to be your new best friend.

The people you relate to as parents might not be the same ones you would have picked out as friends before your baby came along. You may not even get a chance to find out, for example, that the mom you've been bonding with at the park is into show tunes when you're into speed metal. And if you did, it might matter a lot less than how she feels about breast-feeding, sleep training, or whatever baby-related issues matter to you.

The bible of our youth, *Free to Be . . . You And Me,* may have said it best: "Parents are people . . . people with children." And some people are just not that nice (or clever or interesting or funny) whether they have children or not. Just because someone has a baby doesn't mean you're going to like them! The idea that parenthood should unite all people in some kind of collaborative solidarity is lovely, but it's also total crap. Parents share some parts of their physical and day-to-day lives. Beyond that, we've all got about as much in common as we did before we had kids. You may well come across some parents you don't like along the way to finding some you do. If you find that you have nothing in common but reproduction, keep looking!

the balancing act

The balancing act is about balancing the needs of your baby with whatever else you have going on in your life:

- **The job that keeps you afloat**
- **The housework that keeps your home in some semblance of order**
- **The creative expression that keeps you from losing your mind**
- **The ambition that gets your heart pumping**
- **The needs of your other family members**

Juggling demands and priorities is part of every adult's life. What makes the balance so challenging for new parents is the giant-size demands of little tiny babies and our complicated views about who takes care of them.

who's doing what?

- **Slightly less than 25 percent of new moms work full-time.**
- **Slightly less than a third stay home.**
- **The rest (44 percent) do some kind of part-time work while their babies are still infants.**

can women "have it all"?

"Having it all" is a phrase that's been thrown around a lot since the seventies. In the beginning, it was meant to be empowering: Women should be able to have families *and* careers, just like men. More recently the expression is often invoked as a criticism of working mothers. "Having it all" can sound greedy, like women are asking for more than their fair share. But in so many situations, women are just doing what life demands of them. The majority of working women are more concerned with making ends meet than making perfect pie charts of their lives—or striving toward some supermom fantasy. This is not to say that there isn't a sense of accomplishment involved. But balancing a job, a family, and a life takes planning, support, and often some sacrifice.

Having it all is sort of an unreasonable expectation, at least on a day-to-day basis. There are a finite number of hours in a day, and something will always get short shrift. But if you view time management as something spread over weeks rather than hours, it may be easier to picture an even distribution of energy for all your needs. Think of your time like a seesaw—at times the weight may seem heavy on one side; at others, another. If you take a snapshot of your life at any given point, it's likely that someone or something will be getting less of you than you'd like. A "balanced life" needs to be judged over time, not on a moment-to-moment basis.

Think back to before you had a baby. Did you ever wish you had more time to work, or work out, have a "life"? As parents these feelings can get way more intense. Not just because time has become scarce, but because what you do with it is suddenly under a lot more scrutiny. If you don't get enough hours of exercise in, no one is going to think you're a terrible person. If you don't spend enough time with your kids . . . that's another story.

As anthropologist Sarah Hrdy discusses at length in her book *Mother Nature,* women have been struggling with the right balance since the beginning of time: "Female primates have always been dual-career mothers, forced to compromise between maternal and infant needs."

For the modern primate, these compromises are rarely easy or obvious. They are personal and change over time. They are often determined by the reality of our homes and workplaces. The perfect balance—just like "having it all"—is always going to be an unrealistic goal, provoking more anxiety than empowerment. What makes the cut and what gets the boot (housework, manicures, vacations, lunch hour, friendships, sleep) helps to make us the people and parents we are.

to work or not to work
(and why this isn't really the question)

Should a mom go back to work (and abandon her children)? Or stay home (and abandon her career)? Such is the gut-wrenching dilemma posed to modern mothers. But does choice even enter the picture? Single parents usually don't get to choose whether or not to work. Nor do parents who need two incomes to support their families, a growing segment of the population. Child-care costs are often equal to or more than a take-home salary (see "Doing the Math," page 244). Corporate America does not make it easy for parents: Workers are expected to put in as much time as possible, upwards of 50 hours per week for full-time. Parenting responsibilities are considered a distraction from work. A day "off" caring for a sick child is equal to a day off skiing. Decent part-time or flex-time work can be hard to find and almost never provides benefits. The high demands and lack of flexibility of most jobs make it difficult for parents who want to be even somewhat available to their children. So, often, mothers are really forced out rather than "opting out," as we are led to believe.

The fact is that for the most part women are not abandoning children for careers, or flaking on their jobs for their children. They're just taking on way more work. According to Ann Crittenden, author of *The Price of Motherhood,* "Working mothers put in longer hours than almost anyone else in the economy. On average, they are estimated to work more than eighty hours a week."

To be a mother, I must leave the telephone unanswered, work undone, arrangements unmet. To be myself I must let the baby cry, must forestall her hunger or leave her for evenings out, must forget her in order to think about other things. To succeed in being one means to fail at being the other.

—Rachel Cusk,
A Life's Work

Seems that the prevailing attitude is that a mother should only work because of financial need and if she does so because she wants to, she's selfish. Don't hear that much about the father's decision to work, though.
—anonymom

I think it is a disgrace that we don't have mandatory paid maternity leave and a way to have our children taken care of that doesn't rely on a wish and a prayer some days. I wish that I could really have a *choice* as to whether both parents work.
—anonymom

I feel pressure from many directions all the time. I feel pressure from moms who stay at home that working isn't the right choice. I feel pressure from people at work who don't have kids and don't seem to understand why I want to rush home and leave the office right at 5 P.M. so I can see my daughter for more than thirty minutes before bedtime. I feel pressure on myself because I want to stay home, but I also don't want to put negative energy out on my child and my family because we can't do that right now.

—anonymom

All of this anxiety about women not working is not an option for most black women, both professional and nonprofessional. For the most part we all work, we all have always expected to work, and in most cases our mothers worked. There are always exceptions and now as we (black people) have access to things we didn't in the past, there are some black moms who can stay home if they wish and they do. But more of us choose not to. Love for a child can come from more than one source and that someone else, if you have chosen well, can be an asset in your child's life.

—anonymom

the mythical "mommy wars"

If you believe what you see on TV, you'd think working and stay-at-home moms were lobbing grenades at each other all day long. There may be some defensive posturing here and there, but down in the trenches this seems to be sort of a *Wag the Dog* war. For those who haven't seen the movie: It's a fakeout, a scandal concocted to distract us from the real issues. All mothers grapple with their choices. Working mothers love their jobs, or need the money, but miss their kids. They might worry about their child's care. Moms who stay home love being with their kids, but may miss the respect and different kinds of stimulation that come with a job. They might worry about their independence and how/when/whether they'll get back into the work world. Moms in *both* groups just hope that they're doing the right thing. And they both want the best for their kids. Spinning a war out of mothers' ambivalence doesn't solve any of the problems moms on either side of the fence are facing. Mostly, it makes for good media and a lot of wasted energy. If we are told to turn our aggressions on each other instead of advocating for change, we're not going to be improving our situation. We're just telling the powers that be, "There's no need to make things easier for parents. We'll work out our differences among ourselves."

Yes, I feel guilty sometimes, like I'm not supposed to want to work. Some people (I've seen websites, books, articles, etc.) actually think I'm evil, and am sending my kid to hell. Most people don't think that, but I don't know any working moms or dads who think stay-at-home moms are going to hell or destroying society. They may joke, but no comments about hell.

—anonymom

My own mother thinks I'm a money-hungry, selfish person for returning to work. Her views about staying home with your children are 180 degrees from mine.... Culturally, other Latinas (in my world) are not as driven or earn my salary and therefore don't feel the pull to stay in the corporate environment. However, after growing up poor, I'm more motivated than ever to take advantage of my earning power.

—anonymom

I feel support when I am with other mothers. Otherwise, I feel there is not a realistic understanding of what it takes to raise children in our society.

—anonymom

Mommy Wars: Stay-at-Home and Career Moms Face Off on Their Choices, Their Lives, Their Families by Leslie Morgan Steiner

The Motherhood Manifesto: What America's Moms Want — And What to Do About It by Joan Blades and Kristin Rowe Finkbeiner

Perfect Madness: Motherhood in the Age of Anxiety by Judith Warner

The Truth Behind the Mommy Wars: Who Decides What Makes a Good Mother? by Miriam Peskowitz

Families and Work Institute: familiesandwork.org

Activism for a better balance: momsrising.org

Support, education, and advocacy for all mothers: mothersandmore.org

(in)equality, (in)dependence, and other perks of parenthood

We grew up thinking women could do anything. We got great educations, made our own money, kicked a little boy butt along the way. We were encouraged to play team sports, ask men on dates, explore our sexual appetites. Things were starting to look pretty damn good from where we sat— fun, fearless, free females that we were. Then we became mothers. Suddenly, the playing field didn't look quite so level anymore. Motherhood can be a gigantic *"What the ????"* for people who considered equal rights a given. A lot of the women's lib progress we've been enjoying has been more about fitting women into a man's world—and pushing aside the "traditional" role of mother. Topics of affordable quality day care, job-sharing, flex time, breastfeeding-friendly policy, and improved maternity leave benefits were not given much airtime around the bonfire of the brassieres. It's only recently that activism about mothers' issues has moved into the mainstream, and there's a lot of work to be done.

how moms get skewed

Employed or otherwise, moms are expected to do the bulk of the work needed for their kids' care. In rare exceptions, the father is defined as an equal or primary caregiver. (See "Shared Parenting" on page 233.) This makes it difficult for mothers to be competitive in the work force.

When women leave the work force to care for their kids, they lose financial autonomy: both in the short term, while they aren't bringing in income, and in the long term, if they take a career hit from taking time off. This might not matter at all. But it can alter the power balance in a couple. You're both working, but only one of you is being paid.

And whose money is it, anyway? Legally, the person who makes the money controls it. Families count on the breadwinner to act in everyone's best interest, but there is little obligation. In most families, mothers do have some access to the finances, whether they work or not. But there is no law protecting this access to the "family" money.

If the couple splits up (over a third do), a mother's decision to stop working can have serious financial consequences. The compensation a stay-at-home mother is entitled to in a divorce settlement varies: She may be assumed to be as marketable after ten years out of the work force as she was when she left her job to care for her kids and denied alimony as a result.

My employer is very supportive but culture and government . . . blech. If they really cared, they would set up low-cost, quality child care so I don't have to worry about my child during the day and wonder if we can afford to have another kid because where am I going to find another seven hundred dollars a month for day care?
—anonymom

I plan to continue working because I want to and feel I have to. I could probably afford to stop working but in the long term I think the penalty would be too high. My skills would be out of date if I stayed out of the work force completely and I would have to start at the bottom again. I will continue working, probably part time, just so that when I am ready and able to resume my career properly, I will be able to.
—anonymom

The government and society need to get it that most of us not only want to work but *have to* and develop better after-school programs and make insurance more affordable for working families.
—anonymom

resources

The Price of Motherhood: Why the Most Important Job in the World Is Still the Least Valued by Ann Crittenden

Get to Work: A Manifesto for Women of the World by Linda R. Hirschman

staying home

People stay home with their babies for lots of reasons: to be intensively involved in their kids' day-to-day upbringing, to focus on child care without the distraction of managing a career at the same time, to enjoy time with their babies. They may be compelled by their own desire, by a sense of responsibility, by the expectations of others, or because no other option seems reasonable. Some have had it with bad jobs, or feel fulfilled by years of good ones.

Caring for a child full-time can be challenging, creative, and satisfying. But it can also involve lots of busy, boring work. Parents who stay home are usually expected to deal with housework and running the household in general. They will probably spend more than an occasional day focused on things like arranging an appointment with a plumber, dealing with clothing returns, buying groceries, and ordering a replacement for a broken door-knob. They may or may not be expected to have dinner ready (or at least considered) by the time the employed parent gets home. For many people this is a fine balance; they are happy to take on housework as a part of their contribution to the family. Others shudder with Stepford Wife anxiety at the mere thought. Some stay-at-home parents resent the assumption that they're just sitting around "playing with the baby" while their partners are *very busy* with Big Important Job Stuff. It can become increasingly difficult to relate to each other's stresses and accomplishments when you spend your time in such different spheres. And since the employed partner often has to put in extra hours in order to support a family on a single income, couples may find themselves seeing less and less of each other.

If you're leaving the workplace to stay home with your baby, you will have some adjusting to do. Caring for kids involves more work than many jobs, but it's work of a different sort. You may find it way easier and more gratifying than what you used to do with your time, or you may find it terribly taxing and dull. It's more than likely you'll feel moments of each. Your feelings will probably evolve as your child grows, so don't panic if you've quit your job to stay home and you start out hating it.

One of the biggest complaints of stay-at-home moms is the isolation. Depending on your situation, you may feel more or less cut off from the world of adults and ideas. If you feel really claustrophobic or isolated at home, it's worth thinking about how things can change. Sometimes small adjustments help—find a way to take some time off each week, or go out more at night if you can, or meet up with interesting mothers or fathers. Talk to your partner about redistributing the housework—remember, you both work during the day.

> We chose Mommy at home vs. real financial security until now, but this will have to change at some point. Can't continue living inside our major city and have a second kid without me earning decent bucks, too. This is a sad thing.
> —anonymom

resources

Online communities for stay- and work-at-home mothers:
clubmom.com
homewiththekids.com
mochamoms.org

> I do feel guilty for not contributing to the household financially. I am a very independent person and was self-supporting for so many years before I got married. So being in this position was new for me.
> —anonymom

> I really like connecting with other mothers and actually knowing people in the neighborhood.... I feel like I'm in a community. This never happened when I worked— I'd get in there and leave at night.
> —anonymom

> I guess I always knew mothers worked hard. What surprises me is how challenging it is to be a mom. How intellectually challenging. I find I apply the same rules of logic and the same analytical rigor at home that I applied at my consulting firm. Different subject but same mental energy.
> —anonymom

> For the last two years I have gone to sleep with a happy feeling about things that happened during the day—something funny or something he'd done on his own instead of thinking about some concerns or stresses at work. It's nice.
> —anonymom

For me,
being a stay-at-home mom
wasn't a political statement. Nor do I
think it is the "right" thing to do or the
"best" way to raise kids. I am just a woman
who used to work outside the home and now
work inside the home. In many ways, my
new life is harder than my old life.
—anonymom

What I do miss is
the adult conversation and
interaction that I had in my office
jobs. But every time I find mothering to
be tedious or boring or repetitive or
frustrating—and I, like any mom, have these
moments frequently—I remind myself that I
had the exact same experiences in my old
jobs. I looked at my watch a lot in those jobs,
too. I rolled my eyes at my bosses behind
their backs just like I roll my eyes
about my new boss (my baby).
—anonymom

I hated my job. I
worked for some
ridiculous, egotistical, high-
maintenance people. It made a
lot more sense to mother a baby
than to mother a middle-aged
narcissist boss.
—anonymom

Staying at home
full-time with my son so far
has been really great, much less
isolating or housewife freaky than I
thought it would be. I really have none of
the issues I thought I might about feeling like
the powerless woman at home because I have
had a career. . . . But I still have some strange
shame about the whole thing and couldn't join
the playgroup of other stay-at-home moms
but instead chose one of career moms so I
don't have to identify as a SAHM (as
they call themselves on the
Internet).
—anonymom

shared parenting: beyond mr. mom

Parenthood is increasingly becoming a shared responsibility. And though fathers who share equally in child care are still exceptional, more dads are taking care of kids than ever, both in terms of what they do and when they do it.

The Census Bureau reported in 2003 that 18.5 percent of fathers with working wives stay at home with their young children. According to a poll reported in *Time* magazine in 2004, 50 percent of dads said they would consider it. Stay-at-home dads can face the same kinds of challenges that moms do when they leave the work force. But dads have some added stuff to deal with. It can be weird being the only dad in the Mommy and Me class (though being a guy can also make you more popular, depending). Men who stay home can also face judgment for challenging traditional gender roles. It seems difficult for people to get it through their heads, but fathers can indeed care for children as well as mothers, and doing so does not emasculate them or indicate that they are not "wearing the pants in the family," whatever that means. People often expect moms to leave their jobs; men who do the same are more likely to be seen as slackers or shirkers. There's also the question of how the time at home will impact future career ambitions: Some say dads are generally less likely to be penalized; others say more so. Most dads (like moms) who stay home do it because they feel that being involved in their kids' lives is worth any trade-offs it might entail or because it's what works best for their families.

Most people say I'm "lucky" (which drives me crazy) that my husband does about half the child care in our house. Depending upon other factors (work, health, etc.), that seems to have changed back and forth a lot over the four and a half years we've been parents. But he absolutely is as involved as I am with the children.
—anonymom

My husband is very involved in our children's care and nurturing. He takes care of the twins the two full days I am at work. He does everything: changing, cleaning, cooking, feeding, homework, baths, tantrums, arguments, etc. The kids get to learn how things are done the "daddy" way. It may be different, but it's not wrong. They get the full male point of view. [But] whenever things are not status quo (i.e., a child gets sick while I'm at work), my husband has no idea how to take care of them or the situation. That means lots of phone calls at work.
—anonymom

I am married and my partner is very involved with our children. . . . He has had a difficult time because our roles are very different—I am the major breadwinner, yet he does not want to be a *stay-at-home* dad. I still do the majority of the domestic work, and this has been the cause of a lot of disagreements between us.
—anonymom

Because both of us have professional jobs that require at least some hours "over and above" the official office hours, there is some pressure sometimes about who gets to "catch up" on work.
—anonymom

resources

Fatherneed: Why Father Care Is as Essential as Mother Care for Your Child by Kyle Pruitt
daddytypes.com
rebeldad.com
slowlane.com

233

going back to work

Here are just a few of the many motivations for working parents: money, insurance, gratification, career stability, setting an example, identity, independence, brain stimulation.

There are also lots of (radically different) kinds of work and work situations:

- Going back to work when you hate your job but need the money is totally different from going back to a career that brings you great joy.

- A job that takes you away from home for more than 10 hours a day is totally different from one that lets you work from home whenever possible.

- A job with tons of responsibility and take-home work is totally different from one you forget about when you leave the office.

It's really hard to know how it will feel to return to work after having a baby. You may be able to get some clues from how you felt about your work to begin with. If you already felt disconnected at your job, you may resent it when you return with new priorities. You may also find that what felt meaningful before feels less so now. On the other hand, you may go back to work expecting to pine for your new baby and find yourself more engaged than before. The intensity of caring for a newborn can leave some people craving other experiences. The mental demands of the workplace can be a welcome change from the physical and emotional demands of babies.

Parents often return to work with a new cut-to-the-chase mentality. When there's a baby to get home to at the end of the day, procrastination may become somewhat less appealing, whether it's shopping online or listening to your colleague's endless staff meeting tangents. Sometimes the challenge isn't handling the workload but the less official parts of a job, like spontaneous drinks with

> I work because I want to save enough money so my son will be able to attend college if he chooses, or travel the world, or start up his own business, or whatever. I also work to be a good example to my younger cousins, especially the girls. I also want to be a good example to my son when he's older.
>
> —anonymom

> I think of work as my investment in the future. It keeps me busy, plugged in to the community, sane, and keeps me from feeling stagnant. I enjoy dressing up to go to work, doing my makeup and my hair; I enjoy working out at the gym or taking power walks after lunch at work. I do enjoy collecting my fat paycheck, so I guess I see work as a job, but I also get emotional satisfaction being part of a dynamic community of working moms and dads, single and dating nonchildren people.
>
> —anonymom

> My "give a f**k" threshold went way, way up. Now when a provider calls with some picayune request at 4:55, I do not stay late to help; I politely take down the concern and tell the caller I'll get right on it . . . "tomorrow." After all, I have a little one to pick up from day care.
>
> —anonymom

coworkers or clients, or the company retreat. The more your work culture revolves around bonding, the more of an issue this is likely to be.

One of the biggest challenges of going back to work is learning to feel comfortable with your child-care situation.

→ See Child Care, page 241.

resources

News and info for working moms: bluesuitmom.com

Online commentary and resources for working mothers: momsrefuge.com

Working Mother magazine's website: workingmother.com

Sometimes I bury myself in work so I don't feel the sadness, fatigue, and stress of having the baby waiting for me at home needing my time.
—anonymom

Some women have only a few weeks before they have to go back to work, so naturally the expectation is to get back to the usual routine ASAP. And that works out some of the time, but I think a lot of postpartum issues are exacerbated by these high expectations.
—anonymom

People don't understand why I don't quit if I don't "need" to work. I often feel conflicted when I am not feeling happy at work—why work if I'm not feeling fulfilled from it?
—anonymom

I am more confident as an employee than as a mother. After all, what is the worst thing that can happen if you make a bad decision at work?
—anonymom

I'm more likely to melt down in frustration at home—at the office, I've had more experience at problem solving the crises that I deal with there.... Some say that I've become more flexible in my "motherhood."
—anonymom

Those people who think I'm disorganized now should reflect on what an organizational disaster I was before I had kids.... I am much more directed with my energy and intellect now than I was before kids.
—anonymom

235

discretion or **discrimination?**

If your workplace is understanding, you may be able to be open about anything that comes up: a feverish baby, sick nanny, sleepless night. But some jobs call for maximum discretion about the way having a kid affects your life. This can make things extra-challenging when inevitable demands arise. You may have to do some research by talking to other parents at your office to see how they've handled things in the past and how it's worked out for them. Often mothers are warned to keep baby conversations to a minimum. Rushing in late with a big speech about an ear infection or teething may remind coworkers or your employers that you have other priorities. A new mom is sometimes unfairly assumed to be more distracted, less dependable on the job, and much more likely to take off time. This kind of subtle discrimination can make mothers feel like they need to work even harder to prove how little motherhood has affected their output. A new father, on the other hand, might be perceived as even more motivated (he has a family to support now). But dads can also be penalized for taking leave to deal with family stuff.

> Everyone knew what was going on—I felt as though I had the scarlet B on my chest. If the baby was up or sick or my sitter was off... everyone knew. My world was completely upside down.
>
> —anonymom

> I feel a great deal of pressure to perform, and very guilty when I have to call out sick to take care of my son when he is ill. Employers say they understand, but underneath their empathy, I truly don't feel they get it.
>
> —anonymom

maternity and paternity leave

The Family Medical Leave Act is the law that grants leave to new parents—both mothers and fathers. A covered employer must grant an eligible employee up to a total of 12 work weeks of unpaid leave for a new baby (adopted and foster kids count, too).

If you are *not* covered by the FMLA (which you may not be if you work at a small company), you will have to negotiate with your employer for time off. Often, the further in advance you raise the subject, the better, but of course every situation has its own variables. You can also consult state laws to find out if you are entitled to any other kind of leave. States can sometimes be more lenient than the FMLA: In 2004, California passed a law that grants some parents paid leave for up to 6 weeks.

Maternity leave often ends up being some combination of sick days (paid), vacation days (paid), short-term disability (some pay), and official leave (often via FMLA and often unpaid). It typically lasts anywhere between 6 weeks and 3 months, depending on how much time a mother can afford to take off (both in terms of salary and job security). You are only required to give 30 days' notice, but advance discussion of maternity leave with your employer can be a good idea, plus your coworkers may notice that you're pregnant at some point.

Many mothers want to take as much time off as they can, but this isn't always possible or desirable. Some people think they can get work done while they're home on maternity leave, and this may in fact be true . . . we have heard stories about moms happily typing or sculpting away while their babies slept peacefully beside them. However, you shouldn't count on it.

Though leave applies to both parents, dads rarely take much time. Many families can't afford 3 months without any income (paid leave is rarely an option). Also, since it's not that common, dads may fear the consequences of extended paternity leave, even if they can afford it. More and more, companies (and parents) are warming to the idea of fathers taking more time for their newborns. Often they use sick or vacation days rather than paternity leave to stay home with the new baby. One possible way for dads to make use of the FMLA is to discuss with their employer the option of intermittent leave (in blocks of time or by temporarily reducing their normal schedule).

short-term disability

Short-term disability (STD) insurance can cover a portion of your salary during the time that you're unable to do your job due to illness, injury, or childbirth. You may be covered through a private plan (through work or personal insurance) or the state. If you qualify, there is usually some cap on the amount of time you can take (6 weeks is typical). Some plans cover up to 12 weeks or may allow more time for bed rest or any complications resulting from a C-section. Talk to your Human Resources department about STD or check your state laws.

> I would have been a lot happier about going to work if I didn't feel so rushed out of that crazy initial newborn mayhem. At two months I was ready to do *some* work, be in the world to *some extent*, but a full fifty-hour work week? I could have used a good six months to ease into the separation. Or a year like in many European countries! Everyone would have benefited: my employer, my baby, me, my husband.
> —anonymom

> I feel that there is much to be said for lack of adequate pay during maternity leave. Women are forced to return to work before they are physically and emotionally ready simply because they cannot afford to take a well-deserved break with their newborn. It is disgraceful.
> —anonymom

resources

Families and Work Institute: familiesandwork.org
National Partnership for Women & Families: nationalpartnership.org
U.S. Department of Labor: dol.gov

part-time and flex time

Part-time work is often a desirable idea for parents (in fact, almost half of new mothers work part-time). But the reality is not always so ideal. Working part-time can mean close to full-time hours for less than half as much pay and no benefits. Corporate culture is based on the model of full-time (plus) work. Many companies are unable or unwilling to break the mold and make room for flexibility. If they do, they often see the flexibility as a benefit in itself, and don't feel obligated to pay well or provide the same benefits that other employees receive. But some businesses are more open: If you're interested, talk to your employer. In "job sharing" arrangements, two part-time workers do one job: The hours and salary are split 50/50. This can be easier in some jobs than others, and is not as common as many new parents would like it to be.

"Flex time" means that your employer is flexible when it comes to your hours. Maybe you come in at ten each day, but take work home on the weekends or come in on Saturday for a few hours. Or work a "compressed work week"—10 hours a day for 4 days. A more casual version of flex time might mean that when something comes up, you're able to make up the work at odd hours without raising eyebrows. If you work sporadic hours, keep in mind that finding child care can be tricky—often the nanny or day care provider needs a baseline time commitment.

> I work part-time to supplement our income and to provide our family with medical insurance, which my husband's work does not provide. I would definitely stop working if I could afford to do so.
> —anonymom

> My employer offered me an abbreviated work schedule of a minimum thirty-two-hour work week. I am very aware that others who may not be aware of my abbreviated schedule may view my short days and varied times in the office in a different light. I think there is a better dialogue happening in our culture-at-large about flex time, etc.
> —anonymom

> I am highly educated with great experience doing a job that is quite "beneath me" in order to give myself the flexibility I need for myself and my family. Once I feel I am ready to go back to a career track, I may make that change. Trying to juggle a fifty- to sixty-hour-plus travel work week (despite the much higher status and pay) would be impossible with my current family life.
> —anonymom

working at home

Working from home can seem like the best of all worlds . . . you can control your hours and see your baby whenever you want throughout the day. Much of corporate culture runs electronically, so if you've got the right job and the right gear, you may be able to do a good bit of your work from home. Most work-at-home parents find that in order to get work done, someone else must be there to care for the baby. So keep in mind that while the flexibility can be wonderful, you'll probably still need to figure out a good support system. You'll also need to establish some boundaries between your work role and your parent role. When your kid is being especially cute or needy but your deadline looms, this may not be easy (take it from us).

breastfeeding and working

If you are going to breastfeed and work full-time, your boss and/or coworkers may need to be reassured about whether breastfeeding will affect your availability and performance. The answer to this is usually somewhere between "minimally" and "not at all." A simple explanation of when and where you'll be nursing or pumping can help clarify the situation and deflect any potential embarrassment. You'll need to gauge for yourself if this is something you want to raise formally with your employer. If you encounter any confusion (or misguided hostility), here's a little more ammo:

- It has been proven that breastfeeding mothers need fewer sick days than those who feed formula. Studies have also shown that companies have saved money by adopting breastfeeding-friendly policies.

- The American Academy of Pediatrics recommends breastfeeding for at least one year and exclusively for the first 6 months. Having your baby nearby for feedings and/or expressing milk during the workday is crucial in order for you to be able to accomplish this.

- A pumping session can easily fit into a scheduled break or lunch hour. If you have a rigid schedule, you can ask to divide your lunch hour into two shorter breaks.

- Some jobs can be done while pumping. If you have a private area with a computer, for example, you can quite possibly work and pump simultaneously. If your work doesn't lend itself to this, let your boss know how you'll make up for any lost time.

→ See Breastfeeding from a Distance, page 306.

> For the first six months I was back to work after a three-month FMLA, I was pumping twice a day and breastfeeding her at day care at lunch. This was a huge time commitment, and I had to reshuffle a lot of work priorities.
> **—anonymom**

> I had trouble when I went back to work. Pumping isn't an option for me at my job, so I had to deal with being engorged and leaking everywhere. As a waitress, I couldn't really stop and pump for twenty minutes . . . customers might wonder what's taking their food so long.
> **—anonymom**

pumping

Moms with private offices often praise the pump for giving them uninterrupted time to work behind closed doors: Few colleagues will bypass a sign telling them what's going on inside. For a mother without a private workspace, pumping during the workday requires finding a clean, private space and time away from her workstation whenever she needs to pump. → See Milk Storage, page 309, for how to chill the stuff.

> I nursed for over a year, pumped at work until ten months or so, and fortunately only had a few difficult juggling episodes. It was a drag, nonetheless, and required constant planning.
> **—anonymom**

> I work in a large room with three men. We have open cubicles. There is nowhere in my building to pump other than my cubicle. I'd turn my back to the cubicle opening, throw a blanket over my shoulders, and pump under the blanket. Not the ideal situation, but what could I do?
> **—anonymom**

> It was very hard to deal with pumping on business trips and having to disclose this to roommates at conferences and other coworkers because I was forced to stay with them. It's also hard to have to stop and pump every few hours on long drives to see clients—finding places to pump, pumping while driving (which my husband would kill me if I told him).
> **—anonymom**

lack of support at work

On top of practical issues, moms do sometimes face hostility about breast-feeding on the job. Negative reactions can range from undermining behavior to teasing to more abusive comments. It may be hard to tell if the negativity is really about breastfeeding (it's certainly an issue about which many people have strong feelings) or about maternal versus career responsibility. Knowing your rights as a breastfeeding mother can help you feel more secure in your actions. Some states have laws protecting a working mother's right to pump, for example. How you deal with these issues is up to you, and will likely depend on what's being said, who's saying it, and any number of other issues at work.

→ See Breastfeeding and the Law, page 315.

encouraging support in the workplace

If your company wants to put their support in writing, they might consider implementing breastfeeding-friendly corporate policy, or initiating a Corporate Lactation Program. These have been shown to boost morale and productivity as well as cut healthcare costs and sick days. La Leche League International offers Corporate Lactation Program packages that include tips for establishing and maintaining an on-site pumping room, educational materials, and a few helpful products such as nipple cream and pads.

child care

Choosing the right child care can be so daunting. If only the perfect nanny really would drop magically from the sky, with umbrella. And without complications, like too high an hourly rate, a penchant for long cell phone conversations, or a rampant addiction to daytime TV. Imagine: no hours of trolling sitter services looking for somebody who seems loving *and* knowledgeable, giving *yet* firm, reliable *and* flexible. No anxious, awkward tours of day cares, putting your baby down on the colorful mat and timing the response of the staff with a stopwatch. Instead, there's a knock at the door, and it's the highly trained, nurturing staff of the world's most trustworthy day care center here to offer a scholarship! Or, it's Mary Poppins herself. Dream away.

The bad news is that ideal child care probably won't be landing on your doorstep. The good news is that you don't actually need magic, or Mary Poppins, for that matter. You need a reasonable, warm, stimulating environment for your child to thrive. When you begin to look for child care—any kind of child care—a formal list of questions and concerns can help you sort out the good from the not-so-good. (We've provided a breakdown of each option in the pages to follow.) We've found that after working out the complex equation of money, time, location, etc., we still had to

> Sometimes it is awkward having him with three different providers during the week, but I trust them all immensely and my son is happy when he is with them. It may not be ideal, but it's what works for us. That's what parenting is all about, doing what you need to do to keep the family functioning well.
>
> —anonymom

> Her close bond with another nurturing adult is most positive. I think this has impacted her ability to easily form relationships—she's never gone through a clingy phase with either my husband or me.
>
> —anonymom

241

I've been having antibiotic overdose nightmares since my son has been in day care. He's not even two and the ear infections have been fast and furious. He is so rarely not sick (or just getting over a sickness), I have a hard time scheduling his shots. Whenever I ask my doctor "How do you get this?" the answer is always . . . "Day care."

—**anonymom**

I know where she goes and who she's with, but only superficially. She lives a huge amount of life in another universe and it's one that I don't share.

—**anonymom**

I think having other caregivers has made my son more flexible and secure. It made separation his first time at preschool a breeze!

—**anonymom**

I felt tremendously guilty leaving my baby with another caregiver, and actually felt rather resentful that fate had dealt me this card that I had to work to help support my family. Once I felt comfortable with my child-care arrangements, I was able to relax and begin to enjoy my work again.

—**anonymom**

rely on our gut feelings. Finding a caregiver is a lot like dating. There are some baseline criteria to go by, but it's the chemistry that helps you make the leap. And, like in any long-term relationship, you may have to make some compromises to make it all work.

Everyone's got a different idea about what makes a good caregiver situation. Here are some basics:

TRUST: Since you are leaving your baby with this person (or people), you need to feel confident that he will be safe and trust the caregiver's judgment. You also need to trust that whoever is caring for your child will respect your wishes about how you want your baby to be cared for.

COLLABORATION: You will be working *together* on the project of caring for your child. This project, and all parties involved, will evolve over time. You and your caregiver(s) may have differences of opinion, but you need to feel like you're on the same basic team and have the same priorities. Too much competition or challenge to your authority can lead to problems. Collaboration is a two-way street: You'll need to get comfortable with this person making day-to-day decisions, too.

COMMUNICATION: You're counting on a caregiver to let you know what's going on with your baby while you're away from him. If communication isn't flowing, you may not be able to get the information you need to feel confident about what's going on with your child. There are lots of ways to convey information, whether or not you speak the same language. Caregivers who keep a log of what your baby does and eats throughout the day, for example, can help you feel connected to what's going on. Being able to communicate with each other is also important for negotiating any conflicts that might come up. It can be helpful to designate a time for more in-depth conversations about her work and/or your child.

A GOOD FIT: You need a situation that will fit well with your family. If you have a nanny, you do not have to enjoy her company, but you do need to be able to handle having her around. If you use a day care, you'll want to feel that the general vibe of the people and place fits with your own ideas, even if they are somewhat different. Caregivers need to be available and reliable enough to meet your needs. And you'll need to be able to meet their needs, too, both by paying appropriate wages and accommodating emergencies. If either side has more needs than the other one is able (or willing) to meet, things can get problematic.

Your baby developing close relationships with others is a good thing. But for many mothers it brings up all kinds of conflicting feelings: relief and comfort that the baby is so happy and well cared for, longing for more time with the baby, and maybe a twinge (or more) of jealousy.

the **mommy-only** myth

"SO WHY DID YOU EVEN HAVE A KID IF YOU'RE NOT GOING TO RAISE HIM YOURSELF?"
Since the beginning of time, women have sought out the help of others to care for their offspring. There is evidence that even the earliest primate mothers (who were nothing if not "hands-on" with their babies) would enlist the support of other trusted females—anthropologists call them allomothers. Making sure everyone is fed, protected, and sheltered isn't easy for a parent, whether single or with a working spouse, foraging in the jungle or multitasking in the suburbs. It's only recently that we've started to expect mothers to handle child care without assistance, even when they can afford help.

Kids need to make a primary attachment in order to develop empathy and trust. Since moms are often the ones who respond first to their baby's cries, most often the mother becomes the primary attachment. But the idea that the mom is the *only* one who can connect with the baby has been dismissed from many angles over the course of many years (and with the backing of many studies)! Even John Bowlby, a founder of Attachment Theory, said the person with whom the baby makes a primary attachment can be a mother or *"a mother figure."* In other words, a father, grandparent, or unrelated caregiver can work just as well.

> I don't know why people assume that the mother is always the best option. I don't have half the patience (or half the experience) our nanny does.
> —anonymom

> We have a fantastic nanny. My children are exposed to a smart, intelligent, creative person who has the patience and strength of character to let them finger paint. And can feed them vegetables.
> —anonymom

> "They" have us convinced our babies will not grow or thrive unless we are giving them constant care and protection. In the long run, I don't think it's healthy for all these kids to grow up thinking their parents' sole concerns are their children. Kids need to see their parents as examples of how to balance the important things in their lives.
> —anonymom

what kind of care?

Is there a best kind of child care? Is a structured center better than informal family day care? Is a nanny better than group care? Each arrangement has its pros and cons, but it's the quality of care that matters most. A fantastic day care with warm, trained caregivers is just as good for kids as an experienced, hands-on nanny. A loving, attentive grandparent can be as valuable for a child's development as a renowned "early education center." Of course, you may not have that many options, depending on where you live, what your needs are, and what your budget allows.

doing the math

COST OF A NANNY: Full-time nannies charge about $300 to $800 a week or more plus taxes. If you live in an expensive area, the price will be on the higher end. Other expenses to consider are benefits, vacations, sick days, meals, and/or accommodations.

→ See The Household Employment Tax, page 252.

COST OF DAY CARE: According to the Children's Defense Fund, the average day-care center charges $4,000 to $6,000 annually for a four-year-old child. Infant and toddler care is more (closer to $7,000 to $18,000 annually). Infant child-care centers in expensive cities can cost over $2,000 a month, full-time.

→ See page 252, for info on taxes and cutting costs.

day care

Day care is out-of-home child care where there are other children and often more than one child care provider. Day care can also be called center-based care, early education, preschool, pre-K, nursery school, or learning center. It might operate through an existing organization like a school, corporation, or church, or it may be independently owned.

BENEFITS OF DAY CARE: Children can become more comfortable around others ("socialized") at an early age. This is especially true for first or only children. Children can benefit from an experienced staff trained in childhood development. They can learn from the other kids and make "friends." They can learn to communicate, cooperate, and play with other children. They can also benefit from an environment thoughtfully geared toward babies or children. It is often more affordable than individual or in-house care, and it can be great if one or both parents are working at home.

POTENTIAL DRAWBACKS: Exposure to lots of kids means exposure to lots of germs. Kids in day care get sick frequently (even when the environment is very clean). Sick days can be complicated for working parents: If the child is too sick for day care, someone has to be home for him.

Some recent (and controversial) studies have shown that children who have been in day care for long periods of time (lots of hours per week, over years) may be more aggressive than children who have not. Experts in this field argue that this is the result of poor-quality day care, not the result of day care in general. Some potential problems from low-quality day-care situations:

- Children may not get enough one-on-one attention. Even babies need to engage in long sequences of back-and-forth "dialogue" with adults.

- Day-care workers can come and go without much notice. Children need some consistency to develop empathy and trust.

- If a day-care center is not focused on productive and creative play (the children are "watched" rather than cared for or guided), the environment can end up very disorganized and chaotic.

- If a day care has too few trained staff and/or unsafe or unclean conditions, it can put the child at risk.

FINDING DAY CARE: A good day care is often found through word-of-mouth: Friends, online groups, neighborhood parents' groups, your local pediatrician, a children's playgroup, or a recreational center may give you some leads.

Sometimes preschools have toddler and infant programs, so check nursery school listings. This may also give you an advantage in the application process, which can be a big plus if getting into a preschool is an issue where you live.

IS IT LICENSED?: Most states license day-care centers and check them for safety and cleanliness. You can find out about most state-licensing regulations at the National Resource Center for Health and Safety (nrc.uchsc.edu). Some programs, such as religious ones, are exempt from state licensing. A license is no guarantee of quality care: Licensed day cares are required to meet only minimal standards to remain in business.

DOES IT HAVE "ACCREDITATION"? Accreditation is when an outside evaluator—the National Association for the Education of Young Children (NAEYC) and the National Child Care Association (NCCA) are the two big ones—determines that the day care meets all the standards for high-quality care.

STAFF: All staff should have extensive experience with children. Ideally, caregivers should have some training in early childhood education. Find out what the staff turnover has been. Meet all caregivers: assistants, part-time staff, and anyone who will be around your child. Try to get a sense of how they feel about children, about their job. Do they seem genuinely engaged? Watch them interact with your child in the space. Ask each of them questions about their experience. And their ideas about children: How do they handle discipline? Playtime? Crying? What are their expectations about toileting? Give them hypothetical scenarios: What do you do about screaming? Refusing to eat? If your baby is young and needs to feed "on demand," ask how this is handled. Ask them questions specific to your child's age about napping, feeding, and appropriate activities. Do they use videos? Do they go outside every day? Are there field trips? Ask about separation. (You should have the option to separate gradually, at least at first.) Can you visit anytime? Ask about the daily routine: What do they do? How is it age appropriate?

The answers to these questions should fit with your own ideas about child care. If they do not, ask to hear their philosophy.

CHILD-TO-ADULT RATIO: The AAP recommends that there should be no more than three infants to one caregiver and no more than six children in a given room (with two caregivers).

POLICY: Policies should be written and given to you; these policies need to include how discipline is handled and how sick children are treated. You should always be given information about the day's activities in advance and you should be able to visit the day care whenever you want to, with or without advance warning.

SICKNESS AND SANITATION: Parents should be required to notify the day-care center if their child gets a contagious illness. Children who are moderately to seriously ill (i.e., with more than a cold) should be required to stay at home. Immunizations are required for entry into licensed day care according to state law. Diaper and food areas must be totally separate. All food-related items (the food itself, containers, cups, bottles) need to be kept clean and not shared. Caregivers should wash hands frequently, between changing diapers, feedings, nose wipings, etc. For young babies, toys need to be washed regularly (since they tend to be touched by mouths as well as hands). Ask who has permission to give medicine and what their qualifications are. If you have a child with a chronic condition such as asthma, ask how this is handled. Where is the medicine kept? Who is monitoring the child? High-allergy foods such as peanut products should be 100 percent banned.

SLEEP: There should be a separate, comfortable, and quiet area for napping. Babies can be encouraged to nap at the same time, but flexibility is important. Babies should be put to sleep on their backs and in ways complicit with SIDS safety regulations → See Sudden Infant Death Syndrome, page 271.

SAFETY: The area should be fully childproofed. All equipment should meet safety criteria.

FINALLY: Drop in unannounced. Do the children seem happy, clean, engaged? Do the caregivers seem overwhelmed or on top of things? Are things organized? Do you have a good feeling about the place? Do you like the other parents? Get all the references you possibly can . . . from previous parents, previous employers.

family day care

Family day care is less formal day care (by a relative, friend, or babysitter) that takes place in the caregiver's home. The casual vibe of the home environment can be part of the appeal. Some family day cares are licensed; most are not. This means you may have to do a little extra investigating of safety and health concerns. For help in assessing a family day care, use the day-care criteria above. In addition, ask who else is around. Are there other family members? (If so, meet them.) Ask about all the other children who attend. Ask to talk to their parents. And ask to hear all the details of the daily schedule. Since home environments usually include a TV and some amount of cooking, ask how that's handled. Does she watch the news? Can her teenage son play video games while the kids look on? You may also want to talk to some neighbors to see if they have any observations they'd like to share.

resources

For more on assessing day care, see the U.S. Department of Health and Human Services report "13 Indicators of Quality Child Care" at aspe.hhs.gov.

in-house care

In-house caregivers are most often referred to as nannies or babysitters (unless the person is related to you). We're always surprised a new word hasn't taken hold. In Australia and England, they sometimes say "carer" or "minder," but these don't roll easily off the American tongue. The anthropological term "allomother" is unlikely to catch on. In any case, you and your child will probably come to think of your "nanny" by her name rather than her job title.

Nannies can provide one-on-one attention and closely supervised care without the distraction of a group of kids. A child may get more undivided attention from a good nanny than even a stay-at-home parent. Many nannies' responsibilities are limited to child care and cleanup, while parents may have more to do around the house while they're with their kids. Often a nanny becomes a part of the family, whether or not she lives with you. Some really appreciate this family feeling—and are especially happy for their child to be at home. Having someone else in the house all the time can also be stressful, especially for parents who are home a lot. In general, nannies cost more than day care. In some parts of the country, in-home care is reserved for the rich, but in big cities, it's common among middle-class working parents. Some parents are eager to have their children around other kids—with a little planning, this is easy to achieve with nanny care. Once "socialization" becomes a priority, the nanny can meet with other kids and nannies, attend classes, or join a playgroup.

HERE ARE SOME WAYS TO FIND A NANNY:

- *Services or agencies:* There are a number of services that place nannies with families. These can be really helpful, as candidates have been pre-screened. There is often a pretty significant fee involved, but you can save a lot of time.

- *Classifieds/job listings:* There are online services for nannies and their potential employers to post job listings. Universities sometimes have online job listings for students. These can be helpful if you're looking for part-time or casual help. General job classifieds (on websites or local newspapers) are also an option. Or try posting online on parents' groups and bulletin boards.

- *Word of mouth:* Tell everyone: Call them, e-mail them. Be specific about what you're looking for. You can also spread the word via any community playgroups or mothers' support groups in your neighborhood. Check bulletin boards at pediatricians' offices or other places where parents congregate.

interviewing caregivers

Since this is all about a personal relationship, you will want to give yourself time to try to get to know any potential caregivers. You can meet with the person privately at first if you prefer, but it's a good idea to have the baby in the room for at least part of the time. Here are some ideas about things to look for and discuss:

- *Watch how she is with the baby.* You need to see that she's genuinely engaged with and interested in your child. If the baby fusses, how does she handle it? Is she a good gauge of the baby's mood? Does she seem upset by the baby's reactions? Does she say things that are positive and reassuring? Even though the baby may not understand words, what she says to the baby can tell you a lot about how she feels about children in general. How does she talk about any kids she cared for in the past?

- *Try to learn about her background and her experiences, both professionally and personally.* What's going on in her life? If she has kids, find out what her own child care situation is like. What's her family support system? Does she have responsibilities to others?

- *Describe a typical day for her.* Tell her about any routines or schedules you've developed, or any you'd like to. If you're struggling with any particular issues (about sleep, feeding, crying), talk to her about your ideas, goals, and concerns. How does she respond? Even if she has lots of answers you like, you want to make sure she's listening to you and is respectful of your (evolving) approach. You'll be working *with* this person as your baby grows, and as you develop skills and confidence as a parent. Discussing problems in a productive way is very important.

- *Be very clear about your expectations.* What will her schedule be? If you're working, how regular are your hours? Will you need her to be flexible in case you need to work late? If you're going to be in the house, be very specific about how involved you expect to be in the baby's day and what you expect her to do while you're with the baby. Make sure she knows how you'd like her to handle feedings while you're home. If you do take the baby for periods of time, what is she expected to do during that time? If you want her to tidy up, be specific about what that means to you. Is it cleaning up the baby's toys, doing laundry, doing her own dishes? What's supposed to happen while the baby's napping?

- *Discuss basic house rules.* If there are things that are off-limits to her or the child, say what they are. What's your policy on phone calls? TV? Visitors? Food? Is she expected to bring lunch? Or do you provide food or money? For live-in nannies, discuss the living arrangements: her room(s), communal rooms, and the issue of privacy—hers and yours. Also talk about the schedule: When is she expected to work? Is she on call at any other times? When is she off? Discuss what happens when she's off duty: Can she have guests over? Is there a curfew? Can she use your car? Watch your TV? Getting these specifics clarified can save stress later.

- **Talk about salary.** It's important to be as up front and detailed as possible from the get-go. How much will you pay? When? What about vacation (hers, yours)? Sick days? Extra time? Healthcare? Talk about procedure. If she misses hours, will she be paid? Can she make up lost hours at another time? Ask her if she has any potential schedule conflicts.

- **Ask her for her ID (license, passport, work visa, etc.) and other personal information: phone numbers, address, emergency contact.** And ask for as many references as you can and call all of them. Ask the previous employers to tell you as much as they can, including any criticisms.

- **If you think you want to hire her, run at least one trial playdate.** Stay at home but try to leave her alone as much as possible to see how it goes.

NANNY QUESTIONS: Postpartum expert and doula Meredith Fein Lichtenberg has held working-mom groups for years and often deals with issues of child care. She came up with these questions for potential nannies. We found them invaluable in our own quests for care—maybe you will, too.

background information

- Where is the nanny from?
- Does she have family/friends in this area?
- What is her visa status?
- How long does she plan to stay in the United States?
- How long has she been here, and does she plan to stay?

experience

- What experience does she have caring for kids? Ask about all her previous child-care jobs.
- How old were the kids at her previous jobs?
- What did the parents do for a living and what were the hours? Ask her to talk about the parents to get a sense of what kind of person she is comfortable working for.
- What were her responsibilities besides playing with the kids?
- What did she like best about them?
- What was most difficult about them?
- Why did she leave them?
- Ask about any gaps in employment.
- If she is not currently working as a nanny, does she have a non-child-care job?
- Does she know CPR?

questions about why she wants to work for you

- What do you like about caring for kids?
- What is your favorite-age child?

- What do you find hard about [the age your child is]?
- What kinds of things do you like to do with kids who are [your child's age]?
- What kinds of things do you do with kids who are [6 months older]?
- What is the hardest thing about dealing with young kids?
- What do you like to do in your free time?
- What kind of family would she find terrible to work for?

hypotheticals (which give you a good sense of how she thinks)

- What would you do if the baby was banging toys and you thought he could break something?
- What would you do if he was playing with another child in the playground and you saw him poking or hitting the other child (also do the opposite scenario)?
- What would you do if you saw he was about to put something dangerous or dirty in his mouth?
- What would you do if you went to the bathroom and heard him crying and came out to find he'd hurt his head badly? (The answer to this should always include "I would call you at work.")
- What would you do if you heard the telephone/doorbell ring while he was in the bathtub (possibly add: and I'd told you I was expecting an important call/delivery)? (Answer *must* be, "I'd ignore it" or that she would bring the phone into the bathroom or not give a bath till the delivery came.)
- What would you do if my mother came over and wanted to take the baby out? (Answer should be that unless you have told her this will happen, she does not give the baby to anyone, EVER.)

things that would probably make me not hire the person even if she seemed otherwise like Mary Poppins

- She hesitates or puts you off about giving references.
- She cancels the interview but wants to reschedule.
- She complains in any way about you or your apartment during the interview, even in jest ("Whoa, that's a lot of stairs!" "You're sooooooo far from the bus stop").
- She seems depressed or notably lonely.
- She refers to a sick relative who lives far away or her own chronic illness.
- She complains during the interview that what you are paying is too low but accepts it.
- She smells like cigarette smoke or perfume that you would not want your house to smell like all day.

the household employment tax

The law requires that both employers and nannies/babysitters pay taxes. After taxes, employers pay around 10 percent more, and nannies take home around 20 percent less. Not all families comply with this law, for a few reasons. Many nannies are not legally allowed to work in the United States. Those who can work legally may not want to sacrifice part of their wages; families may not be able to afford paying the same salary with taxes on top. The marketplace is an issue, too: Why would a nanny work on the books when she could make more money off the books down the street? But it is the law. If you avoid this tax and get busted, you may face fees, back tax payments, and possibly even prosecution. You'll also miss out on any child-care-related tax deductions. (If you have any ambitions for public office, don't even think about paying under the table.) If the paperwork is an issue, you can hire someone to deal with the payroll and tax preparation. Payroll services charge about $35–$55 a month. You can also talk to an accountant or a lawyer specializing in household employment.

To legally hire a nanny yourself, you need to read *The Household Employer's Tax Guide* available on the IRS website (irs.ustreas.gov) or by calling 800-829-3676.

some ways to save

- *Flexible spending plan:* Talk to your employer about the flexible spending plan. If you are eligible, you can deduct child-care costs from your pretax income (thus lowering total taxable income).

- *Child-care tax credit:* Check the IRS website or talk to an accountant to find out what deductions you can take. You cannot use both the child-care tax credit and the flexible spending plan, so see which one makes more sense for you.

- *State-subsidized child care:* You can apply for child-care aid through local agencies. A listing can be found at Child Care Aware (childcareaware.org).

He is a very social and loving child. I think it's because he's been exposed to people from such a young age. Difficult parts have been when he is not feeling well, or just wants to be held—especially when he was an infant. It used to hurt a lot when I would go pick him up and find him bundled up in a teacher's arms being rocked and soothed. I got past it once I discovered that I can soothe him much faster than anyone else.

—anonymom

I returned to work after six months. I was eager to go back because I was getting bored at home. I needed adult interaction and I needed to be challenged in a way that was different from the challenges you face with a new baby. I was starting to feel like a mom and not an individual. I used to be the person everyone came to for advice with how to manage people or how to take on a certain project. Now not even my husband asks me work-related advice anymore. I guess I didn't feel intelligent anymore.

—anonymom

I hated going back at first, but then realized using two hands when eating makes the meal better! The glorious lunch hour helps me get things done.

—anonymom

My daughter is very confident and has very good social skills. She has been described as a natural leader by her teachers. She is highly adaptive, very friendly, and outgoing. I feel these characteristics of her personality have been enhanced by her preschool care. . . . However, she has expressed frustration that she does not spend enough time with me and my husband, nor enough family time together. We have all felt the same way and it is very difficult for us.

—anonymom

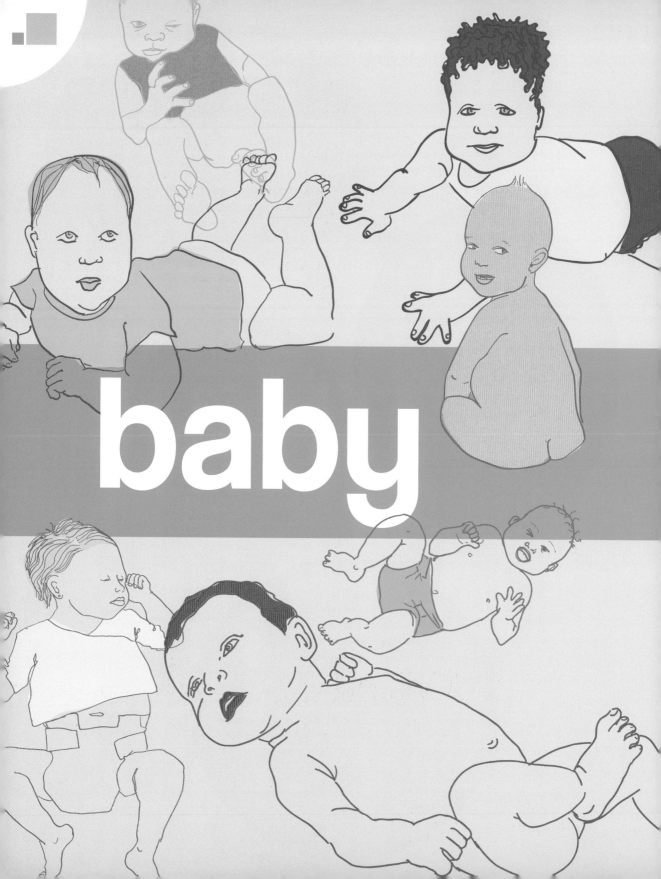

baby

babies. They're adorable. They're precious and miraculous. But they're also kind of intimidating and indecipherable. We found ourselves reading our babies' dirty diapers like tea leaves. Is Dijon mustard a sign of contentment or digestive trouble? Every day with a new baby is like waking up to the world's cutest puzzle. Solve it and you're rewarded with coos and cuddles, as well as sleep, precious sleep. Otherwise, chaos. Is it any wonder new parents are obsessed with finding solutions? In the early months, you may be shocked by the sheer quantity of data you accumulate, most of it revolving around infant feeding, sleep, and excretory activities. Some baby care information really is so basic you can tack it to the fridge: *When does the baby outgrow his car seat? How long can I freeze breast milk?*

But other questions require more soul-searching than check-listing: *Is it a good idea to let a baby cry at night? When should I wean?* These are the questions that had us racking our brains and scouring the Web at all hours of the night. We read lots and lots of books, most of which told us we could solve all our baby problems by following a simple plan (or signing up for a complete holistic lifestyle makeover). But we could never really get with the program. Maybe it's because we aren't really joiners as a rule, but we felt like the only thing that made sense was to find our own way of caring for our babies, taking a little from what others told us, a little from what we read, and making up the rest as we went along. In the end, this may have been more work than just following a script. But for us, it was worth it.

Your own style of baby care will be something you'll define for yourself, whether it comes from your gut, what you learn, or some combination. This part of the book covers not just the practical stuff but the controversies, opinions, and trends . . . so you can figure out what makes the most sense for your baby—and you.

baby care basics

This is a stripped-down primer on taking care of a young baby: basic sustenance-level stuff. You'll find there is very little in here about either major medical issues or developmental milestones. Your pediatrician should be contacted with any health or development concerns. There are also a number of reliable print and online resources; see the box below for some recommendations. In the meantime, here are some of the many things there are to know about babies and how to keep them safe, healthy, and relatively happy.

baby acne

Pimples on the face and back are common in newborns. Acne usually goes away in a few weeks. It can be aggravated by contact with products or by too much rubbing or washing.

baby states

To help parents and caregivers understand newborn behavior, pediatricians have defined six different states of baby consciousness. This information can be helpful in the early months as you are getting to know your baby's cues and behavior. Many infants flow from one state to the next in cycles throughout the day. Some, however, skip certain states or spend the majority of time in the sleeping and crying states. → See Sleep, page 332, for more.

QUIET (OR DEEP) SLEEP: The baby is still, has even breathing, is hard to wake up, and does not move much except for the odd twitch. If you lift up his arm, it will flop back down limply. This is the easiest time to move an infant without waking.

ACTIVE (OR LIGHT) SLEEP: The baby may move a little, have REM (rapid eye movement) beneath lids, make sounds, smile, experience irregular breathing, and is very responsive to internal stimuli (e.g., hunger, gas) or external stimuli (e.g., movement, noises).

DROWSY: In between sleep and alertness, a baby may have irregular breathing, closed or squinting eyes, and show some movement. This is the state before and after sleep.

QUIET ALERT PHASE: The baby seems well rested, able to focus, really taking things in, with lots of looking and listening. This is often when caregivers get the most positive feedback from the baby. This can also be a good time to feed an infant.

ACTIVE ALERT PHASE: The baby is attentive to surroundings and actively moving. May show signs of hunger (sucking fingers, rooting). Babies can be fed and/or coaxed from this state into a drowsy or sleep state. If not, this phase can move quickly into crying.

CRYING PHASE: The baby is crying and has erratic movements and irregular breathing. The crying may indicate hunger, tiredness, or overstimulation (among other things). The baby can be guided to another state by feeding, minimizing stimulus, comforting, or getting to sleep.

bathing

SPONGE-BATHING: Most doctors recommend sponge-bathing until the umbilical cord falls off and circumcision is well healed. Since a lot of babies don't like being totally naked early on, you can wash your baby while semi-swaddled in a towel. A sponge bath can be given with a washcloth or sponge. Water temperature should feel warm, not hot, on the inside of your wrist. Gently wash the baby with attention to the creases and folds. Cotton balls are useful for cleaning between crevices or hard-to-reach spots.

TUB-BATHING: Babies can be washed in a special baby tub (freestanding or in the bathtub) or in the sink, lined with a folded towel or sponge mat. Some babies love the water; some fear it. Baths can be very brief to start out. Check the water temperature, using your wrist or a thermometer (should be close to body temperature). Low lights or singing can help make bath time more relaxing. You can also take a bath with your baby. This can be especially comforting to a baby who gets stressed by the water. To avoid slipping, have the baby handed to you once you are in the tub and hand the baby over to someone before you get out.

And do not forget the fundamental rule for baby bathing: Never leave the baby unattended for even a few seconds.

blocked tear ducts

Babies' eyes usually don't begin tearing until about week 3. Before then, tears drain via the nose. If you see some sticky, yellowish goop around your newborn's eyes, he may have a blocked tear duct. The ducts are beneath the eyes, close to the nose. Talk to your pediatrician, who can show you massage techniques to open the ducts or prescribe antibiotic ointment. Blocked tear ducts can recur over the first six months. Frequent and persistent blockage beyond six months of age may require a minor procedure to help alleviate the problem.

potions and lotions

A newborn doesn't need washing with soaps and cleansers. Though there are lots of products out there, for the most part they should be saved for older kids. Powders, when inhaled, can irritate a baby's nasal passages. Talcum powder has been associated with cancer and should not be used. Cornstarch is safer but can promote growth of fungus. Since moms and babies know each other's smells (and these smells are a part of a whole network of responses), it's a good idea to avoid any perfumes on a new baby and a new mother.

body temperature

The womb is a soft, cozy, airless environment. Babies aren't used to cool air on their skin. They also have a hard time conserving body warmth in the first month. As a general guideline, a newborn baby needs about the same amount of clothing as an adult, plus a hat if it's cool outside. As babies get older, they become better at conserving heat. Overheating can be an issue for all babies. Keep the baby away from direct heat sources (including direct sun) and dress in light layers in warm weather.

burping

If your baby makes a strained expression, cries, squirms after a feeding, or rejects the breast or bottle midway through a feeding, she may need to be burped. Bottle-fed babies may feed faster and swallow more air and therefore require more attention to burping. Breastfed babies may swallow air too, depending on latch or other issues. They may also need to be burped, especially if they are fast feeders or the mother has a strong milk-ejection reflex. Sometimes burping a breastfed baby when switching from one breast to the other can prevent lots of air buildup. Getting a good burp after every feeding is not necessary unless your baby seems uncomfortable or distressed. Burping is less of an issue for older babies, who sometimes learn to "burp themselves."

The basic idea with burping is this: Hold the baby with her head higher than her belly and apply some pressure to her tummy while patting her back. This should help get the air bubbles moving up and out.

some burping positions you can try

- With the baby on your lap, in a sitting position, tilt the baby forward slightly with hand on lower stomach and pat her back.
- With the baby's stomach against your shoulder and his head over your shoulder, pat his back.
- When seated, put the baby stomach down onto your thigh. Hold the baby's head and pat her back.
- Hold the baby, stomach down, along the length of your forearm, with his head supported by your hand.
- Just carry the baby around in an upright position (in arms or a sling).
- Gently push the baby's knees up to her chest to help squeeze out any gas.

colic

The word "colic" comes from a Greek word that means "suffering in the colon," and is often thought to be related to some kink in the baby's digestive system. However, there is really no clear understanding of what the exact kink may be, or if there even is one. What we do know is that the baby is in some kind of real distress.

- Colic is a very specific phase, with very vague causes.

- A colicky baby cries inconsolably, and may flex his body, scrunch his knees up, buck and/or curl up with a tight tummy.

colic happens:

- **three or more hours a day (usually starting in late after-noon or early evening)**
- **at least three times a week**
- **for at least 3 consecutive weeks**
- **from about 3 weeks of age**
- **until around 3 months of age (sometimes longer)**

The stress and emotional wreckage caused by a colicky baby cannot be overestimated. It's hard enough for parents to listen to a crying baby, but when all the usual tricks don't work (feeding, rocking, burping, singing), it can be beyond frustrating. It's hard not to project not-so-favorable personality traits onto a baby who goes ballistic for a few hours every day, but colic does not mean you've got a permanently crabby, "spoiled," or unpleasant kid on your hands. *(And, it is worth emphasizing here that you cannot "spoil" a baby by responding to her cries or by picking her up too much.)* There is certainly a continuum of fussiness. Many high-need babies require more holding and attention, but a colicky baby is at the extreme end, and is often difficult or impossible to soothe with extra TLC. This is not to say that they don't benefit from cuddling and holding and rocking and love, but they may continue crying throughout. Parents have come up with many creative ways to ride out colic or at least shave a few minutes off the hours of torture.

things to try

- Put the baby in stroller, car seat, or carrier as soon as the crying starts and go out for a long walk/drive.

- Put on music . . . and rock, sway, bounce, or dance with baby in arms. Choose music you like since you may end up listening to it every day. And try music with a good beat. Repetitive movements and a steady beat can be far more lulling than lullabies.

- Keep a diary so you can track the crying and see if there are any

the happiest baby on the block
by harvey karp

L.A. pediatrician Harvey Karp is famous for canonizing the idea of "The Fourth Trimester"—the first three months of life, which, he attests, would actually be spent in the womb if the human body were better designed to accommodate birth. But the brain is big, the human pelvis is small, and the result is that human babies, even term ones, are basically born three months premature. So, during these first three months, Karp suggests that the best way to keep babies happy is to mimic the conditions in the womb. *The Happiest Baby* says that crying, even the kind known as colic, can be soothed by triggering a baby's "off switch" or "calming reflex" by creating a womblike environment. Karp offers a simple (and cute, no less) plan involving a lot of S words—swaddling, shhhhing, sucking, and some other stuff. *Happiest Baby* is also available in DVD and video format for parents who want to see the five S's in action before trying them out on their own babies.

> I wish I had known about colicky babies. (Colic, for those who think it means some kind of intestinal problem, is actually just the medical term for "cries a lot for no apparent or understandable reason.") I knew babies cried, but I honestly didn't realize that some babies can literally cry for hours and keep crying even though you pick them up and hold them and soothe them and rock them and do everything you can think of to ease their distress. I felt like a terrible parent because I couldn't soothe my baby. Also, colicky babies tend to nap very little—I didn't understand why my baby napped so little, which left me exhausted.
>
> —anonymom

My second born screamed for about six months straight. It was emotionally draining. It was frustrating and upsetting. There wasn't much to do to comfort her or soothe her. It seemed like she would never stop.
—anonymom

spoiling a baby

There is a long-established, flawed belief that too much cuddling, carrying, and comforting can "spoil" a baby and lead to bad behavior later in life. Babies were meant to be held and comforted. The more comfort they get, the more they are reassured, the more trust they build and the more confident they can become later on. Babies are not grown-ups or grown children who may be crying for a whole range of complex reasons. They are not "manipulating you" in a malicious or calculating way. Crying is their only means of communication. Spoiling is something that happens to food left to rot. Not to a baby who is given deserved love and attention.

common patterns related to environment, feeding, gas, pooping, burping, and sleep. If patterns emerge, you may be able to alter some circumstances.

- See a lactation consultant for help if you are breastfeeding and your baby is often unhappy. Several breastfeeding problems such as a very large milk supply can be associated with colic and are easy to fix.

- Rule out other causes such as gastroesophageal reflux (GER) or food sensitivity. If crying coincides with feedings (spitting up, refusing to feed, watery or hard poops, crying after a feeding) or the baby has a rash, he may be sensitive to something in the formula or breast milk. → See Gastric Reflux, page 264, and Food Allergies and Intolerance, page 264.

- Go to your doctor (both parents and caregivers can attend) to discuss the situation. Let the doctor examine the baby so you can rule out any medical causes of crying.

- Try slower and more frequent feedings.

- Rub the baby's tummy while holding, or try holding the baby stomach down along the length of your arm, thigh, or a big ball: Pressure on the tummy, back rubbing, or some lulling movement can all help.

- Push baby's knees to his abdomen or move his legs in bicycle kicks to help get out any trapped gas.

- If your baby is comfortable in water, give her lots of warm baths—even if only for a few minutes at a time. Sitting with your baby—or breastfeeding—in the tub can be very soothing.

- Carry the baby against your chest in a baby carrier for as long as you can (or care to).

As for your care: Realize that this is **not your fault,** that it will pass; talk to other parents of colicky babies; and get as much help as you possibly can at all hours of the day. → See Emotional Landscape of Parenthood, page 188.

cord care

The cord area can be cleaned with a Q-tip dipped in alcohol, though there is research showing that it will actually heal faster if left alone. The leftover cord will probably fall off in a couple of weeks. Sometimes it can come off earlier due to accidental tugging. If this is the case, continue to clean with alcohol. There may be spots of bleeding on and off for a couple of weeks. A small amount of bleeding is normal. You can buy diapers with a cut-out or cut a space in the diaper so the cord isn't irritated and can "breathe" or try putting a

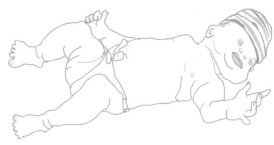

little gauze over the cord and under the diaper. You may see some yellow or green pus drainage at some point. If you notice excessive oozing, bleeding, or rawness, call your pediatrician. He or she may apply some silver nitrate to help dry and seal the cord area in order to promote healing, though this is rarely necessary. Call your doctor about any other signs of infection, including fever, foul-smelling discharge, or redness and/or soreness on the skin around the belly button.

cpr

An infant/child CPR class is by far the best way to learn CPR. You will learn not only lifesaving techniques (which are different for babies than for adults) but also what *not* to do, what the common hazards are, and lots of valuable and general safety information. Educate yourself and all other caretakers about everyday safety risks. → See Childproofing, page 354, for more about protecting your baby in your home.

cradle cap

Sometimes babies develop flaky, scaly skin on their scalp or eyebrows. It may be oily or dry, yellow or orange in hue. This is called cradle cap (officially, seborrheic dermatitis) and it is very common; it may last for a few weeks, months, or occasionally past the first year. Although it might look weird, it's not at all harmful and will go away on its own eventually. If cradle cap persists beyond 6 months and seems to be getting worse, your doctor may prescribe a special shampoo or scalp cream. Sometimes the same condition appears on the baby's skin, around creases, ears, or eyebrows.

> I used olive oil and a gentle fine-tooth comb to comb out the flakes. It worked wonders! But I did have to shampoo afterwards because his hair was so greasy.
> —anonymom

crying

It can be very hard for a new parent to hear a newborn cry. But crying is the only way the tiny, vulnerable baby can communicate with the world. Parents need time to appreciate a newborn's cry as the baby reaching out for care, not a sign of the kind of sadness adults associate with their own crying jags. This is not to say that babies cry for no reason or to strengthen their lungs (that's a myth). Babies cry because they need something. A big part of the learning curve for parents is figuring out what that need is. Some say they can instantly distinguish a hungry cry from a sleepy one (though this may be more about an awareness of the baby's feeding and sleeping habits than an ability to decode the timbre or tone of a particular wail). As babies get older, and parents get wiser, the mystery and stress surrounding every cry starts to lift.

Here are some common reasons a baby might cry and a few ideas about how to cope:

HUNGRY: Crying may be accompanied by rooting, sucking on hands. Milk or formula is the only thing that will help.

> I think she has finally discovered her voice (not in that Women's Studies 101 kind of way, though!) and as a result her cries are more frequent and louder.
> —anonymom

> With the first one, I was a complete mess. I had a nervous habit of singing "Ten Little Indians" super fast every time he cried.
> —anonymom

SLEEPY: A baby may cry because she needs help getting to sleep.

UNCOMFORTABLE: This can be about gas, being too hot or cold, or just a need for a change in position. Move her around, burp her, remove or add a layer of clothes. → See Burping, page 258.

OVERSTIMULATED: Most newborns have a low threshold for stimulation. Crowds, noise, visual stimulation, even eye contact can quickly overwhelm a very young baby.

NEEDS SOOTHING: It can be reassuring to get back to the familiar smells and sounds of Mom's body or another heartbeat. Sucking can be soothing; you can let them linger on the breast or offer a pacifier or a clean, short-nailed finger.

→ See Burping, page 258.
→ See *The Happiest Baby on the Block* by Harvey Karp, page 259.
→ See Feeding Your Baby, page 274.
→ See Sleep, page 332.

the pros and cons of pacifiers

PRO Babies like to suck. It "pacifies" them—calms them and, not insignificantly, keeps them quiet. The pacifier is in many ways a rather ingenious invention, giving the baby exactly what she wants without requiring a breast or a bottle (or a person attached to either). Many adults prefer pacifiers to thumb or finger sucking simply because a pacifier can be taken away. Pacifiers can also help tube-fed preemies develop sucking skills.

The AAP's 2005 sleep report says that pacifier use can help prevent SIDS and will not interfere with breastfeeding if introduced after nursing has been well established, after about a month. (Their breastfeeding recommendations, however, do not fully correspond.) The academy suggests that the pacifier can be put into the mouth as the baby falls asleep but should not be replaced if it falls out during the night. Most pacifier advocates suggest some kind of moderate use.

CON From a purely practical standpoint, pacifiers can introduce a bunch of new problems: lots of hunting, washing, rescuing, and reinserting. Some parents have huge bowls of them in every room to make sure they are always on hand. Some babies are very particular and will take only one, which can cause a lot of anxiety about protecting the precious pacifier. Many babies quickly become used to sucking on the pacifier in order to fall asleep. Even parents who strive for the recommended moderate use end up making lots of trips to the crib throughout the night in order to reinsert an accidentally ejected pacifier. Hygiene can be an issue. And pacifiers can introduce cavity germs as well as increase risk of crooked teeth in bottle-fed babies. Also, there's the matter of giving up the pacifier, which many babies, toddlers, and even little kids find very challenging. Some research shows that pacifiers put children at increased risk of ear infections. For safety reasons, the AAP recommends that parents use only one-piece pacifiers, yet most easily available pacifiers are two or more pieces.

Breastfeeding and Attachment Parenting advocates, including many doctors and sleep experts, believe that a breast/parent comfort substitute is not so great for the baby. They argue that babies need more than comfort sucking; they need to be held close to their parent, surrounded by their warmth, smell, breathing, voice, and so on. Some question the murky science behind the AAP conclusions on pacifiers and safety (wondering how breastfeeding and other factors relate or compare, for example). Constant pacifier use may also prevent a baby from exploring objects with his mouth or experimenting with sounds.

diaper rash

All babies get diaper rash from time to time. Moisture, friction, and a sealed diaper can cause redness and rawness. Tender skin is more vulnerable to bacteria, which can make the rash worse. Diaper rash is uncomfortable for the baby but it can be controlled very quickly with regular rinsing in plain water and liberal use of diaper rash cream.

PREVENTING DIAPER RASH: Change wet diapers frequently and change soiled diapers immediately. Clean the area thoroughly with unscented wipes or water. Use diaper rash cream on sensitive spots (around anus, anywhere else that tends to redden).

TREATING DIAPER RASH: Blot or rinse (don't wipe) the area with water. Let some air in by letting the baby lie on a waterproof pad with no diaper on for a little while. Use rash cream generously.

diapers: cloth vs. disposable

Disposable diapers are convenient, but they do pile up on the planet. Cloth diapers are considered the more environmentally sound choice, though cleaning them requires detergents, water, and energy. New, biodegradable disposables are being developed to help minimize environmental impact. Cloth diapers are less expensive if you wash them yourself, but the cost evens out somewhat if you use a service (or take into account the wear and tear on your appliances).

cloth **pros**

- Use less landfill space.
- Soft on baby's skin.
- Convenient cloth diapers offer Velcro attachments or thicker middle sections.

cloth **cons**

- Babies needs to be changed very soon after wetting or soiling.
- You need to remove poops and deal with cleaning the diapers (or getting them cleaned).

disposable **pros**

- Can stay on baby longer (since liquid is "drawn" away from skin).
- Often come with pictures of cartoon characters.
- Have less poop-bottom contact.
- Sometimes perfumed to disguise smells.

"When your baby wakes up in the middle of the night, you don't need to change her diaper (unless some number two is involved of course)." That, while common sense, was the best advice I had ever heard.
—anonymom

263

disposable **cons**

- Use more landfill space (less so for biodegradables).
- Often come with pictures of cartoon characters.
- Require some trash routine (plastic bags or diaper-disposal trash cans and liners).
- Perfume-disguised smells may prevent a timely diaper change.

food allergies and intolerance

Cow's-milk protein allergy is relatively common in babies. Usually changes in the breastfeeding mother's diet or the baby's formula are recommended. Some premature babies may have a temporary lactose intolerance. This goes away over time and can actually be treated by feeding the baby breast milk. Otherwise, lactose intolerance is very rare in infants. Galactosemia is an extremely rare metabolic disorder (1 in 62,000 babies), in which a baby is born unable to metabolize lactose and, therefore, unable to process human milk (or any milk).

→ See Do I Have to Watch My Diet?, page 296.

→ See Choosing a Formula, page 322.

→ See Starting Solids, page 328.

gastric reflux

Gastroesophageal reflux (sometimes called GER, GERD, or just reflux) is a condition caused by a weak lower esophageal sphincter, the valve connecting the esophagus to the stomach. Affected babies have a hard time swallowing and keeping down milk. A baby with reflux might fuss during feedings, arch her back, and/or wake frequently. A baby with bad reflux may be really uncomfortable and cry a lot—undiagnosed reflux may be behind some of the crying identified as colic. Reflux is not always easy to diagnose. Other signs, which may or may not be present, include wheezing, coughing, and other throat sounds. While mild reflux is common in young babies (many newborns have undeveloped esophageal sphincters), severe reflux is much less so. If your baby has symptoms of reflux, your doctor can help you determine if any treatment is needed. Symptoms usually go away within the first year, as the muscles develop and strengthen. If breastfeeding is a problem, a lactation consultant can look at the baby and help you come up with feeding strategies.

some tips for feeding a baby with reflux

- Give frequent, small feedings.
- Feed in an upright position and keep the baby upright after feedings.
- Ensure regular burping.
- Speak to your doctor about various medications commonly prescribed for severe reflux.

genitals

Baby girls may have a little normal clear/white vaginal discharge that doesn't require cleaning. It is common and normal for a baby girl to bleed a tiny amount from her vagina in the first few days. Any other buildup of secretions or diaper cream around the labia can be gently wiped (front to back) with a cotton ball soaked in warm water. Baby boy parts can be rinsed. If there is no circumcision, just wash the base of the penis (do not pull back the foreskin).

CIRCUMCISION CARE: The doctor or mohel performing your son's circumcision will advise you about how to care for it as it heals. The circumcision site should be protected with petroleum jelly or another lubricating ointment at each diaper change. It usually takes about a week for the site to heal. Watch the area for signs of infection, which include swelling, redness, and pus.

hiccups

. . . happen a lot. You can wait them out, or try feeding the baby from the breast or bottle.

jaundice

Mild jaundice occurs normally in baby mammals. A baby with jaundice will have a yellowish tint to her skin and the whites of her eyes. This is because babies are born with extra red blood cells that the newborn liver can't process fast enough, which creates the yellow pigment (bilirubin). Your pediatrician will check for jaundice at birth—if it seems more than normal, blood tests and treatment with phototherapy may be used. Jaundice is rarely dangerous, unless the baby is not getting enough to eat or is breaking down blood cells faster than usual. Breastfed babies tend to remain jaundiced for a little bit longer than formula-fed babies, maybe up to (or beyond) 3 weeks after birth. Parents are occasionally advised to stop breastfeeding for 24—48 hours to lower bilirubin levels in a baby with prolonged jaundice, but most of the time no interruption in breastfeeding is necessary.

kangaroo care

"Kangaroo care" involves placing a premature baby against a parent's bare chest (with the baby's ear over the adult's heart). In many countries, kangaroo care is continuous, but in the United States most hospitals allow only short periods of contact. Studies have shown both physical and psychological benefits for baby and parent. If your baby is in the NICU, talk to your doctor and the nurses about kangaroo care. Policy often requires that the baby be stable and breathing on her own, but sometimes the baby can be held while still monitored/getting oxygen.

multiples

If caring for one baby is a lot of work, is caring for multiples that much work times two (or three, or more)? Often yes, according to parents of multiples, but the systems and techniques that parents of more than one learn by necessity may actually make some things go more smoothly. Parents of twins-plus often develop routines that allow them to feed their babies and get them to sleep fairly efficiently, simply because if they don't, things will quickly devolve into total chaos. Multiple babies sometimes learn to soothe themselves more easily than single ones since they may have to wait for a parent's attention. Still, multiples are more mouths to feed and more needs to tend to. And multiple babies are more likely to be born prematurely and have medical issues that require more frequent care. Many parents of twins or more say that the first few months and even years may be a lot more difficult than with single babies, but after that, the payoff is great. Not only do multiples provide parents with multiplied benefits, they also provide each other with entertainment.

Although it might be difficult when your babies are tiny, they will definitely begin to express their unique desires and sensibilities as independent babies as well as part of a package deal. Parents of twins and books and sites on the subject can give specific advice about making life with twins as simple as possible. → See Parenting Multiples resources, page 374.

> I haven't had much one-on-one time with each baby so I didn't experience that ideal mother-child relationship full of tenderness; you know, looking into your baby's eyes, watching for cues, bonding deeply from the get-go. Sure, I'm now deeply bonded to my children but not the way I had expected. I was always so busy with baby maintenance, always so preoccupied with remembering everything I needed to do for them.
> —anonymom

> My parenting style is different from what it probably would have been with one. I'm a very laissez-faire type of person. If I had one, I probably wouldn't have imposed a schedule on the baby, we may have coslept. But with two, I've become a real control freak.
> —anonymom

> We got them on a schedule ASAP. Naps in the crib (so they don't sleep in the stroller, which means less flexibility), meals at the same time every day, etc.
> —anonymom

> I have yet to read a book that was helpful, and most twin parents don't have time anyway. When in a crisis or a situation, it's much faster to call another twin parent.... Parents most definitely benefit from a support network.
> —anonymom

> Scheduling is absolutely more important with twins, since if they're not in sync, then the parents never get any downtime.
> —anonymom

nails

Babies' nails grow very fast and since newborns have very little limb control, they tend to scratch themselves on a regular basis. The scratches heal quickly, but to prevent them, try trimming the nails often (about once a week or more) with baby nail clippers, a file, or by gently tearing the long nail off with your fingers or teeth. Some find this easier to do while the baby is sleeping. Try to avoid leaving sharp edges by clipping the pointy sides off first. Don't forget toes.

nicu

If your baby needs special care or observation for any reason, he will be brought to the Neonatal Intensive Care Unit (NICU) after birth. Having a baby in the NICU can be shocking and challenging. The hectic, impersonal atmosphere of the hospital can make parents feel isolated from their newborn. And the anxiety about your baby's health can be overwhelming. But advances in neonatal medicine have made it possible for babies with a wide range of issues to thrive with NICU care. Here are a few ideas that may help you cope:

GET SUPPORT: Ideally the NICU staff will be excellent when it comes to offering support and guidance, though some are better than others. Don't be afraid to talk openly about any anxieties you have. Parents sometimes develop strong bonds with the people who care for their newborn in the NICU.

GET INFORMED: Get to know the people involved in your baby's care and let them all know that you want to be informed and involved. Learn as much as you can from nurses and staff about baby care. This will help you feel confident when the time comes to care for your baby at home. Some recommend writing things down since you may get a lot of new and detailed information in a short time.

VENT: Share your stories in a support group (some hospitals provide these) or go online.

TAKE CARE OF YOURSELF: Try not to feel guilty for getting rest and going home—your strength is important for the baby.

BOND (BUT DON'T FREAK OUT ABOUT BONDING): Do what you can to feel connected to your baby. Sing to her, speak to her, touch her, hold her (see "Kangaroo Care," page 265), participate in weighing the baby, tube feedings, etc. Building a bond with your baby can help build your confidence. But also remember that bonding is a gradual process. As the baby grows stronger, so will the bond.

→ See Feeding a Baby in the **NICU**, page 288.

→ See Preterm Babies, page 269.

I cried a lot. My baby was in the NICU and I just couldn't stop crying. Every time I went in there I wept uncontrollably (and he was by far the healthiest infant in the room).
—anonymom

I have spoken to a few other preemie moms—it was something they discouraged in the NICU because NICU parents tend to compare their babies' status to the point where it can be really upsetting to one or the other parties.
—anonymom

The social worker for the NICU wouldn't give us the time of day, which at the time really irritated me, but looking back on it, there were parents there who needed her services much more than we did. There are a few websites/message boards dedicated to parents of preemies, but I found them to be a little hokey and religious.
—anonymom

peeing

Day 1:	About 1 wet diaper
After week 1:	About 5—6 sopping wet diapers a day

Three tablespoons of water poured into a clean diaper offers an indication of what a sopping wet diaper feels like. More frequent wet diapers may be less soaked. Since today's diapers are superabsorbent, they may feel dry by the time you touch them. Putting a piece of tissue or cotton in a diaper may help you make a better assessment. Newborn babies should have clear, basically odorless pee. Darker urine, or reddish colored dust (urate crystals) in the diaper are normal for breastfed babies in the early days (while milk is coming in), but beyond that they may suggest a hydration problem.

playgroups/mommy and me

Activities for infants are becoming increasingly popular, though it's not clear how important they are to the infants themselves. Babies don't really have a lot of peer interaction in the early months. And though classes may tell you they'll turn your baby into a genius, your child's intelligence will not be defined by his infant coursework. Parents, on the other hand, might really appreciate having somewhere to go with their baby and finding other parents to talk to. Classes and playgroups can help build a routine or just give you a chance to look at a range of other parents and babies in action. This can be good for both of you. They can also provide opportunities for comparing yourself and your baby to others, which can be not so good. Classes are optional. If you like them, great. If not, don't feel like you're missing out on anything important.

pooping

Day 1:	Sticky, dark, tarlike meconium
Days 2—3:	A few greenish brown transitional poops, sometimes bright green, full of curds and explosive
Day 4+:	3—4 dirty diapers a day, each poop larger than a quarter. Poop turns a kind of mustard yellow or orange color, is somewhat runny with what look like little seeds or curds in it (breastfeeding) or runny and tan to yellow (formula feeding).
After 6 weeks:	Breastfed babies can have anywhere from many poops a day to a few poops a week. Formula-fed babies should have slightly bigger tan/brown poops more frequently (about once a day by 3—6 weeks).

All babies make their first poop—dark, black or green meconium—within the first couple of days. Even though meconium is pretty gnarly stuff (hard to wash out, very sticky and tarlike), parents and pediatricians are usually happy to see it because it signals that the baby's digestive system is ready for something other than colostrum. If a baby doesn't pass meconium, there may be a bowel obstruction (this is very uncommon).

DIARRHEA AND CONSTIPATION: Constipation is more common in formula-fed babies. A lack of fluid is a common cause and a few drinks of water can help. Most loose stools are from diet, not infection. If a formula-fed baby has diarrhea, especially if it comes with any vomiting or fever, he may have gastro-enteritis and should be taken to a doctor right away. If your baby has very watery poops, very hard poops, or very few poops, talk to your doctor.

positional plagiocephaly (flattened head)

Positional plagiocephaly is the flattening of the back or one side of the baby's head. It's "positional" because it's caused either by the intrauterine position or by being placed in one position (on the back or with the head to one side) preferentially. It can be prevented or reversed (especially within the first six months) by alternating the position of the baby's head when she sleeps and giving her time on her tummy when she's awake. If you notice a flattening of your baby's head, talk to your pediatrician. In rare cases a corrective helmet or headband may be recommended.

preterm babies

About one in eight babies in America is born preterm. Because premature babies' organs may not be fully developed, they are at risk of medical complications, such as infection, anemia, low blood pressure, difficulty breathing, and intestinal problems. Babies born very prematurely face the greatest risks. By 28—31 weeks, there's a 90 to 95 percent survival rate, and the likelihood of long-term problems is reduced. Babies born after 34 weeks have little risk of serious complications. Premature babies often spend time in the Neonatal Intensive Care Unit (NICU), a facility equipped to deal with the specific needs of premature and low-birth-weight infants. → See NICU, page 267.

When your baby comes earlier than expected, it can be shocking. Your first days as a parent, hovering around an incubator, might not bear much resemblance to your fantasies. And your baby may not look the way you imagined him. He may have thin, reddish purple skin. Due to underdeveloped muscle tone and nerves, he may not curl up and move around like a full-term baby. These things are totally normal for his age and will change over time. Talking to the NICU staff about your baby's appearance can be reassuring.

For the first two to three years of life, preterm babies are measured by adjusted or corrected age, taking into account the date they were due as well as the date they were born. Because premature babies had less

I'm sure every parent has a fear that their baby will stop breathing in the middle of the night. Multiply that by a thousand, and that's how I felt [with a preemie]. I slept in her room for the first few months.

—anonymom

The scary start really threw me off—I am (or I should say *was*) a really compulsive person . . . I had a 6-worksheet Excel spreadsheet listing everything I would need to buy (prices, stores, etc.), everyone who would need to be informed of her birth, address listings for announcements, emergency contact list, etc. Everything was meticulously planned—but you know what they say about the best-laid plans. . . . That was the smack-in-the-face lesson I got at the beginning of parenthood that made me realize that nowadays it's all about flexibility. I think learning that has really helped me as a parent. . . . If everything with my pregnancy/delivery had gone as planned, I think we both would have been a lot more rigid.

—anonymom

time to grow in utero, they may not develop at the same pace as full-term babies. A 6-month-old baby who was born 2 months early may be developmentally closer to a 4-month-old full-term baby. Premature babies often need more time before they can sleep well, take big feedings, or concentrate for more than a few seconds. They sometimes have a hard time regulating body temperature and can easily be overstimulated.

A lot of extra support can really help as you try to juggle the demands of work, life, doctors' appointments, and feedings. Though every baby develops in her own way, other parents of preterm babies can be a source of comfort as well as a lot of specific information.

→ See Difficult/High-Need/Demanding/"Hurting"/Hard Babies, page 198.
→ See Kangaroo Care, page 265.
→ See Multiples, page 266.
→ See Breastfeeding a Premature Baby, page 289.

rashes

Diaper rash is the most common baby rash. Newborns may get a harmless rash that looks like flea bites in the first weeks of life. Babies also sometimes get a rash when they're overheated (known as heat rash or prickly heat). This rash appears as small bumps (sometimes red) in areas where he's likely to be particularly hot: under clothes or in skin crevices. Heat rash is most common in summer and in babies with fevers. Other rashes may indicate food sensitivities, allergies, or eczema or can be symptoms of common childhood illnesses. Call your doctor if your baby has a rash that you can't identify.

→ See Diaper Rash, page 263, and Meet Your Newborn, page 164.

routine and consistency

Both of these clichés are true: Babies are creatures of habit. Babies are very adaptable. Consistency can help babies know what to expect, and therefore feel safe and secure. If the baby knows, for example, that pjs and *Goodnight Moon* mean bedtime, he may be more at ease with the idea of letting go and going to sleep. But routine doesn't necessarily mean adhering to a tight schedule (and freaking out if there is any tiny change). There are many ways to build and maintain familiar associations for the baby without looking at a stopwatch: your smells, the warmth of a bath, a flickering light in the nursery. Familiar feelings are comforting, even if they don't come at the exact same time each day. Building some flexibility into a routine can make it easier on both of you when inevitable interruptions occur. The need for order can change as a baby gets older or goes through a particularly insecure time (such as when they are trying new things). → See Sorting Through the Voices: Everybody's Got an Opinion, page 363.

safety

→ See Sleep Safety, page 336.
→ See Childproofing, page 353.

shaken baby syndrome (sbs)

Shaking a baby violently can result in brain damage or death. Even a few seconds of violent shaking can be dangerous. According to both the AAP and the National Center on Shaken Baby Syndrome, brain injuries are generally caused by an aggressive back-and-forth motion, most often resulting from an adult's frustration with a baby's behavior (typically, inconsolable crying). Playful bouncing, jiggling, tossing, and jogging with a baby do not cause SBS. If you're feeling extremely tense and angry about your baby's crying, it is often recommended that you put your baby down in a safe place and walk away to give yourself a chance to regain composure.

spitting up

It's common for babies to spit up a little bit after a feeding. The baby may have eaten too fast, taken a little too much milk (and/or air) in at once. If your baby spits up all the time, or vomits, talk to your doctor to rule out reflux.

→ See Gastric Reflux, page 264, for more.

to reduce spit-ups, try

- **Good burping**
- **Smaller, more frequent feedings**
- **Calm and uninterrupted feedings**

sudden infant death syndrome

According to the SIDS Alliance:

"SUDDEN INFANT DEATH SYNDROME is the sudden, unexpected death of an apparently healthy infant under one year of age that remains unexplained after the performance of a complete postmortem investigation, including an autopsy, an examination of the scene of death and a review of the medical history."

SIDS affects about 1 in 2,000 babies, according to the National Center for Health Statistics. Even though the chances of a baby dying from SIDS are therefore only about .057 percent, most parents can't help but worry about SIDS at some point . . . or fifteen times a night. Most SIDS deaths happen between one and four months of age. Ninety percent take place before 6 months. Some risk factors include smoking parents, baby sleeping on stomach, prematurity, low birth weight, and a family history of SIDS. There are lots of theories about the cause of SIDS, none proven. One current popular theory is that SIDS is related to a problem with the brain's arousal system. While researchers continue to search for a conclusive cause, the most effective effort toward reducing the threat of SIDS has been the aggressive Back to Sleep campaign, launched in 1994 in the United States. As a result of public awareness about back sleeping, SIDS deaths in the United States have declined more than 50 percent.

→ See The Extreme Vulnerability of a Newborn Baby, page 199.

→ See Sleep Safety, page 336.

→ For more info, see sidsalliance.com.

swaddling

Many newborns (though not all!) like being wrapped up securely. Maybe it's because they're used to being cozy in the womb, or maybe it's because it keeps them from flailing around or smacking themselves in the face when they haven't developed motor control. Swaddling is a little tricky to learn but very easy once you know how. Hospital nurses can bundle babies like burritos with their eyes closed. Sometimes dads become the swaddling experts because they're freer to look over the nurse's shoulders. Here's the most commonly used swaddling technique:

Wrap the baby up snugly, but be sure the swaddle is not so tight that the baby's breathing is restricted.

teething

Teething usually starts between 3 and 7 months and can continue through toddlerhood. Signs that your baby is teething include drooling, swollen or puffy gums (maybe even teeth coming through), fussing, night waking, and gnawing or biting (of fingers, toys, you). Babies will teethe on whatever they can get their hands on. If you want to, you can try (chilled) teething rings. Talk to your doctor if you want to give pain medication including teething gels. Teething pain varies from child to child, and tooth to tooth; it may cause mild diarrhea and/or a low-grade fever (less than 101).

vaccinations

Vaccines have saved countless lives, but they've also provoked a lot of controversy. Almost all doctors believe vaccines are a crucial part of maintaining children's health on an individual and a societal level. Many see vaccination as a social responsibility, everyone doing their fair share to keep dangerous diseases at bay. The current rarity of many diseases may make vaccinations seem irrelevant, but it's vaccinations that have made them so rare. The effects of vaccines are not limited to the individual. If a child who hasn't been vaccinated against rubella contracts the disease, he'll likely be fine, but the unborn sibling his mother is carrying may not be.

Those who question vaccines see them as an unnecessary burden on a young baby's vulnerable immune system, which may lead to disorders or disease. There has been a lot of recent anxiety about a possible link between the MMR (measles, mumps, and rubella) vaccine and autism, suggested by a 1998 study that was later largely retracted. Still, some believe that such a link exists. They also question whether the vaccine industry is providing parents with all the facts. The most controversial ingredient in vaccines is thimerosal, which contains mercury. Since mercury is a toxic element even at low doses, this has been a cause for major concern among child health activists. Although thimerosal use has not been banned as many would like, "thimerosal-free" versions of many vaccines are now available. Some pediatricians offer these by default. Others will do so on request. And some won't, because they do not think there is any danger associated with the thimerosal in standard vaccines.

Vaccines do carry some risk of side effects. Most people firmly believe that the risks are far less serious than the risks of not vaccinating, on an individual as well as a broader scale. But some feel that the arguments against vaccination are scary enough to avoid them. Other parents make compromises by stretching out the vaccination schedule to delay shots or limit the number of vaccines their children receive at once. If you're interested in exploring options beyond the immunization schedule recommended by the Centers for Disease Control (CDC), be sure your pediatrician is okay with this. Some doctors are flexible about vaccines, and some are not.

feeding your baby

choices and considerations

Breast? Bottle? Both? What's the big deal? *"It's just food."* Actually, feeding can be hugely complex. It's more than nutrition. There are logistics and costs and science and stigmas to be taken into account. A few considerations are easy to pick apart into pros and cons; many are much less obvious and far more personal.

Feeding may not be an either/or proposition. Parents who feed only breast milk or only formula are in the minority; most babies are fed a combo of the two in their first year of life. But you should definitely give the matter some thought before your baby's born. Switching from breastfeeding to formula is easy enough, but switching from formula to breastfeeding is not.

Some people are dead set on the way they want to feed their babies (though they may need help to make it happen). Others are torn. This chapter lays out the options, facts, and issues so you can filter them through your own priorities and make a decision that works for you.

I chose to bottle-feed. My husband and relatives could help, which in return meant I was more active and not a walking zombie. My boys are happy, healthy, and wise. *You're* the mom and you do what you want. Your children will be fantastic!
—anonymom

Most of my friends and family didn't breastfeed because they couldn't stand the pain of it. So, they're all surprised that I did. And one friend doesn't understand it because she never did it. She just thinks it's so "primal."
—anonymom

I was convinced I would *not* breastfeed for more than a week, but I vowed to give it a try. It's now been six months. . . . It was a lot easier than I imagined.
—anonymom

I loved breastfeeding and would recommend that every new mom give an honest attempt to do so. However, it is hard to start and not every woman wants to do it (or her husband doesn't want her to do it). But, you cannot tell in a room full of your friends or colleagues who was breastfed and who wasn't, so whatever decision works best for mom and baby is fine.
—anonymom

I definitely wanted to breastfeed. That was the goal. But I got a bad start on so many levels and I think because there were several things going against me that it just didn't work. I tried everything, but the stress was getting to be too much and my milk wasn't coming in. My son was losing weight; we weren't feeding him enough.
—anonymom

what's **great** about breastfeeding . . .

- Biologically best food for babies
- Many health benefits for baby
  → See Benefits Breakdown, page 277.
- Many health benefits for mom
  → See Benefits Breakdown, page 277.
- Changing tastes in milk from mom's diet may promote acceptance of a variety of flavors in solid food.
- Hormones can help mom relax and bond, help with stress.
- Helps shrink uterus to prepregnancy size
- May reduce effect of pollutant exposure in utero
- Burns calories, may promote quicker weight loss
- Physical proximity can encourage closeness.
- Forced "downtime"
- Giant boobs
- Inexpensive
- Convenient, portable, never needs heating or sterilization
- More digestible

what **sucks** about breastfeeding . . .

- Can be painful and difficult in the beginning
- More complicated for others to feed baby
- More complicated for working moms
- Mom's diet can possibly affect baby.
- Very limited margaritas
- Not all medications are compatible with breastfeeding.
- Some level of organic pollutants
- Public breastfeeding can be stressful.
- Hormones can make mom tired during feedings.
- Boobs become the baby's territory.
- Forced "downtime"
- Physical proximity can limit mobility.
- Giant boobs
- More digestible milk may mean more feedings.
- Leaky boobs can be messy.

some other things to **think** about

- If you're thinking of not breastfeeding because you think it will save your boobs from sagging, you're out of luck. Sagging is primarily the result of pregnant boob swelling (and deflating), not of breastfeeding.

- If you're thinking of not breastfeeding because of squeamishness or weirdness about using your breasts in a functional way, or having other people see you breastfeed, please see "Public Opinion: Attitudes About Breastfeeding" (page 313) for a deeper look at these issues.

When asked if I was going to breastfeed, I always said that I was going to try. I knew from hearing from friends/family that it wasn't an easy thing, and I didn't know exactly what to expect. Not to mention, I wasn't sure if I was going to physically be able to. I thought that my inverted nipple was going to be an issue. Then my first goal was to make it to six weeks, then to six months, and now my son is eight months and I'm having a hard time with the thought of weaning!

—anonymom

I think people put too much stress on breastfeeding. Yes it's nice if you can do it, but I was made to feel like I was harming my baby by stopping. I also felt so guilty, because everyone says it's best for the baby, and I felt like my baby would immediately get sick once I stopped. I felt like a terrible mother. But I was so miserable breastfeeding, that it was making me resent my baby. I was a much happier person once I started formula-feeding. I wish people would just realize that breastfeeding is not for everyone and that giving a baby formula is not going to slow down your baby's development or make him/her sick. My baby is actually much happier on formula and so am I.

—anonymom

what's **great** about bottle-feeding . . .

- More physical freedom
- Other people can feed the baby=more bonding for others.
- Diet unaffected by feeding
- Margarita intake unaffected by feeding
- Medications don't interfere with feeding (most medications are compatible with breastfeeding).
- No pumping is required.
- Takes longer to digest than breast milk/can mean less frequent feedings

what **sucks** about bottle-feeding . . .

- Fewer health benefits for baby
- Fewer health benefits for mom
- Expensive
- Sterilizing equipment required, etc.
- Prep/cleanup time longer
- No immune boosters
- Initial pain from engorgement
- Harder to digest than breast milk; may cause digestion problems
- Moms miss out on calorie burning of milk production
- Risk of bacterial/chemical contaminants from water, bottle, formula
- Does not help uterus return to normal size
- Formula goes bad after 1 hour at room temperature.

breastfeeding: benefits breakdown

Breastfeeding is good for babies and good for moms. But just how good is it? Many benefits have been proven through thorough research, but some oft-cited advantages of breastfeeding are not as definitive as others.

Here's a list of the proven (or probable) benefits of breastfeeding, as well as a few that are more controversial or difficult to quantify. Please keep in mind that future studies may have an impact on this list.

benefits for **babies** . . .

- Fewer infections in the middle ear, upper respiratory system, and gastrointestinal tract
- Less diarrhea and constipation
- Faster recovery from sickness
- Boosted immune system
- Improved response to vaccinations
- For premature babies: reduced NICU time, increased protection from illness
- Reduced chance of diabetes and obesity later in life
- Lowered risk of SIDS
- Less colic
- Reduced risk of allergies, asthma, and eczema, need for tonsils out
- Strengthened facial muscles, perhaps reducing future need for orthodontic treatment

benefits for **moms** . . .

- Decreased postpartum bleeding, more rapid uterine involution
- Reduced chance of postpartum hemorrhage
- Earlier return to prepregnancy weight
- Decreased risk of premenopausal breast, ovarian, and uterine cancer
- Lower risk of hip fractures and osteoporosis later on
- Relaxation while breastfeeding

is the **bottle** half-empty or half-full?

If breastfeeding has health benefits, does that mean *not* breastfeeding has health risks? The argument against focusing on the downsides of formula is that it will just make a lot of formula-feeding parents feel anxious and guilty. Formula is also a zillion-dollar business with its own interests at heart (and promoting breastfeeding isn't one of them). It's hard to say whether thinking in terms of formula's risks rather than breast milk's "perks" would change how we all feel about our various feeding options. What is clear is that parents should have all the facts before deciding which feeding method to pursue, and then feel supported once they've made their choice.

and a few more controversial benefits . . .

HIGHER IQ FOR BABIES: Studies have pointed to slightly higher IQs in breastfed babies. Some people question whether these studies effectively control for various interfering factors, and other research suggests no IQ boost.

STRESS RELIEF FOR MOMS: Some say breastfeeding mothers are more relaxed. Research indicates that hormones released during breastfeeding can reduce a mother's stress levels. But not everyone finds this to be true in practice.

INCREASED BONDING: The skin-to-skin contact and cuddling necessary for exclusive breastfeeding can certainly help build a bond between mother and baby. But it's arguable that a similar physical connection can be achieved in a bottle-feeding relationship as well, if a parent makes it a priority.

where we are now

Breastfeeding is more popular now than at any time since formula became widely available. The AAP has been steadily increasing their endorsement of breastfeeding in recent years. Their 2005 policy recommends breastfeeding "for at least the first year of life and beyond for as long as mutually desired by mother and child." According to CDC data, in 2004, more than 70 percent of women attempted breastfeeding. But only 17 percent were still breastfeeding at one year.

A (VERY) BRIEF HISTORY OF BABY FEEDING

- Clay bottles found circa 3,500 BCE.
- 1 C.E. Jesus is breastfed. Extended breastfeeding is common.
- **MIDDLE AGES:** Babies are commonly breastfed for two to three years. Taboos about women's bodies (no sex during breastfeeding) encourage aristocrats to send babies to wet nurses for suckling.
- **1600S:** In Europe breastfeeding is discouraged, as it "spoilt the figure," was "noisome to one's clothes," and "interfered with gadding about." Sick infants fed directly from goat's teat. First breast pump invented.
- **1700S:** French aristocracy thinks breastfeeding is bad for mother's health, body, and ability to produce heirs. Wet-nursing continues. Only 10 percent of Parisian babies nursed by own moms.

- Bacterial infection from container-feeding leads to soaring infant mortality rate. Campaign begins to encourage breastfeeding. In England, Mary Wollstonecraft urges moms to breastfeed.
- **1800S:** Condensed and evaporated milk means baby can get cow's milk without access to actual cow. Pasteurization (invented in 1860) greatly improves safety of milk, but distribution is slow. Infant mortality still high. Wet nursing on the wane.
- **EARLY 1900S:** Most U.S. women breastfeed. Strict feeding schedules introduced. Infrequent feeding leads to low supply for many moms; new formulas flood market. Breast pumps, bottles, nipples in 1902 Sears, Roebuck catalogue.

- **1940–1960S:** Formula feeding on rise, along with women in the work force. Strict breastfeeding schedules now considered unhealthy: "demand" feeding introduced.
- **1972:** Formula embraced by feminists seeking freedom from traditional female roles. Only 22 percent of U.S. moms attempt to breastfeed.
- **LATE 1970S:** New research, "back-to-breast" movement, and growing La Leche League all raise awareness about breastfeeding. In 1978, the American Academy of Pediatrics announces that exclusive breastfeeding is ideal for the first 4 to 6 months. Breastfeeding rates begin a slow climb.

New moms get a lot of mixed messages about how to feed their babies. It's sometimes less a matter of choice than a matter of circumstance. Some examples:

- The all-time low point for breastfeeding in America was around the time our moms were having kids, so many breastfeeding women can't turn to their own mothers for support.

- Pumping in the workplace requires space and time—not much, but more than some jobs allow. Many (maybe even most) moms have work environments that make breast-feeding difficult or impossible.

- Nursing is not very common in public or in the media, so women feel weird doing it.

- Doctors' advice and/or hospital policy may not be ideal for breastfeeding. So when a new mother wants to breastfeed, she may find that her efforts are thwarted by bad advice she gets along the way. → See Doctors and Breastfeeding, page 293.

- Breastfeeding can complicate extended (and extensive) family child care that many women rely on.

When we give mothers misinformation, minimal support, and make it hard for moms to breastfeed and do the other things they need to do, it doesn't seem so much like a "personal choice." Hopefully as our culture relearns what it takes to breastfeed (and changes policies accordingly), women will be free to actually make choices instead of getting pushed into them by crappy circumstances. But until that happens (and even when it does), remember, what you feed your baby doesn't make or break you as a parent.

> My mom wasn't very supportive in the beginning. We were all formula fed, so she just didn't understand it. She kept thinking he wasn't getting enough to eat because he was hungry so often. She eventually came around once I explained how it all worked.
> —anonymom

> I was a formula-fed baby, my mother kept reminding me, and turned out fine. Stop anytime, she would say.
> —anonymom

> [My mom] was actually okay but made lots of comments like "The breastfeeding is okay but I hate to see you work so hard. You should give yourself a break" (i.e., formula).
> —anonymom

> It's so annoying that breastfeeding is described in terms of "success" and "failure": "Were you successful at breastfeeding?" or "Did you *fail* to produce enough milk?"
> —anonymom

resources

At the Breast: Ideologies of Breastfeeding and Motherhood in the Contemporary United States by Linda M. Blum (fascinating history of modern infant feeding trends and ideas)

Fresh Milk: The Secret Life of Breasts by Fiona Giles (collection of stories about breastfeeding)

Milk, Money, and Madness: The Culture and Politics of Breastfeeding by Naomi Baumslag, M.D., and Dia L. Michels (a history of infant feeding with an emphasis on the rise of the formula business)

Mother's Milk: Breastfeeding Controversies in American Culture by Bernice L. Hausman (a look at cultural issues surrounding breastfeeding)

The pollutants in milk are troubling, but, apart from women who for some reason have been exposed to very high levels of dangerous chemicals, the health benefits of nursing far outweigh the potential hazards. So, even allowing for the problem of persistent organic pollutants, breastfeeding is a better alternative than formula.

—Dr. Gina Solomon, M.D., M.P.H., senior scientist at Natural Resources Defense Council (nrdc.org)

Babies get most of their pollutant burden during pregnancy. Even though breastfed babies are exposed to a small increase in pollutants, they actually suffer far fewer effects of having toxins. In other words, breastfeeding has a mitigating effect on our polluted world.

—Catherine Watson Genna, B.S., I.B.C.L.C.

resources

Having Faith by Sandra Steingraber

MOMS (Making Our Milk Safe) website: safemilk.org

Natural Resources Defense Council: nrdc.org

toxic milk?

There have been a number of disturbing reports in recent years about the presence of toxic chemicals in breast milk. These environmental pollutants get into us through the air and water, the products we use, and the food we eat. Because many chemicals are fat soluble, they accumulate in our fat stores over time and are drawn out when we nurse our babies. This is obviously concerning. But is the presence of these toxins a reason not to breastfeed? The answer, from child-safety advocates and environmental experts alike, is no.

The fetus has already been exposed to toxins in utero. Some studies suggest that breastfeeding may actually have a protective effect against any damage from these chemicals. It's also important to note that although formula contains much lower levels of the persistent organic pollutants found in breast milk, it may contain other toxins. Formula may contain higher levels of heavy metals like aluminum, cadmium, manganese, and lead. Soy formulas contain high levels of phytoestrogens (see page 66 for more info). When formula is mixed with water, it passes on the chemical contaminants found in the water supply. Since regulation of bottled water is less strict than tap water, bottled water may actually contain higher levels of pollutants. There are also questions about the safety of the polycarbonate plastic used in many baby bottles.

The real question is not whether breast milk or formula is safer. The science clearly favors breast milk. Here are some better questions: Why is there no way to feed our babies without subjecting them to some manner of chemical contamination? Why must our babies pay the price for the "Do it now and ask questions later" mentality of the modern industrial age? And what can we do about it?

We need to let people know that while breast milk is still the healthiest food for our babies, continuing to pollute our milk is not okay. It is possible to make a difference. European regulation of flame retardants, for example, has successfully (and rapidly) reduced levels of these toxins in breast milk. The United States needs to follow suit; our levels are climbing.

→ For more on toxins in utero, see Fear of a Toxic Planet, page 72.

We strongly emphasize that the mere presence of an environmental chemical in human milk does not indicate that a health risk exists for breastfed infants.... All information gathered to date supports the positive health value of breastfeeding for infants.

—Cheston M. Berlin, Jr., M.D., Penn State University professor of pediatrics and pharmacology

"breastfeeding nazis"

Consider this scenario: A struggling nursing mom reaches out for help. Instead of getting straightforward advice, she gets an earful about the seemingly endless benefits of breastfeeding and the undeniable risks of formula-feeding. The problem isn't the unarguably true content of these speeches (Breastfeeding is really great! Breast milk is sooooo much better for babies than formula! Really!). The trouble starts where the reality of breastfeeding meets . . . the rest of reality. Instead of supporting a woman in weighing all her decisions and needs—or at least giving her the mental space to do it herself—some very well intentioned advocates just can't stop toeing the party line. The reality is that new mothers face a range of challenges and have different priorities, levels of commitment, and access to resources. A "no ifs, ands, or buts" position about baby feeding negates the uniqueness of each woman's situation.

Now for the other side of the story. The champions of breastfeeding—often volunteers—offer their advice and support because they know that we live in a world where breastfeeding is not always encouraged and breastfeeding information is not always available. They know the statistics about the low rates of breastfeeding and believe that these rates represent a serious lack of support and education in this country. For every mom who gives up breastfeeding for a really good reason, there are many more who give it up due to misinformation or cultural bias. We're still a generally formula-friendly society and breastfeeding is still pretty marginalized. Breastfeeding advocates are providing what they see as a needed counterbalance. They may think that saying it's okay for one individual woman to give up on breastfeeding is like saying it's okay for the whole world to give up on breastfeeding. This can-do cheerleader attitude pumps some people up, but it turns other people off. If you get an unwanted earful, try to remember that the person with the bullhorn is probably just more keyed into the general story of breastfeeding than into the specific story of your life.

breastfeeding

Whenever we mentioned that we were writing a book about having a baby, people all but shook us by the shoulders and said, "I hope you're going to write about this breastfeeding insanity!" We promised everyone we'd do our best to tackle all the issues, but it hasn't been easy. Breastfeeding's like a lightning rod for parenting anxiety plunked in the middle of a mess of hyper-charged concerns: privacy and personal freedom, sexuality and mothering, your baby's needs versus your own. We both breastfed our babies. Sometimes it was an alienating (and alienlike) experience, isolating us from the people, places, and things we loved. Other times, it kept us connected to our babies (and the planet) in what felt like a truly psychedelic swirl of new and raw emotion. Within the course of an hour we could go from feeling like all-giving goddesses to dairy cows shackled to the sucking machine. We were both pretty bowled over by the experience, and by all the confusion and misinformation and weirdness we encountered about breastfeeding. We've tried to break it all down for you here.

the basics

Breastfeeding depends on a combination of factors: confidence in your ability, straight-up luck in the biology department, education about how it all works (as well as what could go wrong and what to do about it), tolerance of pain and inconvenience, support from the people around you, and patience with yourself and your baby.

GETTING OFF TO A GOOD START: Breastfeeding is your first joint project as a mother/baby team. It's new for both of you. Remember: The beginning is the hardest part . . . making it over the early hump(s) is most of the battle.

> My milk didn't come in until day four. Luckily I had a postpartum doula who knew that was normal, because otherwise I would definitely have been swayed by the chorus of family telling me my baby was starving and needed formula! (He was totally fine.)
> —anonymom

> My milk came in at 3 A.M., twenty-four hours after birth, and I spent an hour crying in a hot shower with the nozzle pointed at my breasts trying to figure out how to self-express!
> —anonymom

colostrum and first milk

Colostrum is a sticky golden substance that usually appears around the time of birth and stays for a few days, until the milk comes in. It oozes rather than squirts out of the nipple. Colostrum comes in small doses but is superpotent: high protein, low fat, and crammed with immunoglobins and antibodies. Some moms leak a little colostrum toward the end of pregnancy while others never even see it (though it is there). Milk usually comes in within the first 5 days. Many moms describe their newly milk-filled boobs as rock hard or like "bags of walnuts." Other moms never get painfully engorged. When milk takes a while to come in, moms (and others) can get anxious. There can be concern about whether the baby is getting the nutrition he needs in these early days—checking diapers can help you monitor the situation. Supplementing with formula is sometimes suggested. If you're concerned about your milk coming in late, talk to a lactation specialist or your doctor.
➔ See Supplementing, page 304.

Here are some ideas to get you off on the right foot (boob):

BE PREPARED: Educate yourself. Read books, watch DVDs, take classes, get advice from other moms, or watch some breastfeeding in action. Consider these products to make breastfeeding easier in the beginning:

- A nursing bra (or a bra with stretchy cups)
- Soothing nipple ointment
- Soothing gel nipple pads
- Breast pads for leakage
- A breastfeeding pillow
- A breast pump: If you wait until after your baby is born, you'll know your needs better. But find out where you can access one quickly and easily.

→ See Choosing the Right Pump, page 307.

MAKE BREASTFEEDING A PRIORITY . . . AND MAKE SURE EVERYONE KNOWS IT: Tell everyone involved with your birth (OB, nurses, pediatrician, midwife, doula, and/or family) that you intend to breastfeed. This means:

- If possible, the baby should be given his initial examination on your chest/in your arms.
- The baby should be brought to you for frequent feedings or room with you at all times.
- The baby should not be given bottles or pacifiers in the hospital. → See Bottle-Feeding a Breastfed Baby, page 311.

BREASTFEED EARLY: The "quiet alert" state that newborns often enter soon after birth is a prime opportunity to breastfeed. If a baby is placed on his mother's chest right after birth, he will sometimes start sucking immediately to get colostrum (and help induce milk supply). Circumstances don't always allow mom and baby to be together immediately. Missing this window doesn't mean breastfeeding won't work! Not in the slightest. But in general, the sooner a mother can get her baby to the breast, the better.

BREASTFEED OFTEN: Women who nurse around twelve times a day (or more) for the first few days are more likely to have success with breastfeeding than those who nurse less frequently. Eight times a day is the absolute minimum for the newborn period. We're not just saying this to torture you—frequent feedings really are crucial for establishing supply. Sleep and eating schedules (if desired) can be established later, once a good milk-making rhythm is under way (after about 6 weeks). → For more on this dynamic, see Supply and Demand, page 290.

It took five days for my milk to come in, and lactation consultants told me not to worry, not to give the baby anything else, but to keep nursing him, which would help my milk come in. . . . So he basically screamed twenty-four hours a day for those first five days . . . and then did my milk ever come in! I have always had small breasts and in a matter of hours I looked like Pamela Anderson. None of my clothes would fit (including the few pieces of maternity wear that I had). The milk would come spraying out so fast that the baby would choke and gag on it and would have to pull away and then milk would just go shooting across the room like a firehose—and it was like that for months, not just the first few days.

—anonymom

resources

Bestfeeding: How to Breastfeed Your Baby by Mary Renfrew, Chloe Fisher, and Suzanne Arms

Breastfeeding Made Simple: Seven Natural Laws for Nursing Mothers by Nancy Mohrbacher and Kathleen Kendall-Tackett

The Nursing Mother's Companion, Fifth Revised Edition by Kathleen Huggins

The Real Deal on Breastfeeding DVD

So That's What They're For! The Definitive Breastfeeding Guide by Janet Tamaro

Spilled Milk: Breastfeeding Adventures and Advice from Less-Than-Perfect Moms by Andy Steiner

breastfeeding.com (resources, videos, forums, and more)

kellymom.com (a wealth of information, links, and studies about breastfeeding)

International Lactation Consultant Association: ILCA.org

La Leche League International: LLLI.org

AVOID FORMULA: Studies have shown that moms who feed formula—or even have it in the house—during the early days of breastfeeding are more likely to stop sooner. → See Supply and Demand on page 290 to understand how formula-feeding can affect supply.

STAY CLOSE: Proximity between mom and baby is a key part of establishing breastfeeding. Learning what baby-hunger signals look like and making your breasts available (day and night) will give you more flexibility (and reduced hassle over supply issues) later on.

how to tell if a newborn baby is hungry

- **Rooting around with mouth open or puckered**
- **Sucking on hands**
- **Fussing first, then crying**

GET SUPPORT: Ask for help from the nurses and lactation consultants at the hospital. Arrange to have someone supportive to help out with the baby. Your big job is to get nursing going—let someone else do the other stuff if you can. It's especially important to get help if you're having a lot of pain. → See Getting Support, page 293.

POSITIONING
New babies need a gentle touch, but they also need a firm hold to keep their bodies and heads in the right place for feeding. Later, when you both loosen up, babies can be breastfed while you are standing, bathing, vacuuming. . . . Below are some ideas to help you with basic positioning in the early days.

POSITIONING: MOM

Sit up straight to protect your back and give the baby good breast access. (Pillows and/or a footstool can provide additional support.)

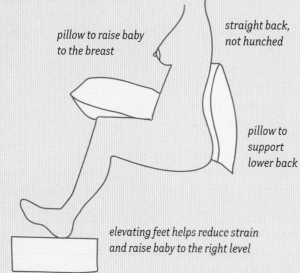

pillow to raise baby to the breast

straight back, not hunched

pillow to support lower back

elevating feet helps reduce strain and raise baby to the right level

POSITIONING: BABY

Use a pillow to raise the baby to the breast if needed. Turn the baby's body to face the mother's (baby's belly to your rib cage). Align head with breast. Baby should not be twisted (with a turned head), which makes it harder to swallow.

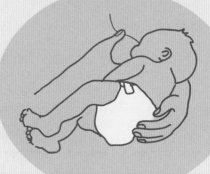

SOME BREASTFEEDING POSITIONS

Since all breast/baby combos are different, you'll probably need to experiment to find your own favorite positions and comfort zones.

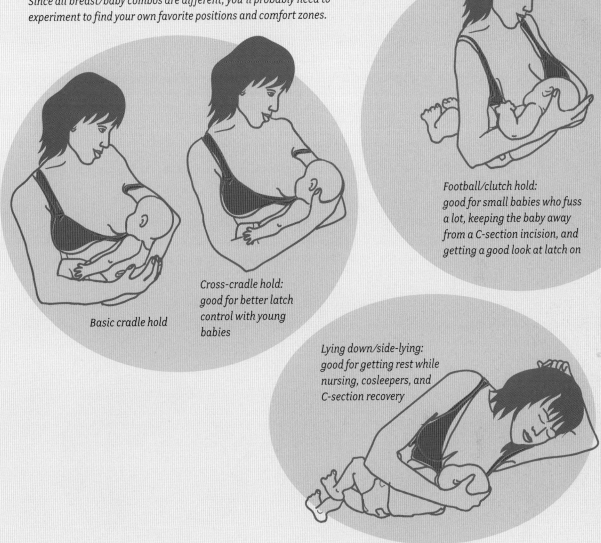

Basic cradle hold

Cross-cradle hold: good for better latch control with young babies

Football/clutch hold: good for small babies who fuss a lot, keeping the baby away from a C-section incision, and getting a good look at latch on

Lying down/side-lying: good for getting rest while nursing, cosleepers, and C-section recovery

LATCH-ON: The way a baby's mouth grips onto the breast is called the baby's latch or latch-on. A good latch is the key to efficient breastfeeding. A bad one can lead to soreness, inefficient nursing, and a potential domino effect of breastfeeding problems.

It's much easier to get an understanding of how a good latch-on looks and feels from your own body than from a picture in a book, so we highly recommend getting someone with experience to eyeball your baby's early attempts at latching on. The basic concept is this: Babies do not suck on the nipple. Babies suck on the whole areola (or as much of it as you can get into their little mouths). Sucking on the nipple will not stimulate enough milk flow and will cause lots of nipple pain.

how to get a good latch

- Make sure the baby's mouth is open wide enough to get around at least a good bit of areola. Do not try to latch on a baby before his mouth is open.

- You can try to tap or tickle the baby's upper lip with the nipple to encourage the baby to open his mouth.

- Point your nipple toward the roof of the baby's mouth, not toward the center. You want him to latch on asymmetrically, taking more of the breast below the nipple than above.

- Don't be afraid to be firm when putting the baby onto the breast. Confident movement encourages a solid latch.

- A good open-mouth cry can provide a prime opportunity for getting the breast in fast, but if the baby gets too worked up, you'll need to calm him down and try again.

- Support your breast (more important with large breasts than small ones).

- Try squeezing your breast by cupping your hand into a U or C shape. Or try making a flattened "sandwich" out of the areola, to help your baby get more of the breast in his mouth instead of just the nipple.

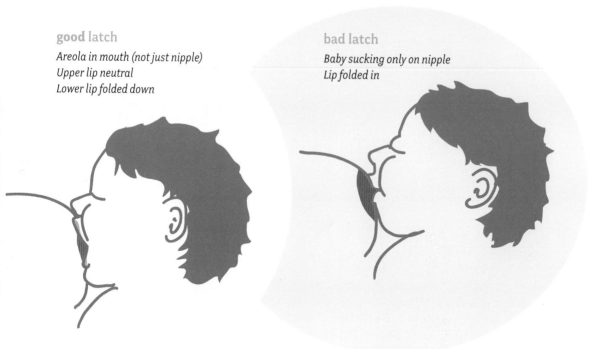

good latch

Areola in mouth (not just nipple)
Upper lip neutral
Lower lip folded down

bad latch

Baby sucking only on nipple
Lip folded in

If a baby gets a bad latch, and you can tell, it's best to remove the baby from the breast and start again. See "Unlatching," opposite.

If breastfeeding hurts for all or most of each feeding, get help quickly so you can make it better before it gets worse! → See Getting Support, page 293.

→ See Getting Support, page 293.

ways to tell you've got a good latch

- If you're not in pain, and your baby is nursing well and gaining weight, your latch is probably not a problem. It may not look like the pictures you see here (or elsewhere), but if it ain't broke . . .

- You may not be able to see the mouth at all. A newborn baby's cheeks should touch the breast and hide the lower lip. If you can see the baby's mouth, it should be opened to a greater-than-90-degree angle (a good latch is more like 130—140 degrees). Both lips should be turned outward.

- The tip of the baby's nose should not touch the breast. He should be able to breathe out of the sides of his nose. Hugging the baby's bottom closer to you can help rotate the nose away from the breast. If you have large breasts, you can also push down on the breast with your thumb or finger to free up more space around the nostrils. Try to alternate where you push to avoid blocking the same duct repeatedly.

UNLATCHING: To unlatch a baby who is actively sucking, gently insert your finger into his mouth to break the suction. Do not try to pull the baby off the breast without unlatching! If you try it once, you will understand why.

FLAT OR INVERTED NIPPLES: Flat or inverted nipples sometimes make latch-on more difficult for a newborn, especially if the baby is small or weak. You can check your own nipples by squeezing your breast about an inch behind the nipple to see whether the nipple protrudes. Any related problems usually diminish in time with continued breastfeeding. An experienced lactation consultant can help you figure out techniques and products to try.

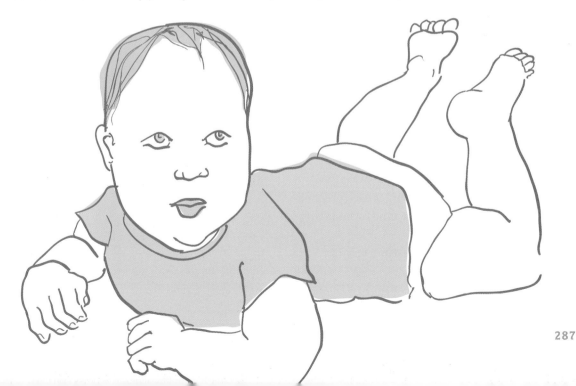

feeding a baby in the nicu

The basic, "normal" breastfeeding scenario involves a superfast learning curve as well as pretty much constant feeding in the first few weeks. In special-care situations, this can become a totally immersive 24-hour job. It may involve not just constant feeding, but constant pumping, on top of huge mounds of stress and exhaustion. Get help. Lots. Get really good advice so that your breastfeeding time is spent wisely. And do whatever you need to do to stay as healthy and sane as possible, which may mean evaluating whether breastfeeding is the right choice for your situation. → See Choices and Considerations, page 274, for more on this.

If you have a baby with a specific and/or serious health concern, you will need to seek specialized support to help overcome any resulting challenges. Some resources for common conditions are listed at the end of the book.

Feeding a baby in the NICU comes with its own set of challenges. Here are some ideas to help make breastfeeding in the NICU easier (although depending on why your baby is hospitalized, your situation may vary):

MAKE YOUR INTENTIONS KNOWN: Since you're not in constant contact with your baby while he's in the NICU (you've got to sleep sometime . . .), you'll need to be sure that the people around you know you mean business about breastfeeding.

START PUMPING: A premature or hospitalized baby may not be able to nurse directly at the breast, so it's important to start pumping within hours after birth to get the ball rolling on supply (and to decant valuable colostrum). You'll need to pump every few hours to keep up your supply. If you end up with more milk than your baby consumes, the remainder can be frozen to feed later. It's important to pump enough milk for a full-term baby, to tell your breasts to make a big enough milk factory. The NICU often provides new mothers with access to the hospital-grade equipment necessary for optimal pumping as well as milk-storage facilities. Pump rental may or may not be covered by insurance.

MAKE CONTACT: While you may not be able to nurse your baby at first, you can still experience periods of skin-to-skin contact. → See Kangaroo Care, page 265. Tender mommy-baby contact not only boosts milk supply but also introduces the baby to the special and comforting feel and scent of his mother's skin, which will eventually whet the baby's appetite for

In that hospital, it is routine to (a) give preemies formula before the mother's milk comes in and (b) feed them with bottles. We had major nipple confusion issues.
—anonymom

I've had babies as young as 32–33 weeks in my practice and as small as 3 pounds and change breastfeed exclusively and do very well. And, I have had other babies who are bigger not be able to breastfeed exclusively yet. So, we have to treat each preemie—each baby—individually. There is no formula that works for everyone.

—Catherine Watson Genna, B.S., I.B.C.L.C.

milk and set the sucking reflex into motion.

FOR MAXIMUM CALORIES: Since premature or hospitalized babies benefit from maximum calories per feeding, lactation experts often recommend separating the hind milk (the fatty, creamy milk that comes at the end of a feeding) and offering only that portion to the baby. The technical term for this is "lacto engineering." A preemie who weighs less than 2 or 3 pounds may be given a special Human Milk Fortifier (HMF) in addition to breast milk. HMF is rich in phosphorus, calcium, protein, and other substances crucial for rapid growth and development.

HOME LACTO-ENGINEERING: HARVESTING HIND MILK:

- Switch bottles midway through a pumping session. The second bottle will get the fattier, creamier hind milk.
- Pump right after nursing the baby.
- Let expressed milk sit in a bottle in the fridge for a day until the fat rises to the top. Skim the cream and serve.

AVOID THE BOTTLE: As with all breastfed babies, it's best to avoid any bottles. In the NICU, the health and vigor of a baby is sometimes measured by his ability to bottle-feed. If a baby is strong enough to take a bottle, the logic goes, he's strong enough to move out of the incubator, off a respirator, or even to breastfeed. But from a breastfeeding POV this is flawed logic. Breastfeeding is often easier for preterm babies than bottle-feeding because the baby can control the flow. To avoid the bottle, you can try to bark up the chain of command beyond the tending nurses to the surgeon or your own doctor. They might be able to forgo this "test" and use other methods to measure a baby's strength.

TAKE IT SLOWLY: Once the baby is ready to nurse, get an experienced nurse or lactation consultant to help you. Start gently and slowly. If your baby won't take to the nipple right away, give it some time. Gradual and positive associations with cuddling and skin-to-skin contact will eventually help the baby feel safe and comfortable nursing. Also, preemies or sick babies tend to be very sleepy and can easily shut down when the environment is too stimulating. With special handling—such as dimly lit, quiet nursing environments and smaller, frequent feedings—hospitalized babies can thrive beautifully at the breast.

breastfeeding a **premature** baby

Mother's milk adjusts for each baby's needs, including babies born up to 3–4 weeks early. Preterm milk contains extra proteins, fats, calories, calcium, nitrogen, lipids, fatty acids, and vitamins. It's also easy to digest, helps fend off a whole range of infections, and can protect a baby from necrotizing enterocolitis, a particularly serious intestinal inflammation common in premature babies.

breastfeeding biology

HOW IT WORKS: The milk-making machinery inside the breast looks a little bit like an exotic tree, with branches and clusters of berries. The milk gets made in these clusters (milk glands) and then moves through the branches (milk ducts) to the trunk (larger ducts) right under the areola. When a baby sucks on the areola, the ducts are triggered and milk squirts out of four or five tiny openings in the nipple. This process is known as the letdown. Sometimes the milk has such a strong ejection it will spray out in all directions like a wacky sprinkler. When let-down is less strong, the milk may dribble rather than spray.

> Make sure your own milk supply is solidly established before you supplement—I thought this rule was for the baby's sake and was endorsed by crunchy judgmental granola moms, but actually I find it is meant to protect the mom's milk supply from running out.
> —anonymom

SUPPLY AND DEMAND: In an exclusive breastfeeding relationship, the amount of milk a mother produces is directly determined by the amount of milk her baby needs. If a baby feeds often, the breasts will refill often, to replace what was taken out. If a baby is fed less often, her mother's breasts will make less milk. In order for babies to effectively regulate the supply and be sure milk production meets their needs, they need unrestricted access to the breast from the start and for (at least) about 6 weeks.

BREASTMILK COMPOSITION: Breast milk varies from woman to woman, and changes over time to meet a baby's evolving needs (this is part of the reason it's so hard to duplicate). It even changes from the beginning to the end of a feeding. The first flow of milk, the fore milk, is watery and thirst quenching, while the milk at the end of a feeding, the hind milk, is creamy and packed with protein and fats. Hind milk signals the baby to stop feeding (kind of like the dessert at the end of the meal) and often has a sedating effect.

Fresh breast milk can range from slightly yellow to bluish. It tastes sweet (people often say it's like the milk at the bottom of the cereal bowl). It can also contain hints of garlic, vanilla, or whatever else a mother might have been eating. Food affects the flavor of the milk more than the quality: a well-fed mom does not have fattier or "healthier" milk than an underfed or "junk" fed mom.

BUILDING A SUPPLY: The first weeks of breastfeeding are what lactation consultant Catherine Watson Genna calls market research for the breasts. Here's how it works: In the postpartum period, a nursing mother has ample milk supply; she's producing lots of the milk-making hormone prolactin. Meanwhile, her body is determining how much milk her baby will need and setting up shop accordingly: If the baby feeds a lot, her body will build a big milk-making factory (with lots of prolactin receptors); if she nurses very little, she'll build a small one. At around 6 weeks, the factory is ready to take over production. From now on a mom's body produces extra prolactin *only when the baby nurses.* The amount of milk she makes depends on how many receptors were activated in the early weeks. If a mom didn't fire up a lot of prolactin receptors, she may find she has a supply problem. This is one reason women find that their milk "dries up" after a few months, or that their babies' needs begin to exceed their supply.

FIL (FEEDBACK INHIBITOR OF LACTATION): Feedback inhibitor of lactation (FIL) is a protein in milk that stops the breast from making more milk as it fills up. This protein is in the breast at birth and must soon be removed (by breast-feeding or pumping within 6 hours) to tell the body that the baby was born safely and the milk is needed. FIL and prolactin work together to help regulate milk supply. Once milk supply is well established, leaving the breasts too full tells them to stop making as much milk.

DOES SIZE MATTER? The size of a woman's breasts doesn't matter when it comes to milk production. But women do have different "milk storage capacities" based on their ducts. Almost all women have the potential to produce plenty of milk over 24 hours; the difference is in how much milk they can provide in one sitting. Moms with a large storage capacity can make a lot of milk to fill up a lot of space. Moms with a smaller storage capacity, on the other hand, must make milk, and feed the baby, more frequently. This shows why some women have no problem with feeding schedules, while others have to feed more often to make enough milk. An experienced lactation consultant can palpate the breast to get a sense of how much supply space you have. However, if breastfeeding is going well, there's no real need for this information.

scheduling

We've made a pretty big deal out of "demand feeding" during the first 6 weeks or so, because it really does have a hugely positive (if not crucial) effect on milk supply. But many moms are understandably anxious to bring order to the unpredictability of demand feeding. Schedule or not, frequent feeding is an inevitable part of having a young baby. Since a baby's growth and appetite fluctuate early on, flexibility is important. As long as the baby is fed eight to twelve times in a 24-hour period, loose scheduling can work. Some babies actually fall into relatively regular feeding "schedules" all by themselves. What is not recommended (for babies or for a mother's supply) is the old-school, ironclad 4-hour schedule. → See Sorting Through the Voices: Everybody's Got an Opinion, page 363.

breastfeeding **after** breast surgery

IMPLANTS Breast implants generally don't interfere with nursing. (The famously enlarged actress Pamela Anderson breastfed her babies.) Sensitive nipples and more severe engorgement are the most common, and typically minor, hurdles to breastfeeding with implants. If implants were inserted under the areola, there may have been nerve and/or duct damage, so a mother with this type of implant should monitor her breastfeeding—with the help of a lactation consultant—for the first 4–6 weeks. There have been concerns about silicone leaking into milk, but there is no evidence that leaking silicone presents a danger to the baby. If supply seems to be compromised, consider "supplementing supply" options (page 304).

BREAST REDUCTION Because it involves removing milk-making tissue and repositioning the areola, reduction surgery can pose more of a challenge to breastfeeding. Women who have had breast reductions may find that their supply is compromised. It is possible to maximize the potential of only a few milk ducts while supplementing in other ways (such as with a nursing supplementer).

For support and information about breastfeeding with a breast reduction, go to BFAR.org, Breastfeeding After Reduction's website.

vitamin supplements
for breastfeeding babies?

The AAP recommends that breastfed infants (who are drinking less than 16 ounces of formula a day) be given daily supplements of 200 IU of vitamin D. The problem is not a lack of vitamin D in breast milk, but the fact that the sun, our major source of vitamin D, is no longer considered healthy for babies. If a baby doesn't get enough vitamin D, he may develop rickets (a serious bone disease). Babies with darker skin are at a higher risk of vitamin D deficiency. Breastfeeding mothers need to take 3,000–4,000 units of vitamin D a day to provide enough for their babies in their milk. Speak to your doctor to find out whether she thinks your baby needs supplements.

is the baby getting enough milk?

Most breastfeeding mothers wonder at some point about their milk supply . . . and wonder easily turns to worry when you are your new baby's major (only) source of sustenance. Here's how you can tell if your baby is getting enough milk:

- *Happy:* A sated baby is usually quiet, alert, and happy, or quiet, calm, and fast asleep. The main thing to look for is an absence of rooting and sucking.

- *Gaining Weight:* Starting at 1 week, a breastfed baby should be gaining about 4—8 ounces a week for the next 3—4 months. After that point, weight gain usually slows down. If there is some concern about weight gain, electronic baby scales (available through a pediatrician or lactation consultant) can be used to weigh a baby before and after feedings to determine his milk intake. Weighing a baby on any other type of scale will not give a reliable read. If your baby has dirty diapers regularly, she is likely getting plenty of fat and calories.

→ See Diapers: Cloth vs. Disposable, page 263.
→ See page 268 for more on peeing and pooping.

breastfeeding more than one

The rules of supply and demand apply to multiples as well: Many moms build a huge milk supply from the stimulation of two babies sucking. Feeding multiples on demand is a huge time commitment, so most experts suggest a flexible nursing schedule for multiples, balancing the babies' different hunger patterns and nursing abilities with a mother's needs. Babies can be breastfed simultaneously, which can be a great time-saver if it works for you, but it's not for everyone.

resources
Mothering Multiples: Breastfeeding and Caring for Twins or More by Karen Kerkhoff Gromada

HOW LONG DOES A BABY FEED? Younger babies tend to feed for longer periods of time (sometimes up to an hour). Older babies can sometimes get what they need in 5 minutes. Length of feedings can depend on the baby's sucking strength and the mother's ejection reflex and supply. Breastfed babies are very good at taking exactly what they need and will not overfeed. If the baby still seems hungry after one breast, offer the other. Try to alternate which breast goes first to be sure they're both getting adequate stimulation. Whether you feed from one breast or two at a particular feeding depends on your own body, supply, and your baby's appetite.

Babies may suck for comfort as well as food. → See Human Pacifier, page 344.

getting support

When problems come up, an educated eye and some understanding can make the difference between getting past them and giving up. Here are some people you can turn to:

Hospital nurses: If you give birth in a hospital, the attending nurse may be the first person to give you breastfeeding advice. A good nurse can be a gold mine of info or she can call in someone who is.

Family/friends who have breastfed: Women with firsthand knowledge can be an incredible source of support for breastfeeding mothers. But as always, it's important to take into account different bodies, circumstances, and experiences. A friend who had a particularly difficult time with breastfeeding may project her anxieties; others may not be able to relate to your pain and may make you feel like a whiner. If the advice is not jibing with your reality, look for someone with a wider range of experience.

Doctors: Most of us turn to a physician when it comes to questions about the body. But breastfeeding is an area that falls outside of many M.D.'s expertise. Some ob-gyns and pediatricians have made a commitment to educate themselves about breastfeeding, but at this point, doctors with extensive breastfeeding knowledge are the exception.

If you suspect your doctor may be giving you outdated or incorrect information, try contacting a lactation consultant, La Leche League (LLLI.org), or another breastfeeding support group for a second opinion or a recommendation. It can be stressful to challenge a doctor's advice, but when it comes to breastfeeding, your doctor may not be the most authoritative voice. Once you know you have the facts, you can make an educated choice for yourself and your baby.

doctors and breastfeeding

Considering the medical community's strong support of breastfeeding, it's surprising how little some doctors seem to know about the nuts and bolts of nursing a baby. How can doctors tell women that breastfeeding is imperative for their babies' health if they are unable to help them manage the inevitable challenges? We spoke with Nancy Wight, the president of the Academy of Breastfeeding Medicine, about this inconsistent message. Here's what we learned:

Doctors want to encourage breastfeeding, but they don't always know enough about it, largely because it hasn't been a priority on the education level. Breastfeeding training is not required in medical school, and although there are advocacy groups working to increase breastfeeding education—adding questions about breastfeeding on exams, for example—there is stiff competition for med students' time and attention. A movement is at work to help doctors understand the issues that breastfeeding mothers face, but change may be slow.

Lactation consultants: International board certified lactation consultants (IBCLCs) are trained breastfeeding professionals. The bulk of the LC's job is identifying breastfeeding problems, finding solutions, and providing support for the breastfeeding mother. LCs work in different ways: The majority make house calls, but some see clients in an office or a center. The downside of working with a lactation consultant is that it's expensive (up to hundreds of dollars per home visit). The financial outlay may be an issue (and annoyingly, lactation consultants are covered by only some insurance plans), but if you're having a breastfeeding problem, an LC can usually identify the issue and help you remedy it quickly. Lactation consultants are individuals with individual approaches. Try getting a personal recommendation or talk to a few on the phone before you hire one. You can find local LCs through hospitals, ob-gyns, breastfeeding support groups, birth centers, or LC organizations. You may be able to get some free LC support while in the hospital if there's one on staff.

Breastfeeding support groups: Many support groups are led by lactation consultants, so they can be a great way to get professional guidance without paying for an individual consultation. Group settings are also vital in terms of show and tell. The confidence that comes from seeing that you're not the only one having issues can be invaluable. Observing a good latch-on and getting hands-on guidance are very helpful. Sometimes leaving the house can be logistically difficult (or at least intimidating) in the early days. Going online for support can be a good way to get and process advice in the comfort of your own home.

Doulas and baby nurses: → For more, see The Support Team, page 170.

la leche league

La Leche League International is the oldest and largest breastfeeding support group in the world. Founded in the 1950s by a group of middle-class moms who met through a Christian family organization, the group took its name from the Spanish word for "milk" (direct mention of breastfeeding was considered socially unacceptable at the time). With support available in sixty-five countries, more than seven thousand volunteer leaders, and the world's largest library of lactation information, La Leche League is now the go-to group for most questions and concerns about breastfeeding; even the American Academy of Pediatrics considers them the ultimate authority. Most women who get involved with LLLI find it enormously useful and positive, both as a resource and a support system. But their aggressive agenda is controversial. LLLI is committed to helping women breastfeed, not to helping women feel better about *not* breastfeeding. Supporters feel their strong stance helps women succeed and pushes our culture to become more breastfeeding-friendly—particularly important when it comes to slow-moving medical institutions:

We need organizations that are true advocates with regards to breastfeeding, with regards to the rights of children to receive the health benefits they deserve, as well as with regards to the rights that women have over their own bodies. Many of the positive changes in breastfeeding policy today have occurred in no small part due to the efforts of those outside of the institution of medicine who have cared dearly about these rights, and who have pushed physicians and administrators to look beyond accreditation requirements and budgetary imperatives.

—Prantik Saha, M.D.

resources
International Board of Lactation Consultant Examiners: IBLCE.org
International Lactation Consultant Association: ILCA.org
La Leche League International: LLLI.org

how to support a breastfeeding mother
(especially during the early stages of nursing)

- **DO** give her time to herself between feedings, but be there for her if she needs you.

- **DON'T** expect her to easily switch gears as soon as she puts down the baby.

- **DO** offer to help in any way she wants.

- **DON'T** pressure her to give bottles before she's ready.

- **DO** try to make frequent feedings as comfortable as possible. Ask her if there's anything she needs while nursing. Bring her water—nursing makes many women incredibly thirsty. Help her arrange herself a comfortable nursing place with pillows, etc.

- **DON'T** suggest that the baby shouldn't be feeding so often. Comments like "She's eating *again*?" may be an attempt at sympathy but can come off as criticism.

- **DO** offer to help with nighttime duties: burping, changing, rocking to sleep, etc.

- **DON'T** start in with lots of pressure and advice about a newborn "sleeping through the night"—nighttime feedings are normal for breastfeeding babies.

- **DO** provide privacy for a nursing mother to feed (or pump) if she wants it.

- **DON'T** make a new mom feel pressured to breastfeed in private. If she's comfortable where she is, but you feel uncomfortable seeing her, don't look. It's much easier for you to adjust than for her to resettle elsewhere.

- **DO** be sensitive to a new mother's need for the time and space for breastfeeding.

- **DON'T** expect a nursing mom to feed *you*! Or to be flexible with social arrangements, going out, and entertaining. Nursing a baby is a full-time job in the beginning.

can i ????? while breastfeeding?

CAN I TAKE MEDICATION? Most medications are considered safe while breastfeeding. Although medication does pass into the baby's body through the breast milk, it does so at very low percentages, usually less than 5 percent of the amount the mother ingests. A few medications pass at higher rates, however, and a very few are not recommended at all for nursing mothers. If your doctor suggests a medication, ask if it is compatible with breastfeeding, and if not, whether there is a comparable breastfeeding-friendly medicine you can take instead. You may also be able to delay treatment. The course of action will depend on how serious your medical situation is, as well as the potential impact on both your condition and your child. Medical professionals are not always familiar with the current breastfeeding research. If your doctor says you can't medicate while you breastfeed, you may want to get a second opinion before submitting to what may be outdated advice. → For info on finding a breastfeeding-friendly doctor, see Getting Support, page 293.

→ For info on finding a breastfeeding-friendly doctor, see Getting Support, page 293.

resources

The Complete Guide to Everyday Risks in Pregnancy and Breastfeeding by Dr. Gideon Koren

Medications and Mothers' Milk by Thomas W. Hale, Ph.D.

Dr. Hale's Breastfeeding Pharmacy: neonatal.ama.ttuhsc.edu/lact

Motherisk Program website: motherisk.com

drugs *not* recommended while breastfeeding (according to the Motherisk Program, Canada)

- Lithium
- Iodine
- Radioactive drugs
- Tetracycline/doxycycline
- Phenobarbital
- Street drugs

DO I HAVE TO WATCH MY DIET? Although breastfeeding mothers are sometimes told that they need to watch what they eat for their baby's comfort and/or safety, most nursing mothers don't need to restrict their diet. In fact, variety in a breastfeeding mother's diet may translate to a baby with an open attitude toward new and interesting flavors later in life. Nursing mothers are not as vulnerable to food-borne illnesses (like listeriosis) as pregnant moms, so you can indulge your cravings for smoked fish, artisanal cheese, and other yummy bacteria-prone stuff. Sushi is also fine with one big caveat: mercury. The mercury-related recommendations for pregnancy still hold true for nursing moms. Eating an organic diet low in animal fats may help reduce new input of pollutants. Some breastfed babies do have sensitivities or allergies that seem tied to the food their mothers eat. But this is the exception, not the rule. → See Food Allergies and Intolerance, page 264.

→ See Food Allergies and Intolerance, page 264.
→ See Guide to Mercury in Sushi, page 74.

WHAT ABOUT BEAUTY PRODUCTS AND TREATMENTS? Beauty treatments, including hair dye, self-tanner, and mani/pedicures are considered safe while breastfeeding. There's no evidence that any beauty product negatively affects a nursing baby, either. Chemicals commonly used in beauty products have been found in mothers' milk. No harm has been shown, but many of the ingredients have not been tested for use on infants (or possibly adults, for that matter). At any rate, it's best to keep creams and other beauty products (except ones specifically designed for breastfeeders) away from the boob/nipple/areola. → See Beauty Products and Treatments, page 76.

CAN I DRINK COFFEE? Less than 2 cups of coffee a day rarely has any effect on a nursing baby, especially after the newborn period. But some babies are more caffeine-sensitive than others (and some coffees more potent than others). Caffeine stays in a young baby's body for a lot longer than adults (2—6 days for newborns). Caffeine in older babies has a half-life closer to an adult's (3—7 hours). A baby who's bugged by caffeine will be wakeful and fussy (not unlike an adult bugged by caffeine).

CAN I DRINK ALCOHOL? We can't really get a straight answer about drinking and breastfeeding. When we were breastfeeding a few years back, we were told a drink or two was fine—in moderation. According to La Leche League, "Occasional or light drinking of alcoholic beverages has not been found to be harmful to the breastfeeding baby." But now, the AAP, which has long suggested that alcohol is not incompatible with breastfeeding, has added a warning against drinking in their 2005 policy: "Breastfeeding mothers should avoid the use of alcoholic beverages, because alcohol is concentrated in breast milk and its use can inhibit milk production."

Moms have traditionally been told to drink dark beer to increase milk supply, but recent studies show that alcohol may actually reduce supply and inhibit letdown. This issue alone motivates many breastfeeding experts to discourage nursing mothers from drinking. Then there's the question of what alcohol can do to a nursing baby . . . a question people don't seem to know the answer to at this point. Alcohol passes into the breast milk and stays there for the same amount of time it stays in the mom's blood. Inconclusive studies have shown some evidence of mild motor delays in babies whose mothers drank regularly. (This is especially evident in heavy drinkers, but some studies have shown a possible impact of light drinking as well.) It's just not clear. So the current recommendation is that nursing mothers who want to drink alcohol should wait 2—3 hours per drink before nursing.

pumping, dumping, and other drunken myths

After ten long booze-free months, we were pretty eager to get back to our vices. We knew that whole "pump and dump" thing was useless: Since alcohol stays in the breast milk in the same quantities as the bloodstream, the alcohol doesn't get siphoned out with the milk you pump. So there's nothing you can do but wait until you sober up to get rid of spiked milk. No problem, everyone told us. You'll just feed the baby a bottle until the alcohol's metabolized. Right. We're not sure whose babies these people tried this out on, but they definitely weren't ours. We remember the first time we gave this a try. There we were, a couple of glasses of New Zealand Sauvignon Blanc under our belts, baby on lap, bottle of defrosted breast milk in hand. Result: red-faced, square-mouthed shrieking. Take two: Daddy takes the bottle. Nope. Who wants silicone when the real thing's in the other room, trying not to trip over the furniture? After many (noisy) unsuccessful attempts, it became clear that our plans for the bottle were unrealistic—on both counts.

HOW ABOUT SMOKING? Cigarette smoke is bad for babies, period. Smoking increases the risk of SIDS as well as other problems (see Sudden Infant Death Syndrome [SIDS], page 271). If you're a nursing mother who smokes, your baby is likely to be exposed to cigarette smoke, whether it's in the air or on your clothes. Nicotine passes through breast milk in concentrated quantities. Studies have shown that breastfed babies of smokers can be exposed to the nicotine equivalent of an adult who smoked twenty cigarettes a day, even if the nursing mother smoked less than half a pack. Cigarette smoking has also been linked to milk supply problems, although it's hard to know whether smoking is the direct cause. But even if you can't quit, breastfeeding is the best food for your baby. One study showed that breastfed babies of smoking mothers were less vulnerable to the effects of cigarette smoke than bottle-fed ones.

Marijuana (as well as all other "street drugs") is on the list of substances contraindicated for breastfeeding. Since breastfeeding and marijuana use is a fairly unstudied area, there's not much data on the subject. There is research showing that breastfed Rastafarian babies (who have been exposed to marijuana through breast milk and smoke) are no worse off than their nonpot counterparts. But there are also studies showing that babies whose moms smoked pot regularly while breastfeeding have more developmental delays. In any case, THC is fat-soluble, so it enters the breast milk in higher concentrations than the bloodstream. And since pot has a long half-life, it won't be out of the mom's milk for quite a while. A baby who drinks his mom's milk after she's smoked pot will test positive in drug tests for weeks afterward, which can (among other things) have legal implications.

WHAT ABOUT MEDICINAL HERBS? Some herbs, like fenugreek, are used to increase milk supply. Others, like mint and sage, can decrease it. Herbs can be extremely powerful, and more than a few are potentially dangerous. It's a good idea to consult an herbalist or other knowledgeable person before taking medicinal herbs while breastfeeding.

pain and problems

Stories about the miseries that can befall breastfeeding women are pretty easy to come by. Your cousin had mastitis. Your best friend had cracked nipples. Your neighbor had thrush. You may have a hurdle or two to deal with, too. If you do experience pain that makes it difficult to feed your baby, you can usually do something about it. Early pain is pretty common as you and your baby learn the ropes. Pain that persists beyond the first week or two usually requires some attention. Pain can be caused by any number of things: latch problems, an infection, even the way your baby holds his tongue. Many problems can be helped with changes in positioning or other techniques, and others resolve on their own in time.

Every night for those first ten days, I'd cry and tell my husband, "Tomorrow, I'm calling the pediatrician and asking what formula to buy!" I never actually did it, but the urge to do so was strong. We visited the hospital's lactation consultants three times and hired a doula to come to the house for a few weeks. Finally, one day it just worked with no pain.
—anonymom

NIPPLE PAIN

	WHAT IT IS	WHY IT HAPPENS	WHAT IT FEELS LIKE	WHAT TO DO ABOUT IT
NIPPLE SORENESS	sore nipples in the early days or weeks	Most women experience some soreness as they and their babies learn good positioning and latch.	Mild to extreme pain at latch-on. Pain should dissipate quickly as nursing session continues.	Continue nursing, always ensuring that baby is positioned and latching well. Expose nipples to air between feedings. Try lanolin cream. Avoid contact with harsh soaps or rough fabric. If soreness continues, investigate other possible causes.
POSITIONING OR LATCH PROBLEMS	pain that lasts beyond the first few days	Improper positioning or latch-on causes the baby's sucking to irritate the nipple.	Major pain at latch-on and possibly throughout feeding. Scabbing and bleeding.	See a lactation consultant or find an experienced breastfeeder who can help you learn to position your baby properly. A large percentage of nipple-pain problems are caused by positioning/latch issues and resolve themselves once these issues are corrected. Seeing an expert is ideal because the problem may also be caused by the baby's sucking technique, which may be difficult to diagnose. Wash cracked nipples twice a day to avoid infection of the breast.
INFECTION	fungal (yeast) or bacterial infection of the nipples	Thrush (yeast infection of the nipples and mouth) and bacteria thrive in the wet environment of a baby's mouth and on damaged nipples.	Intense burning pain, sometimes accompanied by itching. Shooting pain in the breast is also possible.	If you suspect thrush, see a doctor for a culture and diagnosis. It is usually treated with topical or oral antifungal medication. Natural products such as grapefruit seed extract and gentian violet are also sometimes used, but should be discussed with your baby's doctor as well as your own to ensure that treatments are safe for feeding.
NIPPLE BLANCHING	blanching and pain in the nipples and breasts immediately after a feeding	Usually attributed to a spasm in the blood vessels, blanching is sometimes called vasospasm or Reynaud's syndrome.	There is a shooting or throbbing pain in the breast, which may be preceded by a burning pain in the nipple.	Apply warm compresses (dry heat is preferable) to the breast after feedings. Vitamin B_6 has anecdotally been shown to be helpful. If pain continues or is interfering with nursing, see a doctor for possible prescription treatment. A lactation consultant can work on the baby's sucking technique, which can also help.

BREAST PAIN

	WHAT IT IS	WHY IT HAPPENS	WHAT IT FEELS LIKE	WHAT TO DO ABOUT IT
BREAST FULLNESS	heavy breasts full of milk	There is often an excess of milk in the early days before a feeding rhythm is established. Later, breasts get full when a regular feed is missed.	Feelings range from discomfort to pain. Leaking is common, especially in the beginning.	Nurse soon after birth, on demand, and as often as baby requires. Establish a good latch-on. Feed from both breasts.
ENGORGE- MENT	extreme fullness	Swelling builds up in the breast when milk is not removed frequently.	Painful, hard, sometimes lumpy breasts. Skin can be tight. Nipples can flatten out, causing difficulties with latch-on.	Follow the instructions for Breast Fullness, above, plus . . . To encourage milk flow, use a warm compress (or take a hot shower) briefly before feedings. Massage the breasts in the direction of milk flow. Cold compresses can help with swelling and pain between feedings. Hand-expressing milk can help relieve pressure and help baby to get a good latch-on, but pumping may stimulate more milk production, so should be done sparingly.
PLUGGED DUCTS	a clog in one of the milk ducts in the breast, preventing flow	Engorged breasts are prone to plugged ducts. Tight, constricting clothing and underwire bras can also restrict milk flow and cause clogging. Improper latch can prevent some ducts from being properly stimulated, resulting in clogs.	Small, hard, and sore lump or lumps in one area of the breast. Pain tends to come and go. Skin may be red in affected area.	Follow the directions for Breast Fullness and Engorgement, above, plus . . . Try different feeding positions to help drain milk from all areas of the breast. Wear a loose bra, if any. If possible, feed rather than pump as the baby is more efficient at removing milk.
MASTITIS	an infection of the breast	Backed-up ducts make the breast vulnerable to bacterial infection. Bacteria can enter through the nipple, usually from the baby's mouth, the mom's nose, or the hospital environment.	Fever, aches, pains, red and painful breasts. Usually happens in one breast.	Feed frequently from the infected breast. Fevers can be treated with Tylenol (acetaminophen) or ibuprofen. Rest. Although mastitis can respond to home treatment, it is a good idea to check in with your doctor. Some cases will need to be treated with antibiotics. Untreated mastitis can lead to a breast abscess, which may require surgery.

I keep thinking about how breastfeeding is supposed to be this beautiful mama/baby bonding experience, but I find at moments I actually feel a bit angry at my baby for causing me so much pain. Obviously I know he's not doing it on purpose, though!
—anonymom

I will share with you my (and many other women's) truth on breastfeeding. It HURTS! Not just "Ouch that's a little sore" but "Holy crap, my nipple is going to fall off!" Bleeding, cracks, mastitis, engorging, screaming hungry baby, shivers down your back, tears of pain and frustration, guilt ("Why can't I feed my own baby?") . . . I do know some mothers who found breastfeeding to be a piece of cake and very pleasurable. And breastfeeding is a wonderful part of being a mother but it's hard for many of us. All the above does pass with time and gets easier. So, please don't feel alone if it's really hard for you. Just do your best.
—anonymom

I had big troubles with engorgement, and yes, did spend a painful amount of time expressing—a hot bath helped, but the best remedy I found was cabbage leaves, freshly applied until they went too soggy and limp; they were wonderfully cool—it's a grandma remedy that worked well for me (even if it did seem a little strange).
—anonymom

Ouch! at first it really is tough. *Warning!:* When nipples are scabbed (yes, scabbed) *carefully* remove breast pad!!!!!! I lost a small chunk of nipple while removing a breast pad once! My nipple is fine now but it hurt!
—anonymom

Stay focused; the uncomfortable part only lasts a couple of weeks and then you can feel good about the fact that you made it!
—anonymom

tongue-tie (short frenulum)

"Tongue-tie" is a condition that affects 3–10 percent of newborns. This happens when the frenulum—the little, stretchy piece of skin that attaches the bottom of the tongue to the floor of the mouth—is too short or tight. A short frenulum can restrict the ability of the tongue to move properly to effectively breastfeed. In many cases, tongue-tie goes undetected until a feeding problem crops up. A baby with tongue-tie often has a shallow latch and sucks continuously but not very effectively. Sometimes the problems disappear after about 6 weeks as the entire mouth grows. Breastfeeding experts sometimes recommend clipping the frenulum, an in-office procedure that has been shown to remedy problems associated with tongue-tie. Babies who have been "clipped" are able to latch on right away, and more effective breastfeeding can begin at once. Not all doctors perform this procedure. You can consult a lactation consultant for a referral.

TONGUE-TIE
SYMPTOMS

- Failure to latch on
- Failure to stay latched on
- Clicking or air-sucking noises during feeding
- Continuous feeding
- Colic
- Slow weight gain
- Painful feedings
- Sore nipples
- White stripe across midsection of nipple after feedings

My son didn't latch at all in my three days in the hospital. . . . They discharged me and my poor son hadn't had any milk yet. I was so concerned I started cold-calling lactation consultants. . . . This amazing woman . . . comes to my house, takes one look at our son, and says, "Of course he can't latch, he's tongue-tied," which means that the frenulum under his tongue was too close to the front and he couldn't extend it properly. I was shocked that the hospital didn't notice this rather critical piece of information. She assured me that we could work through it.
—anonymom

He bit me once when he was eight months old. I yelled *No!* without thinking. He pulled off, shocked, and crumpled into tears! It was the first time he had ever cried like that, seeming sad rather than needy or angry. Then I tried to nurse him again, but every time he turned into the breast, he got that sad lower lip thing and started crying again. I was so afraid I'd hurt his feelings! But he definitely didn't bite me again. . . .

—anonymom

breastfeeding when sick

A simple cold or upset stomach can add stress to breastfeeding (and parenting in general) but when the illness is more serious, the impact can be more serious, too. With few exceptions, continuing to nurse (when possible) is the best thing for both mother and baby. Many mothers are concerned about passing a contagious illness to their babies while nursing. The baby has usually already been exposed to germs before a mother even realizes she's sick. Antibodies in breast milk may actually help a baby from getting infected, or help fight the infection if one manifests. Everyday illnesses such as colds, flu, and food poisoning cannot be transmitted through breast milk. Use common sense (wash hands, don't cough in baby's face, etc.) to keep germs away from the baby. If you have a serious contagious infection such as tuberculosis, speak to your doctor about breastfeeding. Hepatitis doesn't preclude breastfeeding, but opinions vary. Mothers with HIV are currently advised to not breastfeed unless no safe alternative is available.
→ See Can I Take Medication?, page 296.

resources
Centers for Disease Control and Prevention: cdc.gov
Another look at breastfeeding and HIV/AIDS: anotherlook.org

BITING: When babies start to get their teeth, they do sometimes experiment with biting the boob that feeds them. Some people panic and take this as a cue to wean, but biting can usually be controlled pretty quickly. Distractions can cause babies to bite, so feeding in a quiet, calm place will sometimes discourage it. Giving the baby other things to teethe on, especially near feeding times, may help, too. But the important thing is to teach the baby that biting has an undesirable outcome.

Here are some ideas to try:

- When the baby bites, simply and firmly remove him from the breast (using your finger to pry open his teeth first!). The baby will probably want to eat more than he wants to bite, though it may take doing this a number of times for him to get the message.

- Show the baby it hurts, saying "Ow!" or whatever other exclamation comes to mind. If the baby reacts with shock and cries at your expression, she may quickly make the connection that what she's doing is causing it. Some suggest saying "No!" to the baby, but others think this is unnecessarily punitive. Some babies will think a loud exclamation is funny, however, so if your baby doesn't seem to be making the association, try another technique.

- Smush the baby's face in toward the breast. This is not easy to do when you'd rather be ripping her off, but people say it works: She will have to unclench in order to breathe through her mouth. If this happens repeatedly, she will begin to associate biting with being smushed.

FOOD SENSITIVITY: A small percentage of babies have obvious reactions to certain foods in their mother's diets. Reactions can vary in intensity and may show up immediately after a feeding, though typically appear about 4—24 hours after exposure. Keeping a food diary can help isolate the culprit. You can also try eliminating common irritants and allergens from your diet to see if anything changes. Research on allergies is inconclusive: One theory says that avoiding allergens may prevent or reduce the severity of an allergy later in the child's life, and other studies show that exposure to some allergens through breast milk can actually make a childhood allergy less likely.

common problem foods

- **Dairy products**
- **Eggs**
- **Tomatoes**
- **Nuts**
- **Shellfish**
- **Citrus**
- **Wheat**
- **Corn**

signs of food reaction (many of these have other causes)

- **Rash, hives, eczema**
- **Fussiness**
- **Sleep disturbances**
- **Dry skin**
- **Congestion**
- **Raccoon eyes**
- **Constipation or diarrhea**
- **Green stools with mucus or blood**
- **Diaper rash**

→ See Food Allergies and Intolerance, page 264.
→ See Gastric Reflux, page 264.

SUPPLY ISSUES: Supply issues are some of the most common breast-feeding concerns. Sometimes supply anxiety is purely the result of not being able to see what your baby is consuming. Sometimes what seems to be a supply issue may actually be something else entirely (like a problem with latch or sucking). Or, latch problems may mean your breasts are not being sufficiently stimulated and are responding by making less milk. (For more on this, see "Latch-on," page 285.) If you do find you're not making enough milk, try not to stress out—stress can affect milk supply and/or the letdown reflex (and lead to panic-inspired choices that may sabotage your efforts to boost production). The best thing to do if you're having a problem with low supply is to start trying to build it.

→ For more on establishing a good supply from the start—which can prevent issues later on—see Getting Off to a Good Start, page 282.
→ See Breastfeeding Biology, page 290.

My baby was very small. My breasts were ridiculously engorged. He couldn't latch on. I hadn't slept in days. I had to pump milk around the clock and feed him with a tube and syringe. I was so determined that he never have a drop of formula. I succeeded but at the cost of exhaustion and massive stress.

—anonymom

supplementing

If your baby is dehydrated and/or not gaining enough weight, you may need to give him supplemental formula. But if you're trying to up your supply, giving bottles of formula can be a double-edged sword. A bottle provides the nutrition your baby needs, but it also takes him away from your breasts, which need all the stimulation they can get to make more milk. If your baby gets lots of milk from the bottle, and your breast milk supply is low, your baby may become discouraged by the effort of nursing. An alternative milk delivery system, such as a cup or supplementer, will help minimize this risk and keep your baby coming to the breast to suck, stimulating your production. Frequent pumping while the baby gets nutrition elsewhere can help, too.

→ See Bottle Alternatives, page 311.
→ For more on bottle/breastfeeding combo, see Breast to Bottle, page 327.

I was told I'd have to constantly have the pump on my breast between having my son on the breast (switching every fifteen minutes or so). Okay . . . when am I supposed to sleep and eat?? Add to the stress please.
—anonymom

if you need to increase milk supply

- *Breastfeed as much as possible.* The more your baby nurses, the more milk you make (nurse at least ten times a day). If you can't nurse, pump.

- *Pump between feedings or after feedings.* The more milk you take out of your breasts, the faster they make more milk.

- *Rest up as much as you can.* Delegate. If you're exhausted and overwhelmed with outside responsibilities, you'll have less energy to spend on increasing your supply.

- *Take time to eat.* Rapid weight loss and dieting are not good for milk production.

- *Try spending a weekend at home (or even in bed) with your baby and have nursing be the number one priority.*

- *Switch sides often while nursing (two or three times during one feeding).* When the baby's sucking begins to slow on the first breast, switch to the second, and repeat this process as many times as your baby will go for it. Or try 5 minutes on each breast, at least twice per session. Done regularly, this can help stimulate production.

- *Discontinue or reduce the use of bottles or pacifiers.*

- *Avoid substances known to decrease milk supply.* These include antihistamines and decongestants, alcohol, hormonal birth control, and cigarettes.

- *Get support.*

GALACTAGOGUES: These are substances that increase milk supply. Chemical galactagogues (found in prescription medications, such as domperidone) can increase prolactin levels (and milk supply) by blocking dopamine. Many people have had success with these drugs, although they are not effective in all situations, and may have side effects. Fennel, oatmeal, blessed thistle, and fenugreek are also used to increase milk supply. → See What About Medicinal Herbs?, page 298.

TOO MUCH MILK? Oversupply is most common in the early days while milk production is established. The main problem with making too much milk is the likelihood of engorgement (which can lead to other problems). If a mother's letdown is very active and she has a lot of milk, her baby may have trouble dealing with the flow. Some babies sputter and cough briefly at the beginning of feedings until the initial letdown passes. One way to help a baby handle a fast flow is to lean back so he's lying on his belly. If oversupply is a persistent problem, you can try nursing from one breast per feeding, or even switching breasts every other feeding (left, left, right, right, left, left . . .). But beware: Efforts to regulate a strong supply sometimes work too well, creating an undersupply instead. Watch your baby (and diaper count) closely to make sure he's still getting enough milk.

when a baby won't take the breast

"nipple confusion"

What it is: Baby rejects breast in favor of bottle. This is often called nipple confusion but can also be described as nipple preference. From the baby's point of view, there is no confusion: He prefers one to the other.

Why it happens: Feeding from a bottle requires different sucking skills from those required for breastfeeding. If a baby gets a bottle or pacifier very early (or very often), he may become accustomed to sucking an artificial nipple. Many artificial nipples deliver more milk with less effort than breastfeeding, which requires the baby to exercise her jaw muscles. When the breast is (re)introduced, the baby can become frustrated and reject it.

What you can do about it: Eliminate bottles and pacifiers. Try to make breastfeeding as relaxed and pleasurable as possible. Spend a few days with your baby cuddling, carrying, and making lots of skin-to-skin contact. Reintroduce the breast when the baby is calm. Try feeding in the bath or while lying down in bed. Focus on reestablishing a good latch. Help speed up the letdown process by expressing a small amount of milk prior to feeding. Changing a baby's pattern is rarely easy, and many babies will continue to resist at first, but with persistence, most will eventually relearn to nurse. If the rejection continues for an extended period, a lactation consultant can help you work on other potential solutions.
→ See Getting Support, page 293.

fussing at the breast

What it is: Baby is restless at the breast, fusses or cries, and cannot settle for a good feeding.

Why it happens: Early on, fussing can be a sign of reflux, fast or slow flow, or, rarely, a response to foods in the mother's diet. Later, when a baby is more aware of the world, he may be too stimulated to be able to focus and feed.

What you can do about it: Eliminate distractions. Try feeding in a familiar and darkened room. Babies can become more relaxed and focused if you carry them around in a sling or baby carrier prior to a feeding.

My baby became "nipple confused" at around four months after I had returned to work full-time. Though I had followed all the advice (only giving him a bottle after about four to six weeks), he just fell for the silicone and started to push me aside. He would scream and scream and buck and crane his head away from me when I offered the breast. The rejection was devastating. I would be pumping milk as fast as I could, only to hand it over to my husband, who would feed the baby. He was taking a few bottles a night but I wasn't getting up to pump; supply issues loomed on the horizon. I wasn't ready to wean. So, I spent a long weekend lolling around the house with no shirt on (for easy boob access). The beginning was very hard—six hours of total rejection—but finally, he got hungry enough to nurse. It was a struggle for days. I came up with my own trick for night feedings: I started with a bottle, then once he was half asleep I slipped the breast in. Within a week he was totally back on the boob. He accepted bottles while I was gone but only while I was gone. What I discovered through all this effort and angst is that my baby was much more adaptable than I had thought. It gave me the ability to see life with baby as a flexible, growing, living thing, not just some banal, Pavlovian cul-de-sac.
—ceridwen

nursing strike

What it is: Baby refuses breast for a period of 1 to 3 days.

Why it happens: Nursing strike is usually a response to some kind of upset: a change in home environment, an ear infection, or a cold. If Mom (understandably) screams after being bitten on the nipple during a feeding, a baby might react by avoiding the breast for a short period.

What you can do about it: Try to nurse when the baby is very relaxed. Cuddle lots and make skin-to-skin contact. Try a variety of feeding positions. Express milk during the strike in order to keep supply up and relieve overfull breasts.

What about self-weaning? Rejecting the breast is often seen as a sign that a baby wants to wean. Many experts on breastfeeding suggest that a baby under twelve months old will not self-wean and that breast rejection at this time is probably a developmental stage that will pass. However, a baby who isn't breastfeeding much anyway (getting a lot of bottles, sleeping through the night) may be more likely to wean early. Sometimes babies are too excited by the world to turn in to nurse. A dark, quiet room can help the baby focus. If you are feeling fed up with breastfeeding, this "window" may be an easier time than others to wean. But since your baby's actions may not represent a real readiness to give up nursing, it makes sense to proceed with caution, or at least sensitivity. ➔ See Weaning, page 317.

breastfeeding from a distance

PUMPING: When people see a breast pump for the first time, they're often reminded of something from another era . . . or even something from another planet. Woody Allen's *Sleeper* comes to mind. We probably didn't see our mothers pumping, and we definitely don't see a lot of women with plastic suction cups over their nipples on TV! Pumping is a mystery to those who don't pump themselves.

Many women see the pump as their "ticket to freedom" . . . freedom to work, sleep, or down a couple of cocktails. For moms feeling chained to the couch, the pump really can be a miracle. And though those weird-looking contraptions can be daunting at first, pumping is actually fairly straightforward. Private time spent pumping can even feel strangely luxurious after a stretch of full-on momming, especially if it's possible to read or relax while expressing milk. But plenty of moms just flat out hate the pump, regardless of the time, place, or circumstance. Some find it tedious, some find it torturous.

If you will regularly be spending long stretches of time apart and want to feed only breast milk, you need to be pretty vigilant with a regular pumping schedule to keep up supply. It's harder to maintain supply with pumping, largely because the pump lacks the built-in supply-and-demand cycle of the baby, who will want to nurse more often if the milk supply is a bit low. A baby's sucking mechanism is also often more efficient than a pump. Lots of "in the flesh" nursing

> I absolutely loathe having to pump milk at work. . . . However, I am proud that I have made it a priority and even to this day our daughter is growing and thriving on breast milk alone.
>
> **—anonymom**

time at night can help make up for the lack of daytime nursing sessions. Many moms (especially those who spend a lot of time away from their babies) find having a backup milk supply in the freezer reassuring, even if they use refrigerated bottles on a regular basis. Others wing it and pump each day for bottles to use the next, maybe giving the occasional bottle of formula if demand trumps supply. Adding an extra pumping session or two for a few days will often increase the supply again.

CHOOSING THE RIGHT PUMP: Some pumps are more complex than others (involving a certain amount of assembly), but all of them are relatively easy to master. Though product descriptions ("vacuum control," "removable motor unit") may sound overly technical, finding the right pump is just a matter of weighing a few simple factors: why you're pumping, how often and where you'll be doing it, and how much you can spend.

Hand pump: Occasional pumping, once a day or less, $, lightweight, labor-intensive.

Battery operated/low-end electric model: Occasional pumping, once a day or less, $$, weight varies, can be noisy, batteries need frequent replacing. Generally the least effective pumps.

High-end portable electric: Daily pumping (up to three times a day) for moms with a baby who is nursing well and a good milk supply, most common pump for working moms, $$$, relatively lightweight, noise varies.

Hospital-grade pump: Pumping all the time (for babies who don't nurse . . . or who don't nurse efficiently), $$$$, can be rented (shop around for best prices), heavy, noise varies.

PUMPING PAIN: Strong, repetitive suction can sometimes irritate the breasts and nipples. The cheapest pumps are most likely to hurt. If pumping hurts or makes the nipples turn purple, the "nipple tunnel" of the breast cup or flange may be too small. The higher end pumps have larger flanges available. Nipple soreness from pumping can be prevented by using the lowest effective suction setting and/or applying lanolin cream to the nipples. Some pumps come with different horn sizes so you can customize the fit to your breasts, which may be more comfortable.

secrets of

hand-expressing

Hand-expressing enough milk for a full feeding can be a time-consuming and labor-intensive endeavor, but it's a useful tool for small amounts of milk, for emergencies, or just to take the edge off when you're feeling uncomfortably full. You can get really good at it, but it takes a bit of practice.

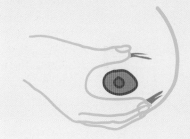

Cup the areola between your thumb and fingertips. Gently press back to the chest wall, trapping milk in the front of the breast. While holding this backward pressure, gently squeeze or roll your fingers toward the nipple. Milk should spray from the breast. Release to let the breast refill, and repeat.

Socially, I always had to consider, "How long am I going to be away from him? Am I going to become engorged? If I am away and don't pump, is my milk supply going to be adversely affected?" As a result, we just didn't go out much.
—anonymom

how much milk will i get?

It totally depends: on your body, your pump, when you pump, how much milk you're making, and lots more circumstances—exhaustion and mood can affect milk yield. Some suggest drinking lots of water or noncaffeinated beverages. Two to four ounces (total) is supposedly average pump production. But, it varies. A LOT.

Remember: The amount of milk you're able to pump is not a reliable indicator of how much milk you are making, nor how much milk your baby is getting. A healthy breastfed baby is usually better at getting milk from the breast than a machine is.

The weirdest place I ever pumped... riding in the back of my (male) boss's Jeep, en route to a customer. Another male colleague was in the front of the car, a female colleague was in the back with me. I plugged into the accessory jack in the back, covered up in a towel, and pumped.
—anonymom

WHEN TO PUMP: If you're pumping to build up a backup stash in the freezer, but don't have any major separations planned, you can be pretty flexible about when to pump. But if you are spending any serious time away from your baby, you'll need to empty your breasts at least as often as your baby feeds. If you typically nurse every 3 hours, for example, you will want to pump every 3 hours. (To calculate how much your baby needs to feed, see "How Much?," page 312.) More short pumping sessions are more efficient than fewer longer ones. The more times you "tell" your breasts the baby is hungry, the more milk the breasts will make.

Consider the timing: Early-morning pumping sessions may produce more milk than evening ones, but this is not universal. Some moms find that their milk flows more readily when their baby is around; others find the baby distracting and have more success if someone else is watching him. If your baby sleeps for long stretches at night, you can also try pumping right before you go to bed.

Pump from one breast, nurse from the other: If your baby is satisfied after nursing from one breast, try pumping from the other. If your baby isn't too distracted and you can comfortably maneuver it, you can pump and nurse simultaneously. This can produce more milk than pumping one at a time (due to extra-high prolactin levels). Since a baby's sucking is best for removing all milk, try to alternate the side you pump from.

Pump after feedings: This assures you that your baby is getting as much as he needs but may not give you much milk, especially at the beginning. It will, however, help you build your supply if you do it regularly.

Pump before feedings: Great if you know you have an oversupply of milk or if you pump on an occasional basis. Not a good idea if supply is a concern. If oversupply is a problem, pumping once in the morning before feeding might help your baby to nurse more comfortably while you work with a lactation consultant to reduce supply.

Pump during your baby's usual feeding time: Best for when you're away from the baby, this might yield the most milk. You can feed older bottles while pumping new ones, or use formula while working to build a stash of milk in the freezer.

PREPARING TO PUMP: In order to relax and encourage milk letdown in the middle of a hectic day, moms are sometimes advised to look at pictures of their baby, smell yesterday's onesie, listen to soothing music, practice yogic breathing techniques. Sometimes the situation can be near slapstick: Polaroid in one hand, boob in the other, phone ringing, e-mails stacking up . . . all to the rhythmic sounds of the pump, pump, pump. In the end, whatever helps you relax in general will probably help you relax while pumping, too.

HANDS-FREE: Hands-free bustiers and bras allow moms to pump both breasts at once, increasing prolactin in the blood to produce more milk in less time . . . even while checking e-mail. You can also just take a crappy old bra and cut holes in the nipples (very sexy)—or cut holes in a nursing bra so you can pump from one side, feed from the other, and check e-mail with your . . . hands.

PUMPING ON THE GO: Pumps are getting smaller and lighter all the time, and they often come with their own cases (combined with/disguised as briefcases or backpacks). With battery packs and car adapters, women can pump pretty much anywhere they feel comfortable doing so. There are even pumps designed to be worn under clothing, undetected!

sterilizing and cleaning

All feeding equipment should be sterilized before the first use. After that, you can use hot soapy water or the dishwasher (unless otherwise instructed by your healthcare provider). If your water comes from a well, you will need to sterilize before each use. Follow the manufacturer's instructions to find out how to clean pump parts.

Be sure to wash all the little flaps and doodads to avoid buildup of hidden bacteria and other icky gunk. Always wash hands before pumping or bottle-feeding and avoid touching the inside of the bottles or parts before feeding. → See Bottles and Nipples, page 324, for info on sterilization and cleaning.

milk storage

Human milk is a living substance: the fresher the milk, the more active, and the more closely its composition will match the developmental needs of your baby. Freezing (and boiling) milk can uncoil proteins, making the milk slightly less miraculous. Vigorous shaking has a similar effect. Breast milk has also been shown to lose some antibodies after several days in the fridge. But even older, "imperfect" breast milk still retains the majority of its benefits. The antibacterial properties in breast milk help keep it fresh for much longer than most other milk. One study showed that milk refrigerated

caregivers and your milk

It's important to make sure that everyone involved with your baby's care considers breastfeeding a priority and understands what it involves. Be clear with caregivers about milk storage and thawing, as well as about how much to offer at each feeding. If you'd like to feed your baby immediately when you get home, make sure this is understood, so you won't walk in the door to find her finishing up a bottle. If you'll be nursing your baby at home while your caregiver is working, let her know what you expect from her during that time. → For more on communicating your expectations to caregivers, see page 242.

309

for 8 days actually had lower levels of bacteria than on the day it was expressed.

MILK STORAGE GUIDELINES*

FRESH MILK	
Deep freezer (below 0°F)	6–12 months
Refrigerator freezer (approximately 0°F)	3–4 months
Freezer compartment within a refrigerator (temp varies)	2 weeks
Refrigerator (32–39°F)	8 days
Cooler bag with 3 ice packs	24 hours
Room temp (66–72°F)	6–10 hours
THAWED MILK	
Deep freeze	Do not refreeze.
Refrigerator freezer	Do not refreeze.
Freezer compartment within a refrigerator	Do not refreeze.
Refrigerator (32–39°F)	24 hours
Room temp (66–72°F)	1 hour
Leftover milk from a feeding	Use immediately or discard.

*New studies can impact guidelines. Check frequently updated websites for current recommendations.

CONTAINERS: Milk can be saved in plastic or glass bottles (some may come with your pumping kit) or in plastic bags designed especially for milk storage. If you want to add new milk to a container of frozen milk, just cool the newer milk first. Saving quantities in 2- to 4-ounce servings means less risk of waste and quicker thawing. Some bags can be frozen flat, which aids thawing and saves space in the freezer. Make sure to label all stored bottles or bags with the pump date. This way you can use the oldest milk first.

THAWING MILK: Milk can be thawed overnight in the refrigerator or by holding the bottle under warm running water. You can also leave a sealed bottle in a bowl of warm water for a few minutes. The smaller the quantity, the more quickly it can be thawed. Commercial bottle warmers can also be used. Do not boil or microwave breast milk.

WHAT DOES STORED MILK LOOK LIKE? SMELL LIKE? Refrigerated milk may be a uniform white/cream color, or it may separate in the fridge, looking clear, white, or bluish with a layer of cream on top. Fat can also be distributed through the milk, yet still separate, kind of like egg-drop soup. Frozen milk can look white or yellowish. After cold storage, milk can sometimes take on a soapy smell due to changes in the milk fats during the cooling process. Scalding (heating quickly and without boiling) then quickly cooling fresh milk before freezing can help prevent this problem, but there is no need to do this unless your baby is rejecting the thawed milk. Sour or rancid-smelling milk should be discarded.

bottle-feeding a breastfed baby

WHEN TO INTRODUCE THE BOTTLE: Although there are stories of success and failure at all ends of the timing spectrum, most suggest introducing the first bottle between 3 and 6 weeks of age. Starting too early can interfere with establishing latch and supply. Waiting too long makes it more likely that the baby will reject the bottle altogether. If your baby gets most of her feedings from a bottle, there's a chance she will grow to prefer it and reject the breast. → See When a Baby Won't Take the Breast, page 305.

BOTTLE ALTERNATIVES: If you need to feed your breastfed baby supplemental milk (or human milk fortifier) soon after birth, the least disruptive choice is to use an alternative "milk delivery system"—one that will not require the baby to adapt to a different way of sucking. Very small babies can be fed with a spoon, dropper, or syringe. There are also specialized infant feeding tools, including finger feeders and the Supplemental Nursing System, which allows babies to suck at the breast while receiving expressed milk or formula from a tube fastened at the nipple. Cups can be used to feed a baby of any age. These methods can feel a little exotic at first, and they can also be more labor intensive than feeding with bottles. But they are far less likely to cause a problem with breastfeeding in the future. Talking to a lactation consultant or a doctor who is experienced with feeding alternatives will help you learn any necessary techniques.

MAKING THE TRANSITION: It's best to give a baby a little time to get used to drinking from a bottle before a planned separation. One to two weeks of adjustment time (at least two bottles per week) is recommended before a mom starts work (or travel, etc.) and her baby is expected to drink from a bottle regularly. Some babies adapt to a bottle right away, but others require a little coaxing.

CHOOSING NIPPLES AND BOTTLES: The best nipples for breastfed babies are the ones that approximate the mouth action required for breastfeeding: A shorter, wide-based nipple will encourage a similar type of mouth position, whereas a narrow one will force the baby to suck with a more closed mouth. If a baby gets used to this kind of sucking, he may try it on your breast (which will hurt) or get discouraged by the different effort required to suck from a breast. Slow-flow nipples (about one drop per second) are typically used for younger babies, and faster flow for older babies. Some moms continue using the slow flow well beyond the first few months, as it's more similar to the flow of a breast and can ease the transition from bottle back to breast.

if your baby resists the bottle . . .

- *Try different positions:* Some babies like to recline as if they were nursing; others prefer to sit up and face out.

- *Feed "in motion":* Jiggling, rocking, or riding in a sling often helps babies transition to the bottle.

- *Change the temperature of the nipple or the milk.*

- *Experiment with different types of nipples and bottles:* Some babies reject silicone but accept latex. Others will take only a certain shape or flow rate. There's even a bottle shaped like a breast specially designed for babies who reject bottles.

- *Have someone other than mom offer the bottle*: Many breastfed babies take to a bottle more easily when it's given by another caregiver. It may be necessary for the mother to actually leave the room, or even the house, until the baby gets used to the bottle.

IF YOUR BABY *STILL* WON'T TAKE A BOTTLE: There are babies who just won't go for bottles in any shape or form. This can be a source of distress for some nursing moms (and pride for others). These babies can sometimes be fed from a cup or one of the other feeding alternatives listed above. Once a baby begins eating solids, he can get much of his milk mixed into cereal or other foods while his mother is away. And growing babies often change their opinions about feeding. If the lack of bottles is stressing you out, don't panic! Keep trying . . . a baby who rejects a bottle one day may well happily gulp one down the next.

how much?

Every baby feeds more or less depending on age, size, and growth spurts. Between months 1 and 6, babies need about 3—5 ounces of breast milk per feeding (newborns take more like 1.5—3 ounces). To get a ballpark estimate of how much milk your baby might drink per feeding, divide 25 by the number of times your baby nurses in 24 hours. These numbers are averages and don't apply to all babies. You know your baby best, so if you think he needs more or less milk, adjust the quantities accordingly. Babies who are used to the breast may drink down a bottle in 5 minutes and still need to suck, though they may not actually be hungry. If your baby is accepting 8-plus ounces of milk in every bottle, you (or whoever's feeding the baby) can try giving him something else to suck on, holding, rocking, or walking to transition away from a feed instead of continuing to top up the bottle with more milk.

exclusive pumping

Some mothers exclusively pump and bottle-feed breast milk from birth by choice, while others resort to full-time pumping when there's a breastfeeding problem. Some moms can pump exclusively for many months with no noticeable dip in supply. Others find that supply begins to fade after only weeks. Many factors are involved, including the woman's milk storage capacity, pumping frequency, and pump quality. Pumps are not as good as babies at getting out milk, but hospital-grade pumps come close. Women who exclusively pump need the strongest possible pump. → See page 307.

public opinion: attitudes about breastfeeding

On paper, mothers are *(strongly)* encouraged to breast-feed. But they often feel *discouraged* from breastfeeding in the real world. If breastfeeding is so great, why are people so weird about it? This has been bugging us since we became aware of the situation—which was when we started breastfeeding our own babies. In fact, we don't know anyone who knew much of anything about breastfeeding before they got there themselves. And it seems like the less people know, the weirder they feel about it. Breastfeeding is still in the closet. We see sexual breasts everywhere we look, but nursing breasts are nowhere to be found. Can you remember the last time you saw a functional breast in a mainstream magazine? The most likely place to see a picture of a baby breastfeeding is, ironically, in an ad for formula or bottles. This is changing, very slowly. Still, a lot of books about breastfeeding don't even show it on the cover!

It's a vicious cycle:

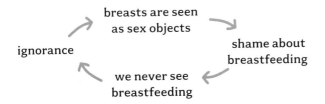

breastfeeding in public

Some people have no problem nursing in public. If you're around supportive people (or if you're the kind of person who just doesn't care what other people think), you may never give it a second thought. But anxiety about breastfeeding in public is a big deal for many nursing mothers, whether "public" means the park bench or the in-laws' house. This can make nursing difficult—at its worst, the stress can discourage women from breastfeeding altogether. Anxiety about nursing in public is a major reason for low breastfeeding rates in this country. If you plan to breastfeed for a while, finding a strategy for public breastfeeding will give you more flexibility and freedom. Here are some things to consider:

> Initially, I was determined never to BF in public and would tote pumped bottles with me. Then the first time I took my son out alone (at about two months), I locked my keys/wallet/diaper bag in my car at Target . . . I had never nursed in public before (or without my nursing pillow) but it was baptism by fire. It was lunchtime at the snack bar and *very* crowded. I thought that would make it worse but it actually made it easier—since we "blended" in better. . . . Since then I have nursed in museums, restaurants, and even at the oil-change place. It just depends on how I am feeling. I have also BF in my car when I did not feel comfortable.
>
> —anonymom

> Of all the places I nursed (which includes while running through the Milan airport) the absolute weirdest was Disney World. There were babies everywhere, but not a single one was breastfeeding. I couldn't find anywhere that felt okay to nurse. In the end what saved us was my son's nursing/sleep association. When the lights went down in the Tiki Room, he wanted to nurse. I nursed him all the way through the Pirates of the Caribbean ride too, and no one saw us but the animatronic pirates!
>
> —Rebecca

> My attitude is ****'em if they have a problem with my boobs. I breastfeed everywhere—on the bus, in the car, at the MET, even in the Neiman Marcus shoe department while trying shoes on!
>
> —anonymom

> I didn't understand people who did it in public. I just didn't get it until I started breastfeeding.
>
> —anonymom

I was not comfortable nursing in public. At first, my baby had a hard time latching on—she was an "eager beaver." Then, she would get so gassy that she'd need to burp frequently, and it was too hard to maneuver without flashing some boob.
—anonymom

I hate it when people come over and throw a blanket on my shoulder. I am very discreet when nursing by not showing any breast or belly (two shirts) . . . but for some odd reason some people think that by making it completely *obvious* that I am nursing less people will notice!
—anonymom

I got comments at the NICU where my first son stayed because they wanted me to use a curtain. I thought that was odd and my husband got furious. There we are trying to feed our premature baby, and some people felt that my breast shouldn't be out. So much for the education of nurses and other adults.
—anonymom

Recently, my aunt walked in on me breastfeeding, and by the look on her face, you would have thought she walked in on me having sex.
—anonymom

I was ushered into closets and bathrooms and backseats of cars. Like I was doing something that people shouldn't see. It took a few too many times of standing in strange and dirty restrooms before I just ignored their comments and fed my son when and where I pleased. I was always discreet. My dad asked one last time for me to feed my baby in the restroom while we were out to dinner and I asked him to take his plate into the bathroom first. He never said anything after that.
—anonymom

AVOIDING IT: Some women choose to bypass the stresses of breastfeeding in public entirely by nursing only behind closed doors. They feed their babies with bottles when out of the house, or don't leave the house at feeding times. This may sound like an easy solution, but lots of bottle-feeding can sometimes interfere with breastfeeding (causing nipple confusion or impacting milk supply). And new moms don't really need more reasons to feel trapped at home: It's hard enough to venture out with a baby without working around feedings. Avoiding public breastfeeding makes moms choose between being out in the world and nursing their babies. One thing or the other is likely to eventually be limited.

THE PRIVACY PROBLEM: If you're a mom who feels better nursing in private, you can try to proactively scan for secluded places to nurse when you're out (before your baby is screaming with hunger). Even if a perfect locale doesn't present itself, assessing the landscape when you enter a new situation can help you feel more prepared to nurse should the need arise.

"DON'T YOU WANT MORE PRIVACY?" Usually, what people really mean when they ask this is that *they'd* be more comfortable if they didn't have to see you breastfeed. This proposal is not only dishonest, but also often unrealistic: a clean, comfortable, private place to nurse is not easy to come by. Dedicated nursing and baby-care rooms are rare, and those that exist are often cramped and smelly. Still, they beat bathroom stalls and broom closets, common suggestions from people who want nursing moms out of sight. Mothers who reject these shameful associations and nurse their babies openly are sometimes seen as exhibitionists. The hostile language people use to describe public breast-feeders, "whipping their boobs out everywhere," makes them sound like flashers—exposing themselves to innocent eyes and even getting off on the act. Anyone who has been there sees the absurdity in this accusation. But not many people have been there.

breastfeeding and the **law**

Most American states have enacted legislation to protect the rights of nursing moms. Many laws have to do with breastfeeding in public. Others relate to jury duty, the workplace, and custody and visitation decisions. ➔ **For a comprehensive and current listing of all U.S. legislation regarding breastfeeding, see LLLI.org.**

nursing "discreetly"

- Lift or unbutton your shirt from the bottom—don't hoist your boob over the neckline.
- Feed in a sling.
- Wear something roomy, stretchy, or specially designed for nursing.
- Use a light blanket.
- Try to teach your baby not to pull your shirt up while nursing.

Some moms swear by nursing clothes, and others think they're unnecessary. One bonus: They let you feed without exposing your belly (something many postpartum moms appreciate).

THE BLANKET SOLUTION: A common answer to the question of how to nurse in public is to use a blanket or shawl to cover up the baby. This method is tried and true, and works well for a lot of moms. It seems like cute new cover-up products are being designed daily. And why not? Baby gets fed, nobody sees anything, nobody gets hurt. Some people, in fact, consider this the only "respectable" way to breastfeed in public.

But actually, that blanket is not quite so simple. Some babies like it fine, but others dislike being under wraps and try to yank off the covers (usually revealing a fair amount of boob in the process).

When a blanket does stay put, it will indeed be modest, but it can also draw attention to the fact that your baby is nursing, not sleeping or snuggling. Some people appreciate the gesture of modesty, but really serious opponents of public breastfeeding think it's inappropriate even when done under layers of fabric. So while a blanket protects you from exposure, it may not always protect you from scorn.

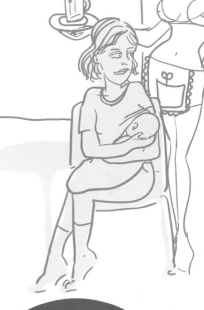

Sorry, You'll have to stop doing that. Some of our customers are offended by looking at you.

I respect a mother's right to breastfeed wherever she wants … but please. A simple blanket!! —anonymom

Maybe I'm a klutz but I find it hard to pull baby over, sit down, get shirt up, bra unlatched, and blanket in perfect position at airports and whatnot, which is why I decided that I would rather fight my awkward feelings about my bazookas than fight the tendency a blanket has to slip all over the place. —Ceridwen

315

ON A DEEPER LEVEL . . . Hiding under a blanket (or in the bathroom, for that matter) feeds the idea that breastfeeding is something shameful and obscene. If people are uncomfortable with breastfeeding because they are not used to seeing it, moms hiding themselves only continues the vicious cycle. Which isn't to say you shouldn't do it. It is up to every nursing mother to decide what level of discretion she is comfortable with. What matters most is that you feel comfortable enough to feed your baby, wherever and whenever you need to. If you feel better under a blanket, great. But don't let someone else pressure you into wearing one. If you choose to nurse only in your home, do it because that's what you want to do, not because others make you feel weird nursing in public. Yes, it is thoughtful to consider the comfort level of others. But it is also thoughtful to consider where their discomfort is coming from, and decide whether you would rather change your behavior or work toward changing their minds.

> I dug those hormonal lovey-lovey feelings you get when you are doing it. I think the boobs are attached to some real "feel good" glands.
> —anonymom

is breastfeeding sexual?

Breastfeeding is a challenge to our ideas about sexuality on obvious and not-so-obvious levels. It can definitely bring up things that *remind* us of sex, both in body and in mind. After all, breastfeeding and sex share overlapping body parts, hormones, and associations. Women sometimes talk about an ambiguous sort of "pleasant rush" while nursing. Some assume this is a simple response to nipple stimulation, but there's more to it than that. When the baby latches on and the milk begins to flow, the hormone oxytocin floods the nursing mother's system. This hormone is also released when a woman has an orgasm. In both situations, oxytocin makes the uterus contract. It can also lull inhibition, generate warmth, and increase feelings of bonding. Some women feel this stuff very intensely and identify it with sexual arousal. Other women don't notice any feelings at all, or if they do, they don't associate them with sex. Hormone levels, and the feelings they produce, can vary from woman to woman and from nursing session to nursing session.

It can be surprising to have these feelings during breastfeeding—and it does freak some people out, or make them feel guilty or ashamed. Pleasant sensations while nursing, whether they are experienced (or described) as "sexual," "sensual," "relaxing," or "bonding," are not only normal, they are an essential part of the cycle of life. It's simple Darwinian logic: The more physiological rewards you get for being with your baby, the less likely you are to abandon it. In some studies, when the oxytocin receptor was blocked, monkey mothers drastically reduced contact with their babies.

But it's hard to escape the idea that anything involving boobs has a sexual connotation. Breastfeeding is sometimes wrongly read as an inappropriate means to a mother's pleasure, indirectly (or sometimes directly) implying a kind of sexual act between a mother and her child. Even the notion that a mother experiences any pleasure *at all* while breastfeeding can be perceived as selfish or hedonistic. The message is that pleasure should never get messed up with mothering—as if feeling good (instead of self-

Maternity is inextricably intertwined with sexual sensations, and it is an infant's business, through grunts and coos, touches and smells, to make the most of Mother Nature's reward system, which conditions a woman to make this infant a top priority.

—Sarah Hrdy, *Mother Nature*

sacrificing) is somehow perverse. Enjoying breastfeeding does not equal sexual feelings about a child. It does not mean a mother is in any danger of treating the child in a sexual way. It simply means that she is responding to her biological wiring, programmed to make this experience a positive one. Breastfeeding may (or may not) provoke sexual feelings. . . . Either way, it is not a sexual act. → See Breastfeeding and Sex, page 213.

weaning

People think of weaning as the end of breastfeeding, but it really starts the first time any other food is put in the baby's mouth. There are many little steps on the road to independence from the breast: bottles, pacifiers, sippy cups, solids, sleeping through the night. By the time a breastfeeding mother starts to consciously think about weaning, many of these steps have probably already been taken. The ideal time to wean is when both mother and baby are feeling relatively ready. But this is not always a point reached in tandem, so some give-and-take is usually involved.

"IF HE'S OLD ENOUGH TO ASK FOR IT . . .": Some people firmly believe that to nurse beyond a certain point is detrimental to a baby's independence, a mother's freedom, a father's fulfillment, and the general order of the universe. For example, many people seem to feel that a walking (or talking) baby is too old to be breastfed. But reaching new milestones—especially huge ones like walking and talking—often actually makes babies more nervous about separation. Despite these cultural pressures, there's a bounty of research that says it's more than fine for a kid to breastfeed beyond toddling.

BABY KNOWS BEST: The other side of the spectrum believes that babies should nurse freely until they stop by themselves, at their own pace, without external interference. Proponents of child-led weaning believe that children know their own needs, and that their need for nursing may not end at babyhood. They also feel that pushing a child to stop breastfeeding before he's ready could make him insecure and/or damage the mother-child relationship. Many families benefit from letting their babies (and later, their kids) take the lead on weaning. But waiting for an older child to wean is definitely not for everyone. Some kids won't self-wean until three, four, and beyond.

> When my daughter was four months old I got an oral infection, and medications needed to be taken that forced me to wean. It was abrupt, and emotionally devastating. I was so crushed to watch her take a bottle, like I was letting her down. I'm still not happy about the way it ended, but know that it was truly the best possible outcome.
> —anonymom

> I weaned gradually by mixing breast milk and cow's milk together, slowly increasing it. I dropped the night feeding first, then the morning. I think my baby was ready, and so was I.
> —anonymom

say when?

There is no threshold after which a baby has effectively stocked up on the benefits of breastfeeding and "no longer needs it." In fact, it seems like the benefits add up as long as it continues. The 6 months of exclusive breastfeeding recommended by the AAP refers to the point at which a baby's digestive system is mature enough to digest other foods, not to a decrease in the value of breast milk.

> The first full day I went without nursing I was really sad. I was looking forward to the freedom I would have, but I knew I would miss that closeness. I'd miss giving him perfect nutrition. I'd miss how excited he would get when it was time to nurse. I'd miss how much it comforted and soothed him. But I was looking forward to no pumping!!! And having the time to exercise again!
> —anonymom

317

> I told him about how tiny little babies can only drink milk, then they get bigger and can have mushy foods, too, and then even bigger and they can have all the foods that big people eat . . . and eventually, they don't need to drink milk anymore because they can eat everything else! He asked for the "little baby" story over and over, and soon he stopped asking to nurse.
>
> —anonymom

FINDING YOUR OWN PATH: If you're not feeling particularly inclined toward either extreme, you can do what the majority of breastfeeding moms do: negotiate your own way of weaning. The first step is to take stock of your situation and your baby's. When do you feel it's time to stop? How big a role does nursing play in both of your lives? What other challenges are you facing? A baby who is under stress—illness, separation anxiety, a change in environment—will probably not deal well with the added stress of weaning. A baby's relationship to breastfeeding changes over time. There are sometimes windows where babies might be less resistant to weaning . . . times when the baby nurses less and/or seems open to breastfeeding alternatives (such as milk in a bottle or cup, cuddling). Observing your baby and following his cues can help you use a "weaning window" to guide the process. But these windows can be subtle and are sometimes followed by a time of more intense attachment. They can also easily close if a baby feels like nursing is an endangered activity.

Many moms find that they move through the weaning process in a gradual, often unpredictable way. There may be small steps forward and huge leaps back or long periods of no progress whatsoever. Weaning can be aggressive or relaxed. A mother can set the pace or let her baby guide her. A baby who is really upset by weaning may become more clingy, fearful, or wakeful. He may act out or withdraw. Some babies show their distress by rejecting food or, more passively, through gastrointestinal upset. If the baby resists, a mom can decide to try again at a later point, slow down, or push on.

> She was down to one nursing a day, and basically, I just put it out there that when she turned two, the milk would be gone. So, every day for a month, I would say this. Finally one night she asked if she was two yet? I said no. She said, "I'm two. Milkies bye-bye. Bye-bye, nursies." I took my cue and the breastfeeding ended very pleasantly.
>
> —anonymom

partners in weaning

Getting a partner involved in the weaning process can be a huge help at every step along the way. Many babies have an "out of sight, out of mind" relationship to breastfeeding, and will adjust much more readily when they're not in the presence of the almighty boobs. Having a partner take over and care for your baby during hot-button nursing times (such as night, bedtime, or early morning) can help the baby get used to a new routine without being constantly reminded of what she's missing.

> I ended up weaning around six and a half months because I was pumping more and yielding less. In addition, I was noticing that he was still hungry after nursing, so I knew I was losing my supply. Last, we wanted to try to have another baby soon, so weaning would help me get my fertility back. All those things conspired to make me wean a little sooner than I wanted.
>
> —anonymom

"extended" nursing

Breastfeeding past babyhood is sometimes referred to as "extended nursing," although considering that the AAP now recommends nursing for at least a year (and the World Health Organization recommends at least two), the term "extended" is a little questionable. Later weaning is the norm in many cultures, and it's an important part of some parenting approaches. Extended nursing and child-led weaning may be a lot more common in America than most people think. Because our culture is not always comfortable with breastfeeding, some moms who don't wean early just keep quiet about it. Many people misjudge extended nursers, suggesting that the mother is somehow using breastfeeding for her own pleasure rather than her baby's needs. And despite the myth that extended nursing is of no biological value, the health benefits continue as long as a mother nurses—new studies show that the milk may actually get more nutritionally potent as time goes on. There's no reason to stop breastfeeding if both people are continuing to benefit and thrive.

A mother can also continue breastfeeding an older baby after the birth of a new one; this is called tandem nursing. The mother's milk will adjust to meet the needs of the newborn baby, and after the colostrum period, it is not necessary for the new baby to feed first to ensure optimal nutrition. The new milk and new baby may increase or decrease the older child's interest in nursing. It can be physically taxing and emotionally confusing to juggle everybody's demands, especially in the beginning. But nursing multiples can also promote feelings of closeness among the trio, and help a mother see, literally, that she can provide for two babies at once. There are some good resources out there to help dispel myths and provide support.

resources

Adventures in Tandem Nursing: Breastfeeding During Pregnancy and Beyond by Hilary Flower

Mothering Your Nursing Toddler by Norma Jane Bumgarner

Most of the advice I heard about weaning was for babies. And all the books about nursing toddlers featured two hundred pages on the joys of nursing to infinity, and two pages of last-resort options to try "if you *must* wean." I felt like I was caught between people who wondered why I'd waited so long to wean in the first place and people who thought trying to wean was a really, really bad idea. But to me, the time felt right. I realized I wasn't going to find the answer somewhere else. So I ended up figuring out my own way of weaning, and it went beautifully. Weaning is a personal choice—the best judge of when and how it should happen is *you*.
—Rebecca

I remember seeing women breastfeeding two-year-olds before my son was born. I thought it was weird. Even the eleven-month-old nursing in my postpartum yoga class looked huge and overgrown compared to my dainty little newborn. But then the months passed, and there was no way my baby was anywhere close to weaning . . . until he was getting close to two. Some women might start out knowing they want to nurse indefinitely. But more often than not, "extended" nursing . . . just sort of happens.
—anonymom

ways of weaning

Don't offer, don't refuse: Let the baby go for the breast, rather than offering it. This common first step to weaning allows the baby to regulate his own needs, and may reduce nursing sessions. It sometimes takes a long time for babies to stop asking altogether. It can also be hard for parents to stop relying on breastfeeding as a tool, so those employing the "don't offer, don't refuse" technique sometimes find themselves making a lot of exceptions. If you're anxious to wean quickly, you might try other weaning strategies at the same time. Trying this out for a little while can help you see how your baby's needs are changing as he grows, whether or not you want to move toward weaning.

Gradual substitution: Substitute bottles or cups for nursing sessions. Most recommend doing this as slowly as possible; one feeding per week or so gives your breasts and your baby time to adjust to the change. Giving up the feedings when your baby seems easily distracted will probably be easier for her than giving up the ones she's come to rely on to get to sleep or to reconnect with her mom after she comes home from work. Many people find that midday feedings are more disposable than morning or evening ones, but every situation is different.

If your baby is resisting the change, try different nipples, bottles, cups, and milks (soy, cow's, goat's, etc.) to see what your baby will take to. If your baby is younger than a year or so, you'll need to use formula to replace breast milk. But breastfeeding is more than milk; substituting other activities that involve close physical contact can help your baby transition, especially if she is old enough to want to move around rather than cuddle with a bottle or cup.

Delaying and distraction: When your baby wants to nurse, try to distract him with an exciting activity. This can work particularly well when a child seems to be nursing out of boredom or out of habit. Avoiding familiar nursing places and positions can help, too. If your child nurses only at home, go for more walks or playdates. If your child is old enough to understand the idea of waiting, you can try delaying his requests for breastfeeding, and see if the urge passes, or at least help him see that his need may not be as urgent as he thinks it is.

Cold turkey: If you're done with breastfeeding (or if your baby decides she's the one who's done), you can opt to wean cold turkey—just stop nursing, flat out. One variation is the "weekend at Grandma's" approach, where mom and baby are separated for a few days, or even a week or more, for weaning purposes.

resources

How Weaning Happens by Diane Bengson
Mothering Your Nursing Toddler by Norma Jane Bumgarner
So That's What They're For! by Janet Tamaro
Comprehensive online breastfeeding resource: kellymom.com

This method can be hard on you and your baby, or both, depending on who's initiating the process. If you suddenly stop providing a route for the milk to exit your body, you'll have a period of extreme discomfort, which often involves engorgement and can put you at risk for plugged ducts, mastitis, and breast abscesses. The more frequently you were nursing before weaning abruptly, the more severe your engorgement is likely to be. And while some babies move seamlessly over to a steady diet of formula after cold-turkey weaning, others don't take to a new feeding method so easily. Some suggest that being cut off from the breast all at once is a bad idea for the baby emotionally, too, especially if Mom herself has disappeared along with the milk. Others think babies will adjust to the change just fine. There are times when sudden weaning is the only option, such as in a medical emergency, but in general, weaning cold turkey is not recommended.

Scare tactics: Mothers can paint foul-tasting stuff, or scary images, on their breasts to change the baby's associations with nursing. The idea is that if the child rejects the breast himself, he'll feel better about it. Some women do have success with this technique (whether they use spices, the stuff they sell to discourage nail-biting, paint, or makeup), but it's unclear whether it might have negative physical or psychological repercussions for the child (one could imagine that a baby who sees his beloved breast transformed into a monster might be a wee bit freaked).

WHAT IT'S LIKE . . . PHYSICALLY: Weaning is rarely comfortable, but it can range from merely annoying to nearly excruciating. Generally, the more abrupt the weaning, the more severe the pain. Your breasts will keep making milk for any feedings you've cut out for at least several days before production slows down. The pressure of the milk from one missed feeding will be a lot more manageable than the pressure of ten missed feedings. But even weaning slowly can sometimes hurt.

Unless you are making a very tiny amount of milk before weaning, a feeling of fullness and/or engorgement will probably last for a few days to a week (or in some cases, a little longer). It can be hard to resist the urge to pump when you know it would make you feel better, but your body needs to shut down milk production, and the only thing that will get that message across is not emptying the breasts. When milk production slows, swelling will lessen, and your breasts will probably shrink, at least a little. This may take a few weeks or it may happen right away. You may still have milk in your breasts for a while—maybe months. Some women's breasts quickly return to an approximation of their prepregnancy selves right after weaning. Many get smaller, some stay larger, and most are a little looser than they were before pregnancy.

> Parts of my boobs would get rock hard and sore. And those spots would move around as one part dried up and another became engorged. Advil and warm, moist heat helped a lot. And all of a sudden one day, my boobs just deflated. Smaller than ever. How depressing.
> —anonymom

dealing with weaning pain

- Hand-express just enough milk to avoid total agony (and major engorgement).
- Use cold compresses or cabbage leaves.
- Use sage or other herbs to suppress milk.
- Try pain relievers (like ibuprofen) to ease pain.

. . . AND EMOTIONALLY: Weaning can provoke all kinds of intense emotions: sadness, anxiety, joy, guilt, relief. Breastfeeding has been a huge part of your interaction with your baby, and losing this connection can be sad. But there are so many gains involved as well. Weaning can be seen as a kind of zooming out on your relationship, rather than just cutting out a part of it. When you stop breastfeeding, it makes room for other kinds of intimacy that may have taken a backseat. It may take a while, but eventually most ex—nursing moms feel great about how their relationships with their babies broaden after weaning. Weaning—like many major changes—is often bittersweet. Acknowledging both sides will help you move on with the sweet part.

formula-feeding

Breastfeeding may be the most recommended choice, but bottle-feeding is the most popular one, at least in America. In 2003, more than 75 percent of U.S. babies were fed some formula, and about 30 percent were fed only formula. People have been looking for alternatives to breastfeeding for just about as long as they have been breastfeeding—bottles have even been found from prehistoric times. All kinds of concoctions—from a bread and water gruel to goat's milk and even tea—have been served to babies, sometimes with not-so-great results. These days we know way more about the baby's digestive system, the importance of sterilization, and the properties of breast milk than ever before. And though it's hard to imagine science ever being able to effectively mimic the ever-changing components of a mother's milk, advances have made formula a more than reasonable substitute.

Formula-feeding is pretty straightforward, which is why this chapter is a whole lot shorter than the breastfeeding chapter (and maybe not unrelated to formula's popularity, either). There are, however, lots of physical issues that can pop up for a formula-fed baby, many of which can also apply to breastfed ones (some of these are covered in "Baby Care Basics," page 256). It's recommended that parents seek the guidance of a pediatrician for any digestive issues. Sometimes these kinks work themselves out as the baby grows. Sometimes a change in the type of formula, bottle, or nipple will help. Whether you supplement with formula or use it full-time, keep your pediatrician in the loop, follow guidelines from the manufacturer, and keep an eye on your baby's reactions. ➜ For Spitting Up, Hiccups, Burping, Diarrhea and Constipation, see Baby Care Basics, pages 271, 265, 258, and 269.

choosing a formula

It is currently recommended that all formula-fed babies be fed an iron-fortified formula for the first year. Though our mothers may have mixed their own formulas, the AAP strongly advises against making homemade formula. There are a number of different types of formula available. Always talk to your pediatrician about which kind of formula to use, whether you're starting out or considering switching.

COW'S MILK: The most commonly used formula is based on cow's milk. Since babies cannot digest cow's milk, the milk in these formulas has been modified: Animal butter fats have been replaced with vegetable oils and other fats a baby can more easily process. Extra sugar, vitamins, and minerals are added to meet babies' needs. Organic cow's-milk formula is now on the market.

LACTOSE-FREE FORMULA: Pediatricians sometimes recommend lactose-free formulas if the baby seems to have lactose intolerance or suffers from a bout of diarrhea, which can affect the baby's intestines, making it hard to digest lactose. If the baby is given lactose-free formula for a short time, the enzymes have time to get back to normal. Because lactose has important roles in the brain and gut, it shouldn't be eliminated without consideration.

SOY: Soy formulas use soy protein instead of milk protein, and glucose polymers or sucrose instead of lactose. Soy formula can be given in the instance that a baby has a cow's-milk protein allergy (or in the very, very rare instance of galactosemia, a metabolic problem, tested for at birth). Soy milk can be given to babies sensitive to lactose, but half of these babies are also sensitive to soy. Always check with a doctor before using soy formula. There is no evidence that soy formula can cure a colicky baby. Organic soy formulas are available.

SPECIAL FORMULAS: Special formulas are marketed for babies with reflux or allergies. These formulas are much more expensive and their effectiveness is controversial from a research standpoint, but a lot of parents feel they have been helpful to their babies. If there is a significant family history of allergies, breastfeeding may be recommended as it has been shown to have a preventive effect. If this is not an option and your baby is having digestive problems, talk to your doctor about hypoallergenic formula. Specific formulas or Human Milk Fortifiers (HMF) are available for premature babies or babies with specific disorders or diseases.

dha and ara supplemented formulas

DHA and ARA are fatty acids found in breast milk and believed to help with brain and eye development. They are often added to formulas or can be purchased as supplements. The jury is still out on whether these supplements actually do any good.

what form?

Formula comes in powder, ready-to-use liquid, and liquid concentrate. Each has its pros and cons:

POWDER: Least expensive, lightweight, portable. Opened powder has a 1-month shelf life. Must be mixed with water. Comes in single-serve packets or bulk. Powdered formula should never be given to a preterm infant, because it is not sterile and is sometimes contaminated with bacteria.

READY-TO-USE: Most convenient, most expensive, heavy and bulky in the fridge. Once opened, lasts in refrigerator for 48 hours. Does not supply fluoride. Comes in bottles (you just add a nipple and, voilà!) or cans.

LIQUID CONCENTRATE: Medium price, weight, and portability. Opened concentrate lasts in refrigerator for 48 hours. Must be mixed with water.

bottles and nipples

CHOOSING BOTTLES: You can use a bottle made of plastic or glass. Plastic bottles are inexpensive though eventually wear down and need to be replaced. Glass bottles are durable though not great for older babies who can hold their own bottles (and throw them). People who worry about the safety of heating foods in plastic may prefer glass—polycarbonate bottles have been shown to leach plastic when reused, although it's not clear what the impact of this might be. Some bottles are marketed to promote less gas. Keep in mind that certain bottles only work with certain nipples.

CHOOSING NIPPLES: Any nipple is fine to use if you're exclusively bottle-feeding. Babies who are also breastfeeding should use a wide, deep nipple. Babies should be encouraged to take the whole nipple (to the base) into their mouths, not just the tips. You can buy latex (rubber) or silicone nipples. Silicone is firm and holds shape well. Latex nipples are softer, but wear out sooner. When nipples start to wear thin, become discolored, or let the milk pour out too fast, throw them out.

FLOW: Nipples come in a range of flows, from slow to fast. Slow-flow nipples are recommended for newborns. Fast-flow nipples can make infants sputter and choke if they aren't able to swallow fast enough and are best suited for older babies. Babies may prefer different flows . . . at different times. Some babies, especially if they are breastfeeding, can use a slow flow all the way through.

CLEANING AND STERILIZING: All feeding gear needs to be sterilized before the first use. After that, warm, soapy water or a dishwasher is okay. If you use well water, it always needs to be boiled. And though it can be a hassle, it is very important to be totally meticulous when it comes to cleaning bottles and nipples. Bacteria love to grow near sweet, warm, damp places, such as in the crevices of rubber nipples, and can lead to nasty infections. Always wash hands before mixing formula and avoid touching the inside of the bottles/nipples once cleaned. Bottle brushes, dishwasher baskets, bottle-drying racks, antibacterial wipes, and other accessories can make cleaning a relatively quick, streamlined operation.

sterilizing options

- *Boiling water:* Boil gear in a pot of water for at least 5 minutes, and let it dry on a clean towel.
- *Electric steam sterilizer:* A compact plug-in device that sterilizes gear within about 8 minutes
- *Microwave steam sterilizer:* A compact device that fits into the microwave and takes about 7 minutes to sterilize and dry.

preparation and storage

Follow the preparation and storage instructions on formula packages. Formula is made to give the baby exactly the right amount of calories, nutrients, and liquids. Adding more or less water (or any other ingredients) can tamper with the baby's health and hydration. If water cleanliness is a concern (as in well water), you need to use bottled water with fluoride. If you're not sure about the quality of the tap water in your area or various kinds of bottled water, talk to your pediatrician.

You can store premixed formula in the fridge for 24 hours; after that, toss it. Immediately toss out any formula left over from a feeding. Do not attempt to reuse. Do not leave a bottle out for more than an hour. Always remember to shake the bottle before serving.

It is not necessary to heat bottles but many babies do seem to prefer formula to be at least at room temperature. Microwaves heat unevenly so they are not safe for heating formula. To warm a cold bottle, run it under a hot tap or let it sit in a bowl of warm water or a pan of hot water on the stove for a few minutes. You can also purchase a bottle warmer. Some moms recommend never warming up the formula: Once the baby gets used to it, you'll always need to warm the bottle no matter where you are. To test the temperature, squeeze a couple drops on your wrist. If you use powder, you can mix directly with warm water (clumps dissolve faster this way, but you'll need to use or refrigerate the formula immediately to prevent spoilage). Always check the expiration date before you mix or serve formula.

how much? how often?

It is no longer considered a good idea to impose a feeding schedule in the early weeks. Feed your newborn whenever he seems hungry (he'll suck on his fists, fuss, root around with his mouth, and eventually cry). Try to get the bottle ready before the crying starts, since the baby may get too worked up and then fall asleep before he's had a full feed. Babies (especially formula-fed ones) often slip into a somewhat regular feeding routine, though it changes with every growth spurt and over time. Check with your pediatrician about quantities of formula as your baby grows. Many formula-feeders find that a semiregular pattern of feeding every 3 to 4 hours starts within weeks or months of birth. After some time of observing your baby and getting to know when he's hungry, when he's sated (and monitoring weight gain), you will become the best expert on your baby's feeding needs. Here are the AAP guidelines to help in the meantime:

NEWBORNS+: About 2—3 ounces every 3—4 hours (Sleepy newborns should be woken up to feed if they go for more than 4—5 hours between feedings.)

ONE MONTH+: About 4 ounces roughly every 4 hours

SIX MONTHS+: About 6—8 ounces 4—5 times in a 24-hour period

OVERFEEDING: Because of the rapid flow of milk from the bottle, babies often swallow even if they are not hungry, just to avoid getting milk down the wrong pipe. Slowing down the feeding by holding the bottle more horizontally will put the baby in control and help to reduce overfeeding. If you get the feeling that your baby wants to suck beyond hunger, try offering a clean (short-nailed) finger or a pacifier (see "The Pros and Cons of Pacifiers," page 262). The occasional bottle of water can also be given to a formula-fed baby. If you're concerned about overfeeding, speak to your pediatrician.

diapers

Formula-fed babies should have at least one poop a day by about 3—6 weeks of age, and five or six very wet diapers a day. If the baby has diarrhea, very hard poops, or not enough poops, talk to your doctor (see "Pooping," page 268).

bottle and baby positioning

Hold the baby so that he's in a semiupright position. Pillows can be used for support. The baby should not lie flat for feedings (this can make it hard for the baby to swallow, and also the milk may run toward his middle ear, causing infection). The baby's head should also be aligned with his body (avoid a turned head or a twisted body). Holding the bottle at an angle so the nipple is about half full of milk will allow the baby to control the feeding.

bonding

Breastfeeding depends on physical closeness, and "bonding" is often listed as one of its benefits. But there's no reason bottle-feeding can't be an opportunity for intimacy and connection with your baby.

Here are some ideas to make bottle-feeding a time of bonding instead of just feeding:

- *Never prop bottles:* This is a safety hazard as well.
- *Focus on feedings:* Make your attention part of the experience.
- *Make eye contact:* Some babies will do this more readily with bottles than at the breast.
- *Hold your baby close:* Maximize touch and skin-to-skin contact.

getting support

Formula-feeding doesn't have the learning curve and physical challenges of breastfeeding, so bottle-feeders may not find as many support groups catering to them by name. But there are other ways to find parents who can relate. Online communities often have formula-specific areas. New mothers' support groups might be useful. Working-mother, gay, or adoptive parent support groups can be especially good sources for meeting other parents who supplement or bottle-feed. Since pediatricians are consulted often when making formula choices and for medical issues, they can often help talk about specific health issues related to the baby's diet, etc. . . . and certainly a lot of our mothers can relate to the logistics of formula-feeding, if not the emotional issues of doing it today.

breast to bottle: supplementing and switching

Most babies are fed some combination of breast milk and formula, through supplementing or after weaning. Some women plan to combo-feed from the beginning. Others find they need to supplement. Just one little reiteration (that should be obvious, but sometimes doesn't seem to be): Supplementing is not a sign of failure! A lot of people feel unnecessarily guilty about this. Breastfeeding is great, whether it happens a little or a lot. There are also many good reasons to supplement or switch to formula. If you do opt to supplement and continue nursing, remember the laws of supply and demand: The more you supplement, the less milk your body will produce. A very occasional bottle of formula (one or two a week) is not likely to impact your supply after it is well established.

➔ See Supply and Demand, page 290, for information on maintaining breast milk supply.

➔ For tips on introducing a bottle to a breastfed baby, see page 311.

➔ For ways to gently transition from breast to bottle, see Weaning, page 317.

public opinion: formula-feeding

Formula-feeding may have been the socially accepted norm for decades, but if you're unable or otherwise choose not to nurse your baby, it can feel like you're going against a medical mandate. The pressure can be intense now that there's such a strong case for breastfeeding. Yes, breast milk is better than formula. But that doesn't mean that breastfeeding is always better than formula-feeding. Formula-feeding just works better for some families. If yours is one of them, try not to let others make you feel guilty about it. If nursing makes you feel miserable or—worse—resentful about your baby, the benefits are probably not worth the trade-off.

This is a choice that needs to work for you as well as your baby, not to mention the fact that choice is often not part of the equation. If you get flak about not nursing, keep your eye on the ball: your own circumstances and individual perspective, which no nosy outsider can possibly understand.

> If you can't breastfeed, don't feel guilty (as many women do). You love your baby just as much as a breastfeeding mother.
>
> —anonymom

> I feel that it is completely irresponsible to tell a mother that not breastfeeding is harmful to her baby. That is the last thing a new mother needs to hear when she cannot breastfeed. I read their list of things they feel can be avoided by breastfeeding. My son has had *one* bug (at sixteen months), *one* ear infection (at fifteen months), diarrhea—only had it with that bug— and he's nowhere near obese. And to say it reduces the chance of a fussy eater since the breast milk aroma and taste change daily, there is almost nothing my son won't eat . . . chickpeas, asparagus, olives, mushrooms, artichokes, tomatoes, things most kids don't like.
>
> —anonymom

> Even though some of the La Leche League nurses at the hospital made me feel as guilty as giving crack to my baby, supplementing breast milk with formula made me feel more confident when feeding my newborn baby. I must say, it did discourage breastfeeding in the long run . . . however, it worked for me.
>
> —anonymom

327

I did not breastfeed....
It's still loving and wonderful and
my daughter had only two small colds in
her first year and a half (to discount the "they
get sicker" theory) and she's very sharp, quick,
and clever (to discount that breastfed babies may
be smarter). She was never hooked on her bottle and
weaning was a breeze; we went straight to a sippy cup
for nighttime and morning milk at one year old. She
lies on the couch and enjoys her milk. For my next,
coming soon, I will also use bottle only.
—**anonymom**

I wanted to breastfeed him
desperately, but because my birth went
horribly wrong (I wanted a natural birth,
ended up with a Cesarean), I decided not to be
fanatical about this "issue" as well. If I can't, I
can't, was my approach after that. So I
accepted my situation and tried to make
the best out of it.
—**anonymom**

Baby is formula-fed now. I wanted
breastfeeding so badly for my baby. The guilt was so huge
when I gave my little one formula for the first time, I felt like I had given
her poison. I am so happy that breastfeeding is so well supported today but I
could have used some support when women looked at me like a terrible mother when
I bottle-fed my baby in the mall. It was breast milk but they didn't know that. Now if I
was to have another baby one day, I would absolutely try breastfeeding again. I
know it is the best, but if I felt that I had given it my very best try, I would do
whatever I needed to to feed my baby.
—**anonymom**

starting solids

Our mothers tell us we were eating sandwiches by the time we could hold our heads up. But these days, we're advised to take things a little bit slower. There is some internal disagreement over at the AAP about the right time to start solids. Their book says that food can be introduced as early as four months, though their breastfeeding policy calls for six months of exclusive breastfeeding.

In order to eat solid foods, a baby should be able to sit up on his own. He must also have lost his "tongue-thrust" reflex—the thing that makes babies push things out of their mouths. There's also some concern that before 6 months, a baby's digestive system may not have sufficiently matured to process solid foods, and that early introduction may make him more likely to develop an allergy. One clue that your baby may be ready for solids is his interest: If he starts eyeballing and trying to eat your food, he might be ready to try some of his own.

There's no reason to rush solids, though. Solid foods provide very little nutritional benefit to a small baby compared with breast milk or enriched formulas. There's also no evidence showing that solid foods will have any impact on a baby's sleep either way. It is fun to try new things and see your baby's reactions (both positive and negative). But many parents find early feedings as much of a hassle as a joy, especially moms who are used to no prep, no cleanup breastfeeding. One final note that's particularly true for breastfeeding babies: The beginning of solids means the end of pristine poop. You may have thought your baby's diapers smelled bad before. But solid-food diapers are a whole other ball of . . . poop.

COW'S MILK: Cow's milk does not have enough iron for babies before around a year old, and is therefore not recommended. It can also be allergenic in young babies and possibly hard to digest. After your baby's first birthday, cow's milk can be added to the diet. However, it is not necessary. If cow's milk is given, whole milk is recommended until the baby has turned two, when low-fat milk can be introduced.

JUICE: Do not offer juice to your baby until he is at least 6 months old. Fruit juices can lead to runny and frequent stools and painful diaper rash. Many doctors discourage juices altogether because of their limited nutritional value and high sugar content.

WATER: Breastfed babies who are feeding frequently should not need extra water. They can start taking sips of water from a cup when they start solid foods. Formula-fed babies can be given the occasional bottle of water. Older babies can be given water more frequently. Do not give babies well water without first having it tested.

first foods

STARTER FOODS: Iron-fortified rice cereal is the most recommended starter food. Oat and barley cereals are other options. Mashed avocado and banana are popular starter foods, too. First foods must be totally smooth and pureed; the younger the baby, the more important this is. You can feed from a prepared jar or make your own food by cooking and mashing stuff up (early foods should be strained). Waiting a few days between new foods will give you time to trace a reaction if one should occur.

FINGER FOODS: Once your baby can use his pincer grasp well, he can pick up food with his fingers. Pieces should be smaller than a baby's fingernail, soft and easy to swallow. Little pieces of well-cooked vegetables, beans, and soft noodles are all common finger foods. A baby can start having small pieces of table food once you've determined that he has no negative reaction to any of the ingredients. See pages 330—31 for foods to avoid (for various reasons).

questionable foods for babies

because they may cause allergies . . .

- Chocolate
- Citrus
- Corn
- Cow-milk products
- Egg whites
- Nuts (including nut oils and butters)
- Shellfish
- Strawberries
- Wheat

because they may be high in nitrates . . .

- Beets
- Carrots
- Collard greens
- Spinach
- Turnips

Nitrates can sometimes lead to a certain kind of anemia in infants. The younger the baby, the higher the risk. Since baby-food companies screen for nitrates, you can offer the above-listed veggies in baby-food form. Organic veggies may be lower in nitrates, too.

because they're just not good for you . . .

- Anything caffeinated
- Canned adult foods (they often contain preservatives and salt)
- Refined sugars in sugary drinks, some juices, candy, sweets, sodas
- Salt
- HONEY SHOULD NEVER BE FED TO BABIES UNDER ONE YEAR OLD due to the risk of botulism infection.

common choking hazards

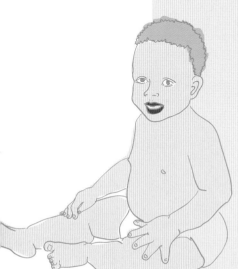

- Anything with a pit
- Anything small and hard (e.g., nuts or candies)
- Hot dogs

- **Overly chunky, stringy, or globby foods**
- **Popcorn**
- **Raisins**
- **Raw vegetables and fruits**
- **Whole grapes or olives**

Babies should always be supervised while eating. Caregivers should learn about choking hazards and safety techniques.

serving suggestions

starting out

- Make sure baby is sitting upright on knee or in chair.
- Avoid feeding while baby is busy playing, moving, or laughing.
- Feed with a spoon (cereal in bottles is not recommended). Older babies can self-feed.
- Try mixing in breast milk or formula with first foods, to help with the taste and texture transition.
- If your baby rejects food, wait a few days or a week and try again. It's more important that your baby enjoys mealtimes than that he start solids by a certain date.

later on

- Set an example—whether this means enjoying a happy social time around food or eating with your mouth closed. . . . Babies are learning all the time.
- Don't worry too much about making a mess in the beginning. Infants can't understand the difference between food and toys. If you want less mess, put fewer messy foods within his reach.
- Avoid distracting games or distressing things while the baby is eating: laughing, crying, and movement all increase the risk of choking
- Some people try to get babies involved in family meals from the beginning, while others prefer to feed them separately. Whenever you decide to feed, try to make mealtimes enjoyable.
- Don't force the issue if the baby turns away. Positive associations matter more than getting down an individual meal, and babies, like everybody, have preferences.
- Don't be afraid of interesting foods. Babies are more open to flavors than many adults. A baby might like green beans or liver more than ice cream or cake! Some suggest saving sweet foods, such as fruits, until after vegetables have been introduced, to encourage openness.

sleep

We both started out with certain ideas about how and where our baby would be getting to sleep and we both ended up doing things that seemed completely unfathomable before we were actually doing them. We both felt the tug of maternal instinct stronger than ever when it came to nighttime crying and feeding, and we both found that same instinct entirely eroded while poring over sleep-advice books all day. The books were all so convincing. And contradicted one another wildly. We became even more confused. Crib or cosleep? Let the baby cry or rush in? Black out the room or train the baby to sleep through light and noise? Impose nap times and protect them at all costs, or let the baby fall asleep whenever and wherever he felt like it? Rock the baby to sleep? Nurse the baby to sleep? Never, ever, either?

It wasn't just that there were too many "sleep solutions" to choose from. It was that each one came with a list of reasons why the other options would not only fail, but how they could actually damage our children permanently. Here are just a few of the nasty outcomes we were told could befall our babies if we made the wrong choice about sleep: lack of confidence . . . inability to handle stress later in life . . . stunted brain growth . . . even a penchant for drug abuse. Our children could end up panicked by the mere thought of bedtime, incapable of trust, and/or afraid of being alone. But not if we chose the right method, of course! Whichever that was. We were flummoxed. These books gave us a hundred more reasons to lie awake at night, even in those precious moments when the baby was sleeping. While parents of sound-sleeping babies were able to muse on the myriad pleasures of parenthood, we were entirely consumed by the (usually fruitless) quest for sleep.

Hopefully, you won't have these problems. But just in case you do find yourself in need of help, this chapter will give you the basic facts, debunk the myths, and give you a bunch of options for helping your baby sleep. You may find a sleep plan that works like a charm

> My son was a good sleeper at six weeks; we were so excited that he could sleep for six or seven hours at a time at such a young age and were certain it would bode well for our future sleep-monster. *No such luck.* I find that it helps to accept one major reality: There is no single formula that will work on all children—they aren't robots.
> —anonymom

> The main thing to remember is the long view—in the end your baby is going to grow into a child who sleeps. The human body needs it. If your average baby had sleep problems, as soon as the kid is old enough to hit the fields, and earn his keep, he's going to sleep at night.
> —anonymom

> The sleep fanatics can get you from all sides: schedule, cosleep, crying, no crying. Even the people who pitch something I do myself can annoy me. There's just this sense that you would be fine if you were not such an idiot moron (by refusing to read X's book or try whatever genius technique). But the only thing that works for me is an inner voice—or really an inner wall of sound—that blocks the BS. I think in the best situations other parents just want to help. In the worst they are like salesmen banging on your door in the middle of dinner.
> —anonymom

right out of the box. But it's just as likely you'll end up cobbling together your own creative (or possibly desperate) solution to whatever problems you encounter. And whatever happens, you can pretty much rest assured—once you're getting rest—that if your baby grows up to become a maladjusted, drug-addicted delinquent, it won't be because of how you handled the sleep situation.

where does a baby sleep?

Where should your baby sleep? In a bassinet? Crib? In your bed? Within each of these options (and between them) there are many variations. Though you may have a strong opinion about where a baby should sleep, your baby may have strong opinions of his own. You may plan on a cradle or bassinet, but the baby will sleep only on your chest or at a certain angle on a particular blanket. If this is the case, you can either try to force the issue or adjust.

In the United States, the majority of babies sleep in a bassinet or crib, but cosleeping is the norm in many other parts of the world. The number of U.S. babies who sleep at least part of the night with their parents is probably somewhere between 10 and 50 percent, according to a 2000 study from the National Institute of Child Health and Human Development. If things like travel sleeping arrangements or occasional stays in the parents' bed are figured in, the numbers are likely higher. There are pros and cons to both sleeping arrangements. There are also safety considerations for each. → For safety information for crib and cosleeping, see page 336.

crib-sleeping

A separate bed can represent a kind of psychic refuge from parenting. Some parents really appreciate this, especially when time away from the baby is scarce. A crib may feel more secure. Night feedings for crib-sleepers may be less frequent than cosleeping babies (though they may also involve greater wakefulness for both babies and mothers). Also, getting a baby used to a crib early on can save the trouble of transitioning him into one later.

what people like about crib-sleeping

- Baby gets used to sleeping alone early on.
- Baby has less risk of SIDS/suffocation if crib is in the parents' room (according to some studies).

> Many sleepless nights with her in our bed have shown me that she likes her crib best (which I really don't understand).... I almost feel rejected by her! By the way, she cannot sleep if I am even in the same room as she is! She loves to "talk" to me if I am around, so it is imperative for me to leave for her to sleep.
> —anonymom

> I tried to put her in the crib, but she just hated it and after a week of trying to force it on her we were both emotionally and mentally drained and that was the end of the crib adventure for us. She has never had a dangerous incident with the covers or a pillow, but she has fallen out of the bed. That was more traumatic for me than for her. Being that I am a solo parent, it made the decision much easier since I didn't have to ignore someone else's opinion on the matter. We bond so much sleeping together.
> —anonymom

- Parents have bed to themselves (and don't have to make sure it fits safety regulations).
- Baby and parents may sleep better when separate.
- Less opportunity for all-night sucking marathons.
- Easier for parents to be away or travel.

what people don't like about crib-sleeping

- More opportunities for all-night schlepping (especially for the person doing the feeding)
- Can be less convenient for demand or night feedings
- Baby may not sleep as well alone.
- Parents may prefer to be near baby.

cosleeping

The practice of sharing a bed with the baby is called cosleeping. (It's sometimes known as "the family bed.") Some people cosleep for convenience; others do it because they believe it has substantial psychological benefits. Cosleeping is popular among breastfeeding mothers. Though cosleeping infants tend to feed more frequently throughout the night, feedings may be briefer and less disruptive to the mother's sleep. Working mothers often praise cosleeping for bringing them close to their child after a day apart. If you're anxious about your baby's well-being, having her nearby can be reassuring. Finally, some babies are just not that psyched about sleeping alone. Parents of these babies may choose to cosleep to avoid distressful nighttime maneuverings. Or they may embrace cosleeping as a natural response to a baby's yearnings for physical proximity.

→ See Attachment Parenting, page 366.

> It's been great having him in bed with us ... and I know he feels content and secure between his mama and daddy and we feel content and secure having him right there with us. And we all get way more sleep this way.
>
> —anonymom

> One of my friends has an interesting sleep setup. At first she refused to allow her daughter to sleep in her bed because she was scared of the suffocation risk, SIDS, etc. After a sleepless three months with her high-need baby, she gave in. She put her mattress on the floor and the crib mattress between the wall and her own mattress and the three of them sleep peacefully at last. She has totally given up on the crib and intends to cosleep as long as possible.
>
> —anonymom

Cosleeping has never been given a hearty mainstream endorsement in this culture (at least not in the last half of the twentieth century). In its 2005 statement on SIDS and sleep, the AAP changed its recommendations on cosleeping from "maybe" to a definite "no," citing that bed sharing can be "hazardous under certain conditions." Yet the practice has always had enthusiastic supporters. Many maintain that babies are actually better off sleeping with their parents than sleeping alone. Some claim it can actually reduce the risk of SIDS.

The controversy on cosleeping safety has been around awhile, to say the least. There's even a biblical story about an "overlaying" death. The recent warnings against cosleeping have been based on studies that do not distinguish between safe and unsafe cosleeping environments. As far as we know, there are no studies of safety formed entirely from optimized cosleeping arrangements, where the parent understands the risk factors and designs the sleep environment for safety. When studies lump a parent who cosleeps with little attention to safety precautions (smoking, drugs, cosleeping on a soft surface, etc.) with a parent who rearranges her entire bedroom around the safest possible sleep environment, it's hard to know how to read the statistics.

But safety isn't the only problem with cosleeping from a cultural (and sometimes personal) standpoint. While parents in other cultures routinely sleep with or near their babies, Americans prize independence, and independent sleep is one of the earliest incarnations of this value. There's also the question of how cosleeping might mess with the parents' sex life—something that lots of bed-sharing parents say is less of a factor than many expect. Cosleeping new parents, it seems from our anecdotal "studies," have no less sex (or worse sex) than those with crib sleepers. Still, a lot of people feel like the bed is the private provenance of the married couple. This may be why cosleeping is also associated with leniency, and in some cases, a slippery slope to letting the baby control your life: "You'll never get him out of that bed!" opponents tsk at parents who have succumbed to the lure of cosleeping. Skeptics say that the baby product industry plays a role, too, as cosleeping is often the option that involves the fewest purchases.

what people like about cosleeping

- Mom's heartbeat can be soothing and regulating for newborn, may mean less risk of SIDS (according to some studies).
- Easy access to breast can mean more sleep for mom, easy demand feeding.
- Time together is good for mothers who are away from baby in daytime.
- More intimacy for family
- Baby may sleep better with others nearby.
- Parents may be more comfortable sleeping with baby nearby.
- Trust and confidence may develop from the comforting environment.
- Can be convenient for travel with baby

I believe that in most cases SIDS is a sleep disorder, primarily a disorder of arousal and breathing control during sleep. All the elements of natural mothering, especially breastfeeding and sharing sleep, benefit the infant's breathing control and increase the mutual awareness between mother and infant so that their arousability is increased and the risk of SIDS decreased.

—Dr. William Sears

what people don't like about cosleeping

- Bedding options are limited for safety reasons (no soft mattress, fluffy pillows, etc.).
- Baby can become accustomed to all-night feedings.
- Parents have less privacy and space.
- Baby may have trouble adjusting to own room (when and if that time comes).
- Babies and parents may not sleep well together.
- It can be harder for parents to go out or travel without baby.
- Drugs, alcohol, smoke are not recommended for either partner.

resources

The Baby Sleep Book: The Complete Guide to a Good Night's Rest for the Whole Family and all other books by William and Martha Sears, askdrsears.com

Good Nights: The Happy Parents' Guide to the Family Bed (and a Peaceful Night's Sleep!) by Maria Goodavage and Jay Gordon

Our Babies, Ourselves: How Biology and Culture Shape the Way We Parent by Meredith Small

The University of Notre Dame Mother-Baby Behavioral Sleep Laboratory: nd.edu/~jmckenn1/lab

→ See Attachment Parenting resources, page 366.

sleep safety

Not too many years ago, babies were routinely tucked in under cozy covers, facedown with a fuzzy teddy bear tucked under an arm. Parents sometimes long for the good ol' days when comfort was king and they weren't asked to put their babies to sleep on their backs on a firm, fluff-free surface. It can be frustrating to listen to parents of previous generations talk about how much better babies sleep on their bellies, or with a crib full of furry friends. But the numbers don't lie: Sleep safety precautions save lives.

POSITIONS: The safest sleeping position for babies is on their backs. The "back to sleep" campaign in the United States has dramatically reduced SIDS deaths. The reasons for this are not entirely clear, but back sleeping may be safer because it allows for unrestricted breathing, both by keeping the nose and mouth clear and by not compressing the lungs and diaphragm. If your baby won't easily settle on her back, here are some things to try:

- *Swaddle your baby:* Many babies who won't sleep on their backs unwrapped will happily do so swaddled. → For more info on swaddling, see page 272.
- *Move him onto his back after he has fallen into a deep sleep:* Keeping a hand on his belly can help ease the transition.

You can also talk to your pediatrician about sleep positioning: the AAP does not endorse any position other than back sleeping, but some individual doctors are okay with side sleeping if the baby's position is secured. Doctors also have differing opinions about sleeping in car seats and strollers (babies sometimes prefer to be at a slight angle or curled up). Research shows that young babies get less oxygen when sleeping in car seats. This has not been shown to have negative effects unless the car seat is used for sleep in unattended situations.

HOME ENVIRONMENT: Don't smoke near your baby, or ideally, in the home at all. Any exposure to smoke increases the chance of SIDS. Parents who smoke should not cosleep. Even if they smoke away from the baby, SIDS risk is greatly increased. Sofas, soft chairs, waterbeds, and other soft, pillowy surfaces are not recommended for baby sleep.

crib/bassinet/cradle safety concerns

- New cribs and cradles are required by law to meet safety standards. Used or antique ones, however, may not be safe. If you're worried, you can check to see that your crib/cradle meets the latest safety standards at the Consumer Products Safety Commission (CPSC.gov). Check hardware frequently and choose a crib without removable decorative pieces or sharp edges/points.

- Choose a firm mattress. There should be no gaps between the mattress and the side of the crib/cradle.

- Sheets and mattress covers should be secured so they cannot be pulled out by the baby.

- Extra padding, such as blankets, pillows, or stuffed animals can be a suffocation hazard. Wearable blankets are preferable to loose ones. Sleeping on sheepskins is not safe for young babies.

- Crib bumpers can prevent babies from getting their legs stuck between crib spokes, though they may be a suffocation hazard. Older babies may be able to use them as a stepping stool for climbing out of the crib. Dangling strings (such as ties on bumpers) are also hazardous.

- Beware of overheating. The ideal temperature for a baby's sleeping space is somewhere between 65 and 70 degrees F.

- Educate relatives, babysitters, and other caregivers about sleep safety.

if you sleep with your baby

- Do not sleep with a baby after using drugs or alcohol.

- Beware of gaps or spaces where the baby could get caught, such as between the mattress and headboard, bed and nightstand, and bed and wall. Beds often move slightly throughout the night, so consider the possibility of these shifts. Some cosleepers put a large, firm mattress in the middle of the floor (away from any place the baby could be trapped).

- Never cosleep on a soft mattress.

- Blankets, loose sheets, and sometimes even pillows are not recommended.

- Be sure there's nothing on your bed or body that could entangle your baby. Nightwear should not have loose strings or flowing fabric; very long hair should be tied back.

- Because studies show partners are not always as aware of a baby's presence, putting a baby between parents is riskier than putting the baby between her mother and the wall or a well-fitting guardrail. Guardrails should be checked for gaps in which babies could get stuck.

- Overheating is a particular risk for cosleeping babies because of the increased body heat from other people in the bed. Take this into account when setting the room temperature and when dressing your baby or yourself. → See Cosleeping vs. Crib-sleeping: The Controversy, page 335.

how sleep works

newborns

Newborns usually sleep between 15 and 16 hours in a 24-hour period. This number looks good on paper, but that sleep can be distributed in all kinds of ways: 30 minutes here, 2 hours there, all through the night and day. Newborns sleep in short cycles, and rarely sleep more than 3 to 4 hours without waking to feed. New parents often find that the baby will fall asleep in their arms, but awaken when transferred to a crib or bassinet. If your baby is not disposed to sleep alone (and you're not disposed to risk waking him up), a good chunk of that sleep may take place on somebody's chest or lap. Also, newborns (unlike older babies) require a diaper change with most feedings, which translates to sleep lost futzing around the changing table at night. So, those 15—16 hours of newborn sleep do not always translate to "free" time for parents.

Just as you need to get used to your baby, your baby needs to get used to you and to life in the world in general. So, during this time of chaos, try not to judge your baby's sleep "patterns." They have yet to emerge. For most parents, this is a time for trial and error and endless, endless, endless feedings.

how much sleep does a baby need?

There's a lot of variation in the amount a baby sleeps. The numbers below are quoted from *The No-Cry Sleep Solution* by Elizabeth Pantley (number of naps in parentheses). Many babies fall outside this range.

1 MONTH	night 8.5—10	day 6—7 (3 naps)	total 15—16
3 MONTHS	night 10—11	day 5—6 (3)	total 15
6 MONTHS	night 10—11	day 3—4 (2)	total 14—15
9 MONTHS	night 11—12	day 2.5—4 (2)	total 14
12 MONTHS	night 11.5—12	day 2—3 (1—2)	total 13—14

sleep stages

All babies, like adults, go through different patterns of light and deep sleep, with periods of brief awakening between them. Babies, however, run through many more cycles than adults and for much shorter chunks of time, lasting about 45 minutes to an hour. (An adult sleep cycle is twice that long.) This means that babies hit in-between stages of brief (or not-so-brief) awakenings every 45 minutes or so. All babies wake up in this way. Some babies go back to sleep; others do not.

sleep temperament

When it comes to sleep, your baby has a mind of his own. Literally: Every baby is born with a unique sleep temperament. That temperament can affect everything from how easily a baby can settle to how much sleep he needs, from where he'll sleep to how easy it is to wake him once he's out. Some babies are born calm and snooze peacefully when they're tired. Others are particularly sleep-resistant. There are lots of ways to describe this kind of baby—"wakeful" and "active" are two common euphemisms. But whatever you call them, babies who don't sleep easily are more common than we are led to believe. When parents say they're lucky because their baby is a sleeper, they are absolutely right! Sleep habits are mysterious things, and the power to change them (as well as the burden of responsibility) is not always in your hands.

sleep disturbances

Parents are often seen *Sssshhhhhhing* everyone in sight so they don't wake the baby, but babies are equally likely to be aroused by some kind of internal disturbance than by something from the outside world. There are lots of funky goings-on inside a baby (particularly a newborn) that may cause wakings. Many disturbances are digestion related. Aside from hunger (see "Night Feedings," page 341), babies can be affected by gas, constipation, reflux, or allergies. They get much better at processing food as they grow. Other disturbances can be caused by rashes (including diaper rash) and teething. ("Teething" often ends up being a catch-all explanation for baby sleep problems.) Developmental changes can also affect sleep. One theory is that babies and kids tend to fall apart just before they reach a new milestone, such as walking. Many parents do find that changes (developmental or otherwise) can mess with sleep. After a day of rampant skill acquisition, a baby might be kept awake processing the changes or too worked up to wind down. Some babies will

> I used to hear about parents with babies who wouldn't sleep and I always thought, They're just not doing it right. They need better routines, more regular naps, etc. Then I had kid number 2. I did the *exact* same things. But this time instead of a cooperative, easy sleeper, I got piercing screams and nonstop night wakings. Now I no longer think it's the mom's fault when a baby doesn't sleep!
> —anonymom

flinging limbs

When a young baby has drifted into light sleep, he might startle himself awake by inadvertently whacking himself in the face. It has been theorized that this common newborn limb flailing, known as the Moro reflex, is a vestigial monkey move—the baby reaching out to clutch the mother's fur for safety. Some babies get little scratch marks all over from Moro reflex–related smacking. It's not dangerous or in any way abnormal, and scratches heal on babies practically overnight, but it can get in the way of sleep. There are little mitts available to prevent this, though not everyone thinks they're a good idea (including the babies who hate wearing them). Some babies seem to experience this reflex more than others, and it can take 6 months or more for it to fade. Swaddling can help control this self-smacking if it's getting to be a problem. ➔ See Swaddling, page 272.

wake up and practice whatever they've been working on during the day.

You may be able to pinpoint a specific reason for your baby's interrupted sleep, but often a baby's waking patterns remain something of a mystery. Your pediatrician may be able to check to see if there's a physical or developmental issue behind your baby's sleep disturbances.

sleep expectations

Since all humans wake periodically throughout the night—and babies wake as frequently as every hour—babies who "sleep through the night" are not actually "sleeping through"; they're getting themselves back to sleep after these brief awakenings. You may also be surprised to learn that the official expert definition of "sleeping through the night" is only 5 consecutive hours—not what most adults consider the night. If your baby goes to bed at seven, and you go to bed after eleven, she may have slept "through the night" by the time you're just falling asleep. And then wake up hourly for the remainder of the night. When will your baby start sleeping through *your* night—the 8-hour stretch an adult craves? The length of your baby's uninterrupted sleep is directly related to her ability to soothe herself—the result of her temperament, things you teach her, or some combination of these influences. (See "Self-Soothing," page 343, for more info.) Some babies are able to sleep long stretches in the first few months; it takes others years to learn to soothe themselves back to sleep when they wake. And lots of babies flip-flop throughout their babyhood between sleeping through the night and waking up intermittently.

I've been reading all the sleep books (my baby is four to five months and apparently there is some crucial window right now where I need to get in and train him to do this and that and sleep through the night). It's making me crazy. Last night I was losing my mind in the dark (nursing) thinking about all that sleeping-theory crap and how it is causing major mommy-baby love interruptus . . . because it all seems so easy when I'm with him and then I think "I should . . ." and it throws my whole mommy rhythm off.
—anonymom

What many parents need to know is that sleeping through the night—that is for an uninterrupted six to eight hours—in childhood or in adulthood is neither a biological truism or a cultural universal.

—Meredith Small,
Our Babies, Ourselves

"is he sleeping **through** the night?"

You'll probably be hearing this question a lot in your first year as a parent. The length of your baby's sleep is a matter of seemingly endless fascination—to friends, family, even to otherwise mostly disinterested strangers. A huge sleep-expert industry has grown around this cultural obsession. Many parenting guidebooks suggest that your baby should be sleeping through the night by 6 months at the latest. So, is your baby sleeping through?? People really want the answer to this question to be a resounding "Yes" and will sometimes go to great measures to be able to say so. They may even lie. And if parents do tell the truth about whatever brutal nighttime reality they've become accustomed to, they often feel like utter failures as soon as they open their mouths. Who wants to be a parent incapable of getting the baby to "sleep like a baby"? Although you may not encounter them in your day-to-day life, there are lots of people who are willing to speak honestly about babies' sleep habits. → See Child-led Parenting, page 364.

night feedings

All babies feed through the night at first. But when is a baby able to take in enough calories during the day to sustain himself through long breaks at night? Depending on who you ask, a baby can outgrow the need for night feedings at anywhere from 6 weeks old to a year plus. There seems to be no one right number and, as always, no average baby.

Breast milk is easier for a baby to digest than formula, so breastfed babies tend to wake more often to feed. Also, night feedings are a part of the supply-and-demand breastfeeding situation—if they are cut out too soon, mothers can experience supply problems. Some moms (especially those from an older pro-early-solids generation) swear that a nighttime calorie blitz—in the form of extra milk or cereal—can eliminate the need for night feedings and get a baby to sleep longer. This has not proven true in studies, so it has lately been discouraged. A bellyful of solids can also disrupt infant sleep with gas and indigestion.

Is it safe to assume that your baby will stop crying to be fed when he no longer needs to be fed? Well, that depends on your definition of "need." Babies may cry to be fed not only to fill their bellies but also to feel the familiar comfort of milk and the person who delivers it. Some argue that comfort is no longer in the realm of the necessary, and that night feeding can become a "bad habit" that needs to be broken. Others think that comfort is just as important to a baby as nutrition, and night feedings are a necessary part of providing comfort. Your doctor may have an opinion about whether your child is big enough or old enough to no longer need the nutrition of a night feeding; you'll have to decide for yourself how to handle the comfort question.

how much sleep do adults need?

Though 8 hours is constantly used as the gold standard, adults usually need somewhere between 6 and 9 hours of sleep to function well the next day. Eight interrupted hours of sleep can be less restful than 5 straight hours, depending on the number of interruptions and where they fall in your sleep cycle. But our sleep needs are not always as inflexible as we think. Some parents find that their sleep rhythms seem to adapt to their baby's waking patterns, and their needs can even adjust accordingly. A parent with a baby who wakes regularly every 2 or 3 hours may find that after a while, her body gets onto this schedule—and it's only when her baby wakes more often than normal that she feels (especially) tired the next day. On the other hand, there's some evidence that sleep deprivation is cumulative, so things may start going downhill eventually if the situation doesn't improve.

SLEEP DEPRIVATION: Sleep can change your whole outlook on life and your baby. Sleep-deprived people often feel depressed and irritable, and generally unhappy. But when things seem to be slumping (or hopelessly unraveling), it can be easy to forget that sleep deprivation might be the reason. People don't always understand how much sleep deprivation has

> All babies don't sleep through the night at six weeks, and sometimes it doesn't matter what you do. They are really their own person. . . . Sometimes you just have to go with the flow.
> —anonymom

messed with their lives until they get to the other side of it. Tolerance for sleep deprivation is really variable. Some people can go for months waking up five times a night; others lose it after one night. But even those with a high threshold need to keep an eye out for the creeping, detrimental effects of exhaustion. → See Coping Strategies, page 345.

Chronic lack of sleep can have the following fun effects on an otherwise happy and healthy adult:

- **Decreased energy, memory, joy, optimism, control of language, ability to problem solve**
- **Increased stress, physical fatigue, pain, weeping, depression, sadness, anger, and early signs of aging**
- **Possible hallucinations and even psychosis in extreme cases**

things to try

Here are some strategies we've culled from parents, pediatricians, and/or sleep experts to help you get your baby to sleep.

understanding sleep signals

Learning to read your baby's cues may give you a better sense of when your baby needs a rest than following a preset plan. If your baby begins to feel hungry or tired, she may seem distracted and stop making eye contact. If she yawns, rubs her eyes, fusses, or begins to cry (and has already been fed), there's a good chance she's tired. Every baby has her own way of expressing herself; yours may rub her nose instead of her eyes, or go straight to manic, bypassing telltale crankiness. Overtired babies are sometimes harder to get to sleep than just regular tired ones. It can be a fine, fine line between the two states (or any baby states, for that matter). You'll start to recognize these signals, though you may experience a fair amount of overtired mayhem beforehand. → See Baby States, page 256.

night vs. day

It takes time to learn the difference between night and day. Here are some ways to encourage your baby to get over the all-night party lifestyle:

- Calm, boring nighttime feedings (minimal fuss, no talking or eye contact) in a dimly lit, unstimulating environment can help a baby remain sleepy. Some suggest changing only dirty diapers during the night and leaving wet ones unless the baby seems uncomfortable.
- A baby can easily get worked up (and wake himself up) if he's left alone to cry. Try to reach him before whimpers turn to shrieks.
- Developing a bedtime routine, vague or otherwise, helps build sleep associations. Night sleep in one consistent place can help distinguish night sleep from naps (if those happen in various spots).

rocking

Newborn babies are used to being suspended in the womb, listening to the thump, thump, thump of Mom's heartbeat (not unlike the sound of a techno bass-line through an overdriven subwoofer). Some prefer being rocked athletically to dance music to being swayed to a lilting lullaby. Rocking doesn't require props, though playing music can make it easier (or more fun) for the rocker. And, it can be done by anyone (unless they've got a bad back or particularly weak arms). In fact, someone other than a breastfeeding mom may be the best option—the smell of milk can be distracting.

Rocking can be great exercise but also thoroughly exhausting and hard to sustain once the baby gets heavier and older. Rocking in a chair can have similar lulling and bonding effects without the back strain. Bouncy seats and swings can reproduce the motion of rocking, but not the human contact.

self-soothing

Many sleep experts (professional or otherwise) recommend putting your baby to bed while awake in order to cultivate an ability to "self-soothe," or to fall asleep alone without rocking, nursing, or coaxing of any other kind. They tend to talk pretty casually about "simply" putting the baby down awake. While some babies adjust to falling asleep alone without too much fuss, some do not. Teaching a baby to self-soothe can involve a lot of trial and error, many steps, and often a lot of resistance (which may mean fussing, crying, or ear-piercing screaming, depending on the temperament of the baby involved). Parents are often encouraged to start babies on the road to self-soothing right off the bat so they can be more independent. But some people discourage self-soothing altogether. They maintain that babies are meant to rely on their parents in the early years of life and that making them rely on their own resources too early disrupts the parent-child connection. ➜ See Interventions, page 346.

routines and associations

Setting up some routines around bedtime can sometimes help a baby feel more at ease with the transition to sleep. A routine can be an elaborate sequence of strictly timed events or a loose framework. What kinds of things work well in a sleep routine? Whatever your baby finds comforting and you can stand doing. Swaying, singing, nursing, bouncing, swaddling, rocking out to Motörhead. As long as your baby knows that this is what happens on the way to sleep, it's a ritual. Trial and error is the best way to see what your baby finds soothing. As they get older, babies can form an association with a particular order of activities (for example, bath, books, bed) or with specific sleep triggers, like a certain song or story.

Associations can be a great help. They can also be hard to break. When considering how to get your baby to sleep, it helps to have a long view and ask yourself: How will this routine work with our lifestyle? How much flexibility do we need? Think not only about what's being done, but who's doing it. With the exception of nursing, bedtime rituals are something anyone the baby trusts can do. Opening up the process to more than just one parent (and/or other caregivers) can be really helpful in the long term, allowing both partners occasional breaks from bedtime duty. You can also think about including more than one sleep association (rocking *and* feeding, for example) so that your baby gets used to a variety of triggers.

Some parents use a structured schedule to define a baby's whole day and night, including sleeping, waking, and eating times. There are a number of experts whose all-around scheduling methods promise flawless naps and restful nights. → See Sorting Through the Voices: Everybody's Got an Opinion, page 363.

feeding

Feeding often has a very soothing effect on babies; sucking is comforting and digestion takes energy. In the early days the feeding/sleep connection can be hard to totally separate. If breastfeeding becomes the primary association with sleep, Mom may need to be physically present for nap and bedtimes, as well as any night wakings. Bottles give more flexibility to the person who's doing the feeding, but can involve more prep time. Bottle-feeding to sleep is more likely to cause tooth decay if the bottle contains anything but water. Some feel that feeding is a perfect sleep-inducing tool and should be used freely. Others argue that keeping feeding and sleep separate from the start prevents parents from having to break this association later.

swaddling

→ See Baby Care Basics, page 272.

human pacifier

Many babies have sucking needs that go beyond hunger. If a baby uses nursing to get to sleep (which is very common, especially early on), she may want the nipple to be there for her if she wakes up. There are lots of phrases to describe this phenomenon; "human pacifier" is probably the one most commonly muttered by nursing moms after a night of constant feeding. Comfort sucking is a part of breastfeeding. It's also part of a baby's development; sucking is one of the only skills a baby is born with. So, really, you're not a human pacifier; that pacifier is a rubber you. But the fact remains that a baby's unrelenting need to suck can really get in the way of a mother's unrelenting need to sleep.

The need to comfort suck may fluctuate throughout a baby's feeding career. One study suggested that sucking through the night might help prevent SIDS. Sometimes an older baby will go through a particularly sucky stage due to some developmental or environmental change. These stages usually pass. If you're overwhelmed by lingering night-nursing sessions, you can try gently removing your nipple and using other comfort measures (rocking, back rubbing, etc.). If your baby insists on constant boob action and you find that the "human pacifier" lifestyle is literally sucking you dry, you can always consider trying an actual pacifier or a bottle (of milk, or even water if your baby's old enough . . . but you may find that waking up to give a bottle is no easier—bottle-fed babies can also get into the suck-to-sleep habit). A lot of babies resist substitutes, at least at the beginning. If you're ready to stop feeding at night entirely, you can try some form of night weaning.

→ See Night Weaning, page 350.
→ See The Pros and Cons of Pacifiers, page 262.

comfort props

The most common comfort prop is the pacifier. Pacifier use for sleep is actually recommended by the AAP (except for breastfeeding babies in the first month of life). But pacifiers are controversial for a number of reasons. (See "The Pros and Cons of Pacifiers," page 262, for both sides of the story.) For safety reasons, security blankets and other comfort objects (dolls, etc.) are usually discouraged during sleep until babies are older. There are varying opinions on what's safe and when; you can ask your pediatrician for her opinion if you're feeling unsure about making a change.

"sleep begets sleep"

This often-repeated baby-sleep theory goes like this: A baby who has had plenty of daytime sleep will sleep better at night. And a baby who has gone to bed early and had lots of nighttime sleep will nap better. The idea is that an overtired baby has a harder time calming down, whether the sleep deprivation is acute (a long, busy day with no nap) or chronic (not enough sleep every night). The concept can give you insight into why your baby gets so flustered after a long afternoon of activity, instead of more sleepy, like an adult. People swear that if you put your baby to bed earlier, he'll wake later and sleep better. This works with many babies, but for some, an early bedtime may mean starting the next day at 4:30 A.M.

coping strategies

Altering your baby's habits is one way to handle sleep issues; altering your life is another. Here are some ways parents change things on their end to make the situation better for everyone.

DIVISION OF LABOR: One thing you can do to increase your sleep is to delegate some of your nighttime responsibilities to someone else. Of course, this assumes that you're able to delegate, which isn't always true, particularly for nursing moms. It also assumes that you have someone else who's able and willing to take on this job, which is not the case for many parents. If you do have someone who can help you with child care, dividing the nights can go a long way toward not letting them conquer you. If your baby's wakings are semipredictable, you can plan who'll be up for which one in advance. Or you can split the night into shifts to let everyone get some uninterrupted rest. Sometimes even being able to count on a break once or twice a week is enough. Another option is to get help in the morning to help you catch up on lost sleep from the night before.

> My husband would go in when she cried and just basically look at her and eventually she found that reassuring. The only thing is now if she wakes up (when she's sick or in a new place or something) I can't do a thing to soothe her. If I pick her up or try to sleep with her she gets really agitated. Now her dad's face is the only thing that will calm her down. I guess he won't be going out or away for a while! (Which is fine with me, I did the first five months.)
>
> —anonymom

> My husband and I are tag-teaming it on sleep. I'll go to bed early while he stays up, then I wake up later and let him sleep late. It's working while he has time off from work; after that, I don't know what we'll do.
>
> —anonymom

> When my wife was breastfeeding, the balance of duties was very different, since she basically had to be with the kid every few hours. I took the morning shift, but she got up with him during the night. Once we stopped night feedings, it was my job.
>
> —anonydaddy

345

When I was leaving the hospital with my firstborn, everyone including the cleaning lady said . . . sleep when the baby sleeps. . . . When I got home, she wasn't sleeping and when she did I thought I would just throw a load of laundry in, or quickly watch a half hour of TV to feel "normal." This was a huge mistake; I got run-down, felt crappy, and was like a zombie at 3 A.M. because I was sooooo tired.
—anonymom

Even a few minutes awake and without the baby clamped on can be so valuable to your psyche—more valuable than sleep? I just don't know.
—anonymom

"NAP WHEN BABY NAPS": Catching up on sleep when the baby's sleeping is an obvious and simple solution to sleep deprivation, and one that's often recommended. But it doesn't always work that well with the reality of many people's lives. It can be hard to nap when other needs are calling—even if it's just the need to be a conscious human being for forty-five minutes without a baby on your lap. While sleep may actually be the best thing for you, there may be times when you want to use your free time for other kinds of restoration.

ATTITUDE ADJUSTMENT: Sleep deprivation has physical and emotional components, and perception definitely plays a role. Can simply changing your expectations be a solution? We have heard from parents who felt a weight lifted once they learned that sleeping through the night is not necessarily the norm. We've also heard from many who felt like choking anyone who suggested that changing expectations could make one whit of difference to the fact of utter exhaustion.

If other people make you feel bad about how your baby sleeps, try not talking about it. You may find that the reality is a little easier to take when you're not worrying about how you measure up. Do you find yourself seething at the clock when your baby wakes up? Try hiding the clock for a couple of nights, and see if the numbers are part of what's getting you down. (This technique is helpful for insomniacs, too.) But if you just feel exhausted regardless of expectations (your own, or anyone else's), more than predetermined ideas need changing.

interventions

Babies do not need to be taught to sleep. But they may need to be taught to sleep in a way that coincides with our own schedules, expectations, or needs. If your baby's sleep (or lack thereof) is making your life miserable, there are more radical things you can do to encourage change. We're calling these more disciplined approaches to sleep "interventions."

Unlike routines, which are pretty universally approved of, interventions are somewhat more controversial, the sort of things parents might get preachy over at a dinner party or discuss behind one another's backs. Because sleep interventions often involve some discomfort (crying) for babies (or for parents), they can have moral overtones. Whatever you believe, there is no shortage of highly motivated experts or parents to lecture you on the pros and cons of any particular method.

when to make a change

New parents have barely wiped away the meconium when they start getting pressure to teach their babies how to sleep. But everyone has a different idea about the right "window" for sleep training: Some say three to six months, some say even earlier, some say once the baby is verbal (some say never). The idea that there's a finite and/or ideal time that applies to every baby and every family is pretty questionable, and way too anxiety-producing. It can be reassuring to remember in the face of any pressure that if you miss one window, there's bound to be another window on the horizon. Initiating change is not always easy. In the dark of the sleep-deprived night, it's very hard to think clearly, and it's even harder to make a move that will very likely result in less sleep in the short term. When it comes to changing sleep patterns, things often get worse before they get better. There's rarely an ideal time to start a sleep-intervention project. The right time, for many people, is when the need for change overwhelms the fear of change, forcing them into action.

THINGS TO THINK ABOUT

- Take a look at your family's sleep situation. Are people functioning? Does everyone seem relatively happy? Or are things (or people) starting to fall apart in one way or another?
- Is there already a lot of crying or unhappiness going on?
- What are your resources for dealing with sleep deprivation? As a person? As a family?
- What's expected of you during the day? Is there any flexibility?
- Does your baby's temperament give you any clues about how he might react to a change in routine?
- Do you have any preconceived ideas about a baby's sleep? Are you open to the idea of letting a baby cry unattended?
- Are you looking for change to happen quickly, or seeing this as a gradual process?

> Sure, they are malleable little beings and sometimes you do need to "help them learn" good sleeping habits (read: Let them cry or whatever), but as a parent, I've never been able to stick to it. Before night three of both attempts, either my husband or I would buckle.
> —anonymom

CRYING IT OUT: "Crying it out" is a commonly used expression for any technique that encourages parents to put their baby to bed while still awake and then leave the baby to put herself to sleep. Some techniques involve periodic visits to comfort the baby; others recommend a cold-turkey approach. These techniques are based on the idea that it is in the developmental interest of the baby to learn to rely on herself rather than be dependent on others for sleep. Once the baby has learned to self-soothe, she may go to sleep with less struggle and be able to put herself back to sleep when she wakes up on and off throughout the night.

Letting a baby cry to sleep has been a longstanding tool in the parental repertoire. But now there are lots of books to all but hold your hand through the process. And the process can be pretty hard. Some babies quickly realize that going to sleep is the only option and are able to make it happen with a minimum of crying. And some parents are able to shut out the sound with a minimum of effort. But many describe it as a grueling experience: "My husband had to hold

> Now that my baby is (finally) learning to fall asleep without me, and consequently not needing me so desperately all the time, I feel sad and a bit lonely. I know it's best for everyone involved but there is still a lot of loss.
> —anonymom

He was already crying all night because he was used to being fed every hour and a half. I was crying because I was exhausted. My husband was crying because I was crying. I figured "controlled crying" would at least put the tears to good use!

—anonymom

I get frustrated when he won't fall asleep on his own. I have tried to "Ferberize" him but feel like I am abusing him. These are the toughest moments because I get pissed off at him and then I realize he is just this little guy who is just looking for some comfort—then I feel bad and like a horrible mother for that moment.

—anonymom

We tried sleep training both our kids in the exact same way. It worked for one and most definitely did not work with the other.

—anonymom

We did Ferber and a consistent routine. . . . It worked out really well, took two nights. I never hear about the child who magically decides to sleep on their own or go to sleep alone after sharing a bed the first year. The parents always have to do some sleep training—it just is a question of when.

—anonymom

me down to keep me from going in there." "We had to put the headphones on full blast so we could tune out the crying." "I was crying, the baby was crying." "I couldn't stand it . . . I had to leave the house." Some babies don't respond to the technique at all, and will continue crying night after night after night. Some say their babies actually got more resistant to sleep after letting them cry. But the techniques are popular for a reason; most of the time, they work—relatively quickly, if painfully. It's a trade-off many parents are willing to make in the interest of more sleep all around.

There is a pretty vocal anticrying camp out there, people who suggest that babies who are left to cry may become aggressive, withdrawn, or insecure. Some say stress levels from uncomforted crying can even kill brain cells. Others dispute these claims. Dieter Wolke, an infant development specialist at the Jacobs Foundation at the University of Zurich, contests: "If you think of the amount of crying babies do, you would think biology would ensure that it doesn't cause brain damage." Many see crying as a necessary evil, without which the baby will be far worse off. They argue that the noisy nights are easily forgotten—a tiny, imperceptible blip in the baby's life.

I never let our baby cry and it was a lot of work. Not much sleep for many months. But I was happy with my decision. I followed my instincts and I felt good about it. What I didn't feel that good about was pressure from others who implied I was letting my baby "walk all over me." My kid is two now and he goes to bed exactly when I tell him with absolutely no fuss. I think partly this is because I never made a big traumatic scene around bedtime.

—anonymom

I just spent two weeks with my sister and her baby who has been trained to sleep by crying it out. I was impressed. I couldn't handle the crying technique. But when I heard my niece's cries, I understood why it worked for her. She didn't really cry per se; she just fussed, like "Eh eh eh." My boy never, ever fussed. He went from 0 to 100 in one second. Total drama queen. If we had let him cry, I swear the neighbors would have called the cops.

—anonymom

GENTLE INTERVENTIONS: Gentle interventions are basically sleep-training techniques that aim to avoid crying. Subtle and gradual changes to a baby's routine are key to this approach. These methods may produce less acute discomfort, but they can be more long-term work and require lots of patience. Gentle sleep training can take months to show measurable results, all the while requiring the parent to assess how to balance the baby's needs with the parents' desire for change. Getting your baby sleeping soundly without trauma or tears sounds appealing. But is it realistic? Maybe, depending on your baby's temperament, as well as your tolerance and expectations. Unless your baby is very easygoing, it's unlikely that you'll be able to avoid crying entirely. Most babies, like most people, resist change when it's forced on them. Even when the change is relatively gentle (for example, switching from rocking to patting as a sleep-inducing attempt), many babies will protest. And protesting, for babies, usually does not involve folk songs and candlelight vigils. Lots of babies will buck and scream at anything other than what they've become accustomed to. The likelihood of this response is not always mentioned in gentle-sleep advice books, so parents sometimes feel like they must be doing something wrong if they're aiming for no tears and getting wails.

Most gentle-sleep advice stresses preventive measures and early sleep associations as much as specific intervention techniques. Experts ("gentle" and otherwise) recommend putting the baby down before he's asleep at least some of the time from a very young age (within the first few months). However, even very young babies know what they like, and many of them don't like being put down awake! → See Self-soothing, page 343.

Here are some basic ideas for building or modifying sleep associations in a gentle way:

BE AVAILABLE: A basic principle of gentle-sleep advice is that babies need their parents at night but can learn (eventually) to need them less and less. In order to feel confident enough to let you go, however, they need to know that you'll come when they cry or call you. This doesn't always mean that you'll respond immediately, just that they won't be ignored.

GO SLOW AND STEADY: Lots of reassurance (physical comfort), calmness, and some semblance of order can reduce bedtime stress and encourage a smooth transition to sleep. → See Routines and Associations, page 343.

SUBSTITUTE: If you have used a certain method to get your baby to sleep for months but want to break the sleep association (or at least reduce it), you can try to very gradually substitute that method with other comforting maneuvers. The weaning from the original to the substitute, however, usually involves some pain of separation (and crying).

> We ended up night weaning at fifteen months, which was kind of a hellish transition but it really worked out well. It probably took about three weeks until he was totally used to getting back to sleep without nursing. It was a long few weeks, there was still some serious crying, but we were always with him and eventually he accepted other methods of soothing from either parent. He also decided that once he wasn't nursing at night anymore, he had no real desire to be in our bed, which was another transition we were worried about tackling at some point in the future!
>
> **—anonymom**

NIGHT WEANING: Nursing mothers often find themselves fed up with night feedings well before they're ready to wean altogether. Babies who cosleep can be especially zealous about feeding at night. (See "Human Pacifier," page 344.) One solution to the problem is to cut out night feedings altogether. This is called night weaning. Night weaning is not recommended until a baby is definitely old enough to be getting sufficient calories during the day. (See "Night Feedings," page 341.) Some people suggest that night weaning is best saved for a baby who can understand language, if not speak it. This way, the baby can be told about day and night, light and dark, or whatever the family decides will differentiate between the time the kitchen is open and when it's closed. The baby may not get it at first and, very likely, won't like it, either. Night weaning can be as excruciating as sleep training. The goal is similar, though not the same. Where sleep training intends to teach the baby to soothe himself without the help of others, night weaning removes one means of soothing (milk) but not necessarily the resource of other people in general. Parents are encouraged to rub, pat, rock, sing, or soothe in any way that helps during the weaning process. The idea is to expand the baby's soothing resources. Night weaning is often easier with the help of a partner or someone who isn't the food source; babies sometimes take to the program more easily if the boobs aren't within smelling distance. Night weaning can also inspire babies to wean altogether, so it isn't something that should be initiated before you're willing to live with that possibility.

resources

Good Nights: The Happy Parents' Guide to the Family Bed (and a Peaceful Night's Sleep!) by Maria Goodavage and Jay Gordon

> My baby only slept through the night once I night weaned (after he was one). As soon as he stopped feeding, he was basically like, you're useless, I'm just going to go back to sleep. I think this worked because the timing felt right to us. If I had tried sooner, it may have been bloody murder.
>
> **—anonymom**

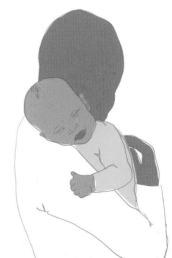

GURU: ELIZABETH PANTLEY
BIBLE: *The No-Cry Sleep Solution*

Elizabeth Pantley's books offer an alternative to the widespread message that crying it out is the only way to improve your baby's sleep. With info for both crib- and cosleepers, Pantley asks parents to carefully assess their children's sleep patterns (as well as their own lives) and gives them tools to try if they're not satisfied with what's going on. She addresses a wide range of sleep issues, including night waking, moving babies from parents' bed to crib, and babies who won't sleep without a nipple in their mouths.

Some parents find her methods hard to implement (they definitely take heaping gobs of patience) and not always effective. But she doesn't promise foolproof results—it's about learning to improvise based on everyone's responses and needs. This book is a good place to start for parents who want to make changes in their baby's sleeping situation, but don't want to do anything drastic.

One caveat: Just because this book is called *The No-Cry Sleep Solution* doesn't mean that your baby (or you) won't cry a bit when you try these techniques! There may be at least a little crying involved, no matter how gentle and slow the going.

GURU: TRACY HOGG
BIBLE: *The Baby Whisperer*

Tracy Hogg promotes an "antiextremist" point of view she calls "sensible sleep," based on her years of experience with real-life babies and their families. Hogg believes babies need to learn to fall asleep on their own, without props, rocking, or elaborate to-dos, but doesn't believe in sending them to their cribs cold turkey. Straddling compassion and discipline, she suggests a gentler sleep-training technique in which babies' cries don't go unanswered, but their needs are not met unequivocally, either. Throughout the book, Hogg offers tips and quips in chummy Anglo-speak, using acronyms to help you plan out your day. While some people find the whole thing a little too cute (and/or bossy), she does provide a compromise.

GURU: RICHARD FERBER
BIBLE: *Solve Your Child's Sleep Problems*

Probably the only parenting guru whose name has morphed into a verb, Richard Ferber is most famous for his system of sleep training, known as Ferberizing. The method involves a timetable in which parents leave their babies alone in the crib for incrementally longer periods of time on several consecutive nights. Trying to get a baby to sleep alone in a crib without a trusty backrub or lullaby is the same as trying to get yourself to sleep on the kitchen floor without a pillow, says Ferber. His technique is designed to help babies break "negative sleep associations" so that they can learn to sleep alone. The result, if all goes as planned, is a baby who no longer needs the breast, bottle, singing, rocking, or any other bells and whistles she had previously relied on to get to sleep. Many parents are zealous about the magic of Ferberization. "It saved our lives" is a refrain heard time and time again from followers breathing a sigh of well-rested relief. While Ferber fans might contest that Ferberizing is not really "crying it out" because they do provide periodic comfort, those on the other side of the spectrum feel that any length of time spent crying alone is effectively a "cry it out" technique.

GURU: MARC WEISSBLUTH
BIBLE: *Healthy Sleep Habits, Happy Child*

According to Weissbluth, your baby doesn't need just any old kind of sleep. She needs the right kind of sleep in the right place at the right time. In fact, she could be as ill served by unhealthy sleep patterns ("junk sleep") as she might be by unhealthy food. Drawing on the popular "sleep begets sleep" theory, Weissbluth urges parents to avoid letting their babies stay awake too long between naps or at the end of the day. Babies who are put down for a nap during their magic window of sleepiness will succumb far more willingly, he argues, than babies who are fighting the artificial stimulation of a second wind. "Perfect timing produces no crying," Weissbluth promises. This optimistic scenario helps frame his book as a holistic sleep program, not simply a guide to "crying it out." While Weissbluth lists several methods for getting a baby to sleep, he suggests that the cold-turkey approach is most effective . . . if only because it's so straightforward, it's hard to mess up. He reassures parents who feel bad about leaving the baby to cry that there is no evidence suggesting that crying to sleep will have a negative impact (though elsewhere in the book, he laments the lack of research on children and sleep). Some see *Healthy Sleep* as an information resource. Others follow Weissbluth's plan religiously, running home to get their babies to bed before their second yawn signals they've crossed the border into over-tiredness. Whether or not you agree with Dr. Weissbluth's prescriptions, if you're interested in the minutiae of infant sleep, this is about as comprehensive as it gets.

nuts and bolts: baby logistics, home and away

fitting the baby into your space

Some parents welcome the apparatus of babyhood as warmly as they welcome the baby itself. And some have recurring nightmares about the Technicolor plastic onslaught. Even the most austere individuals tend to pile on a little more fluff when they bring a baby into their world, no matter how hard they try to resist. Of course, there are people who may be able, through great design, great effort, or great help, to maintain their minimalist sensibilities. Others end up expanding their view of "clean" to include "not covered in baby bodily fluids."

If you have a nursery, you may have no problem keeping the baby stuff in its rightful place. But even those with dedicated children's wings find that baby detritus creeps out into shared space. One option is to relentlessly move things back. You can also try stuffing the unsightly objects into attractive containers.

The recent product-design revolution has finally crossed over into kid stuff. Now, parents who are willing to go out of their way and/or spend several times more than necessary can find items that may be less of an eyesore when plunked in the middle of a high-style household (depending, of course, on the style of your household).

Jennifer Saunders, creator of the British TV series *Absolutely Fabulous*, hilariously captured the inevitable clutter of babyhood in this scene about Bettina, "The Queen of Minimalism." Bettina and Max used to live in a white box decorated only with clear prisms. But now they have a baby, and things have changed. . . .

> Bettina enters, wearing something crumpled. She has the baby on her shoulder, and cloths and bottles in her hand. She looks absolutely fraught all the time. Max enters behind her. He is dressed casually in jacket, denim shirt, jeans and espadrilles. He looks more relaxed than Bettina, and this is a constant source of annoyance to her. With Max comes a mountain of backup baby equipment which they always take everywhere. There are changing bags, nappies, bottles, bottle-warmers, packets of dried milk, clothes, blankets, carriers of every description, pushchair, baskets, collapsible playpen, toys, etc. They have everything the baby might need for the next two years.
>
> —Jennifer Saunders, *Absolutely Fabulous 2*

childproofing

Childproofing is an evolving process. At first your baby won't be venturing far alone, but as he grows and develops new skills (mobility and the pincer grasp), you'll need to up your protection level accordingly. Some kids are more persistently curious while others are content to stay out of your business (and cabinets). Another important factor is your own vigilance; you can leave your edgy coffee table unmarred by foam corners if you're willing to be on the constant lookout for potential pokes in the eye. Some parents take a "better safe than sorry" approach, while others think kids need to learn about bumps and bruises firsthand before they'll get the message to stay away. Consider the stakes involved; you can't predict what the consequences of a bump on the head might be (nor can you always prevent one). But you do know that a swig of toilet bowl cleaner would be B-A-D. Step one is basic household safety: Smoke and carbon monoxide alarms should be tested regularly and toxic things should be locked away safely. Often the best way to learn what you need to do to protect your baby from dangerous stuff in your home is to get down on his level and see what he has access to. Don't forget about things that can be pulled down or dragged over as well as things within immediate reach. Dangling cords, unsecured bookcases, and open(able) bags are all risks to keep in mind besides the obvious poisons, stairs, and sockets. Lastly, remember that babies grow quickly and sometimes make huge developmental jumps without warning. What seems impossible today may be all too easily accomplished tomorrow!

You can find specific information about how to childproof your home from the U.S. Consumer Product Safety Commission (cpsc.gov) or anywhere that sells childproofing products or services.

hidden **toxins**?

Parents know to protect their babies from the bottles of poison under the kitchen sink. But many environmental and child-safety groups maintain that there are actually some baby products that contain potentially harmful chemicals. Companies are not required to list these ingredients on product labels, so it is difficult for parents to tell when they are being used. Some organizations regularly test products and post the results on their websites for consumers.

→ See Fear of a Toxic Planet, page 72, for more information on which chemicals to look out for.

resources
Environmental Working Group: ewg.org
Safe from Toxics: A Project of the State PIRGs and State Environment Groups: safefromtoxics.org

getting out and about

While the first few trips out of the house can take a lot of courage (and planning, and quite possibly arm strength), they are an essential way to build confidence and freedom. Getting around with your baby generally gets easier as you go along, until she gets too heavy, or too squirmy, or too eager to walk, or . . .

Opinions vary on when it's a good idea to take a new baby out of the house. It depends, among other things, on how well the parents are doing, how strong the baby is (premature babies may be more vulnerable to infection, so it's often recommended that parents wait longer before bringing them out in public). The weather is also a factor, though unless heat or cold are really extreme, babies can usually be bundled up or stripped down enough to allow for excursions. Sun protection is a big issue for newborns. Sunblock is not recommended until babies are 6 months old, so shade is the only option. Hats with brims, umbrellas, and other stroller accessories are especially important in the summer.

Before they become mobile, little babies are quite portable and can be integrated relatively easily into many "adult" environments. Use your judgment about what's appropriate. A restaurant doesn't need to be "child-friendly" at this stage, but it's probably better if it isn't pin-drop quiet and romantic, or pounding with dance music and smoky. If you're thinking of bringing your baby to a party, it's a good idea to check with the host first. Taking your baby along to social events can be a mixed bag; you may discover that you prefer having your baby with you to leaving her at home (or staying home yourself), or you might find that the demands of baby care interfere too much with your social time.

A baby is an attention magnet for a large portion of the population. If you happen to come across some particularly enthusiastic baby-lovers on your travels, you may have to decide how much attention you feel comfortable with. Some strangers have no problem asking to hold your baby, or even reaching out for a feel (or a kiss!) without permission. Some parents are not bothered by this and think it's sweet. Others are totally freaked out and awkward about how to address it. Although people may not always like to hear your responses, you are more than within your rights to want to keep strange hands (and germs) off your baby. Feel free to make that clear, in whatever way feels right to you.

I remember when my baby was born, I was so frightened that I would never be able to "get out" that I insisted on dragging my wounded postpartum animal self to the nearest subway—tiny, days-old, crusty-belly-buttoned baby in arms—so that we could enjoy a summer afternoon at the Frick. What could be more civilized? Well, turns out they wouldn't let us in with the stroller, so we spent the afternoon in Central Park. The sun was very healing. We were both squinty eyed, vulnerable, and pale, and fell in and out of sleep under a tree. I was sore and scared, but the trip made me feel that getting out was still possible.
—Ceridwen

I took her out the second week. Logistically, I hated all the crap that you needed to carry around. She also had this amazing gift for crapping her pants the minute we walked out the door. So, I feel like a lot of the early days were me preparing to take her out, only to leave the house for one minute, and then come back in discouraged and ready for a nap!
—anonymom

We took our baby out often, but since he was the type who wouldn't be put down without shrieking, we frequented only restaurants that allowed for eating with babe in arms. The major factor determining entrée choice was how easily it could be funneled from plate to mouth: penne = good, spaghetti = bad. Sandwiches can work depending on their content and volume. Panini are excellent as they hold together well and rarely require the deft extrication of overflow filling from mouth and back into bread, a feature of some sandwiches. Salads work as long as pieces are small enough to not require cutting. In fact, nothing that requires a knife is suitable unless another two-handed party is present and open to spending a good portion of the meal slicing and dicing. I generally couldn't be bothered with this and found the platefuls of bite-size morsels that were handed back to me infantilizing and unappetizing. So I began to crave only manageable foods, and we chose our venues accordingly.
—Rebecca

baby carriers

The simplest way to get out with your baby is to carry him. Baby carriers allow you to do this while keeping one or both of your arms free, and distributing the weight in a more-or-less comfortable fashion. Baby carriers have become popular in America only in the last few decades, but they've been used forever in many parts of the world. The most commonly used carrier is the front-pack type, but sling carriers (which can be worn in many different ways) are getting more popular all the time. The ever-mounting variety of baby carriers available caters to a range of needs and situations. Many carriers are inspired by designs from indigenous tribes, where strollers and infant seats are nonexistent and babies are carried almost constantly. Baby carrying benefits many parents and babies, providing both convenience and closeness. Baby carrying can also help soothe a newborn by putting the baby close to the rhythm of a beating heart and a warm body. If your baby's happy in a carrier, wearing him can give you the flexibility to do things around the house, like cleaning and food preparation. But loading a dishwasher over a tender fontanel may be a bit . . . awkward. People who believe in Attachment Parenting are huge fans of baby carrying (they believe it increases bonding and trust between parent and baby) and can often be a great source for tips on various styles and how to use them. But baby carriers are used by parents with all kinds of philosophical beliefs. Not all babies and parents take to it easily, though; some babies don't like the confinement at first (or when they are older); some parents find it hard on their backs. If baby wearing is important to you, keep trying options at different points in your baby's development; there's a good chance you'll find something that works.

Popular brands are available at any baby store. Check the back pages of parenting magazines or the Internet for some less ubiquitous styles.

strollers: first wheels

Not so long ago, it seemed like every mom had the same baby carriage (black) and then the same stroller (navy). Now, there are as many stroller models available as family cars, and deciding which one to buy can seem almost as mind-boggling. What you need in a stroller depends on your lifestyle and where you live it, as well as the size and age of the kids in your family. What you *want* in a stroller depends on your aesthetics, your love of bells and whistles, and perhaps your desire to shell out lots of cash. You can get a stroller that will cover the basics for a pretty reasonable price. Some parents are cool with strolling around town with the infant equivalent of a compact car, while others have eyes only for the luxury model. Strollers are the most publicly visible baby product and one of the most expensive, some currently topping $1,000 or more (although this is the exception and most strollers are a fraction of that price). They're also one of the most used, especially by parents who walk a lot, which may justify some of the expense if you're considering a major purchase. Some people buy one stroller right off the bat that's meant to last three to four years; others buy several as their child grows. Sometimes one expensive adaptable stroller that covers a baby from newborn through toddlerhood can end up being a more affordable alternative than a couple of strollers for different ages and needs.

Here are some things to think about when facing the dizzying array of stroller options and features:

- Where will you be using it? In the city, suburbs, parks?
- How often? All the time, or only for neighborhood walks?
- Will you need to carry it up stairs, or fit it through many doors?
- Will you be folding it up often? Does it need to fit easily into a trunk? How will it be stored at home?
- Do you need to take it on public transportation?
- How far down do you need the seat to recline? (Newborns need full recline.)
- Do you need it to adapt as your baby gets older? Or if you have another one?
- Are you planning for this to be your primary stroller for several years?
- How important is it to you to have a "fashionable" stroller?

Once you've answered these questions for yourself, you can start asking around to see what strollers might work in your price range. Friends and other parents are a great source of honest info about strollers—if you see someone pushing something interesting, ask for an impromptu review. Salespeople may or may not be helpful—you may want to do some home-work before you hit the stores so you know your options. Models and styles change pretty frequently, so you can sometimes save money by buying last year's model after new ones are released. Gently used strollers are also an option if you don't mind a little wear and tear.

Here are some of the major stroller types. Within each stroller type the features, additions, design, maneuverability, and price vary by brand and model.

standard stroller

- Weighs at least 12 pounds, often more
- Can be very portable, depending on model/weight
- Typically for older babies (above 20 pounds) through childhood

convertible stroller

- Weighs at least 12 pounds, often more
- Can be very portable, depending on model/weight
- "Converts" from reclined baby carriage to upright stroller. Can be used for newborn through toddlerhood and beyond; may adapt with sibling attachments

lightweight or "umbrella" stroller

- Weighs 12 pounds or less
- Very easy to fold, carry, and stow
- Preferable for toddlers or kids, shorter trips for younger ones; little padding and recline, not great for young and/or napping babies; cannot be used for newborns
- Good for public transportation
- Less sturdy, may not last as long
- Often the least expensive

car seat stroller (infant car seat snapped onto stroller frame)

- Weighs approximately 21 pounds (base is 14 pounds; car seat is 7 pounds)
- Offers flexibility (can use in car and on street)
- Can be used only for infants under 20 pounds, 26 inches
- Large storage basket
- Stroller frame is inexpensive; infant car seat price varies

"travel system" (stroller including attachable infant car seat)

- Weighs at least 25 pounds (17-plus pounds for stroller; 7-plus pounds for car seat)
- Adapts to all ages; relatively expensive

all-terrain or jogging strollers

- Not so portable, tend to be around 20-plus pounds
- Big-wheeled easy-glide strollers, designed for exercise or extensive walking; can handle rough roads, curbs and pavement; easy to maneuver (unless front wheel is fixed)
- Sturdy and long-lasting
- Can be on the expensive side
- Not always appropriate for young babies

strollers for multiple kids

The increase in multiple births has also increased the variety of twin-appropriate strollers. Double strollers are also often used by parents with more than one young child. Jogging strollers are available for twins or kids of different ages/sizes. Parents who anticipate a sibling can purchase a convertible stroller with multiple kid attachments.

These are the major multiple stroller styles:

side-by-side

- Kids have same POV, can communicate and keep each other company
- Both seats recline the same amount (often to flat)
- Can be harder to fold up
- Width makes it hard to navigate and fit through doors

tandem (one seat in front of another)

- Easy to fit through doors and can be easier to fold up
- Front seat may not recline as far back as the other seat
- Kids are separate, may both prefer the same seat

double or triple deckers

- Seats are arranged in staggered heights, one in front of the other
- Kids have similar POV but can't communicate with each other
- Many come with detachable car seats
- Smallest footprint is easiest to navigate

car travel

In all parts of the United States (and a lot of the rest of the world as well), babies are required to travel in an approved car seat. Many hospitals won't let you take your baby home unless he's strapped into one. There are portable car seats designed for infants, allowing the baby to be carried around in the seat. They can work well for parents who don't have their own car, since they often don't need to be installed with a base, and can be easily snapped into a stroller base (or "transport system") for street travel. If the baby will be traveling in the same car(s) all the time, car seats can be permanently installed; this makes it easier to get the baby in and out. Convertible car seats, which can be used through toddlerhood, can save parents the money and hassle of buying a new car seat when the baby outgrows the infant seat (which depends on his height and weight, but is usually by about 6 months).

Car seats should be installed facing the rear until the baby is over one year old and is more than 20 pounds. Used car seats are not recommended. Setting up seats can be complicated and is often done incorrectly. Many people we've talked to had a small breakdown over that first car-seat installation. To help ease you through the process, find a resource with explicit information about installing car seats, or, better yet, an expert installer to check your work. Some local police departments will do this for you. Rental car companies usually offer car-seat rentals as well, and will often install them for you. It is always worth doublechecking to see that they are secure, however.

taxis

At this point, cabs are exempt from laws requiring car-seat use in many cities. But taxis, although yellow, are still cars, and cab drivers can be unpredictable. Plenty of people do just hoist kids of all ages into the backseat and pray. Maybe this works if you're a Hope for the Best type, but Imagine the Worst types may not find this solution feasible. Some people schlep car seats on cab rides. This is no big deal in the infant-seat phase, but far less convenient when talking about a behemoth of a toddler seat. There are also a couple of iffy travel car-seat options currently available. Some car services will provide car seats. But be prepared, as car seats may be the wrong size (like a toddler seat for an infant, and vice versa), installed wrong, or not installed at all. Since many people travel without car seats in livery cars (because, legally, they can), drivers are sometimes cranky about complaints. You may be able to find cooperative car services in your area by talking to other parents or checking local parenting resources.

public transport: buses, trains, and subways

Trains have a lot going for them when it comes to baby travel. There's lots to look at, room to move around, and babies often find the noise and movement soothing. But the lights can be bright and the crowds overstimulating. The hardest part of train travel is usually getting to and from the train platform. Parents often end up doing a lot of carrying up and down stairs, sometimes with the help of other passengers, sometimes solo. If turnstiles are the only way in or out, you've got to take the baby out of the stroller, fold it up, and squish both, along with yourself and anything else you've got with you, into an obscenely small wedge of space on the way through the egress turnstile. New York City subways can be particularly stressful for these reasons. Some other cities are more enlightened.

Bus travel is often the urban transport method of choice for people with babies in tow, if only because of the lack of stairs. Generally, strollers must be folded up and babies must be held.

plane travel

Airlines allow babies to travel quite soon after birth, but some may recommend waiting. The biggest concern is exposing vulnerable infants to germs. If you're worried about traveling with a young baby, ask your doctor what she thinks. On some airlines, babies under two are allowed to travel domestically for free, or for a nominal percentage of the ticket price, on the lap of an adult. The safest option (but also the most expensive) is to buy a seat, sometimes at a reduced price, for your baby and install a car seat onboard. Some parents suggest bringing along a car seat even if you don't buy a seat, in the pretty unlikely case that the airline lets you use a spare seat for free. If not, the car seat can be checked. Be sure your car seat is FAA approved before bringing it on board! If it's not, you won't be allowed to use it. A few airlines will provide car seats for children. Since regulations vary, speak to your airline about what they do and don't allow, provide, and recommend for babies.

Young infants are actually relatively low-maintenance air travelers. But still, travel with babies involves a lot of schlepping, a period of limited mobility, and the (fear of) reactions of people around you. In this day and age, air travel is hardly a relaxing experience. Increased security and anxiety put people on edge, and when they see your adorable baby, they see the potential for hours of nonstop screaming. Being the parent with the inconsolable baby on an airplane is a sort of parental rite of passage, albeit a rather unpleasant one, for those who fly. If (when) it happens to you, there's not a whole lot you can do— once you've exhausted your soothing arsenal—except wait it out. Apologize if you're inclined, but keep in mind that your baby does have a right to travel (and that some travelers find the anxiously placating parents of babies more irritating than the babies themselves). Every child travels differently and every individual trip holds different circumstances; the more you travel, the more coping mechanisms and tricks you'll develop.

Here are some things you can do to help steer you in the direction of a pleasant trip:

- Encourage your baby to drink or suck on something during takeoff and landing to protect his ears. A good chunk of baby crying on flights is attributed to ear discomfort.

- Dress everyone in layers for maximum flexibility.

- If you are taking an international flight, "bassinet" seats may be available for the baby. These need to be pre-booked. Your baby might be able to sleep in one or he may hate it, but it's worth a shot.

Traveling by plane has been a real eye-opener for me about how clueless I was before I had kids. Last time we flew our son (one year old) fell asleep in the backpack and a woman on line for the plane said "That kid is dead" and someone else said "Let's hope he stays that way until we land." I'm sure I would have thought this was funny if it wasn't my kid but I found it incredibly rude as the kid's mom. The hostile looks and comments were incredible. A global apology to any parents I insulted in my previous life!
—anonymom

I flew around the world (New York to Australia) alone with my eight-month-old son. It all went pretty smoothly. I kept him in a BabyBjörn for much of the travel, though he spent many hours sitting in the Qantas bassinet making faces at a large and trapped audience of vaguely amused strangers. At various gates along the way, I would spread out a blanket and let him roll around and play for as long as possible. I also revealed toys one at a time, over 24 hours, so there was always some novelty. He got over jetlag much more easily than I did (though we had our share of 4 A.M. breakfasts). All other parents on the flight agreed that traveling with a baby is not nearly as hard as traveling with a toddler (who wants and needs to move just about all the time) and/or multiple kids.
—Ceridwen

- Overnight flights can be easy for babies who sleep, but if you know your baby doesn't sleep well on planes, traveling during the day may be easier on your family (and other passengers).

- Some parents prefer to check their stroller so they have less stuff to keep track of. Others check the stroller at the gate, and pile bags and/or baby on it as they go through the airport.

- A bulkhead row will give you extra space. But it also means no under-seat storage, so you won't be able to access your carry-on, at least during takeoff and landing. If you request one, be sure the ticket agent knows you're traveling with a baby.

- Opinions vary about giving kids antihistamines during long flights to help them sleep. If this is something you're interested in, talk to your pediatrician. Never give medication on a flight without trying it out first to see how your baby reacts. Some kids get stimulated by antihistamines rather than knocked out!

- Consider bringing earplugs: not for you, but for your fellow passengers. The plugs probably won't block out the noise entirely, but they might at least amuse people with a sense of humor.

things to bring on board

- More diapers than you think you'll need, in case of delays
- An extra change of clothes in case of messiness
- Several blankets of varying thicknesses
- A baby carrier if you use one
- Water, especially if you're nursing
- Lots of whatever your baby usually eats/drinks
- Lots of small toys if your baby's old enough to play with them
- Whatever you usually use to clean and care for your baby

sorting through the voices: everybody's got an opinion

One of the greatest challenges for many new parents is navigating the massive barrage of information about parenting. The helpful advice of experts, doctors, grandparents, friends who have been there, and perfect strangers can become a cacophonous mêlée to exhausted ears. The noise starts when you're pregnant: "You've got to circumcise! Immunize! Ferberize!" and keeps right on going through the whole child-rearing process. Whether the ideas come from your own mother, a bestseller, or some whacko on the street, it can start to feel like everyone's an expert . . . except you.

I was walking down the street with [my baby] in a front-carrier thing the other day; he fell asleep and his head was lolling all over the place but I was like, f**k it, we're almost home, I can't worry about this lolling, and at that exact moment this middle-aged *man* walked past me and as he did, he shouted: "You better do something about that baby's neck!" Of course, I felt publicly shamed—everyone heard this comment—and branded Bad Mother. Practically in tears, I turned up a side street, holding his head in my mittened hands.
—anonymom

schools of thought

Much of the advice world can be generalized into two camps—parent-led and child-led. We're summarizing them here not to suggest that you "pick a side" (you might, you might not) but to help you understand some of the ideas out there and see how they sit with you. In reality, most parents, and even most parenting experts, probably take some from each.

parent-led parenting

IN THEORY: The basic idea behind parent-led child rearing is that the baby must learn to fit into the family (society) rather than the family (society) adapting to the needs and wants of the baby. Parent-led philosophies tend to encourage structure and boundaries to help the baby make sense of the world and give everyone in the family a chance to experience independence. Advocates are big on sleep and feeding schedules. Though the specific recommendations vary, what most of the theories have in common is the belief that both the baby and the family need ritual and predictability to flourish.

A baby's world, as many parent-led experts see it, is a chaotic one; it's the parents' job to provide organization and consistency through routine. Mothers who take the parent-led approach talk about the relief of knowing when they can have "my time." Even if they are feeding the baby as often as a mother who feeds on demand, they find comfort in the predictability of a schedule. These methods also stress teaching the baby to separate from her mother and to soothe herself (thus fostering a baby's psychological journey toward independence). Furthermore, parent-led moms and dads believe that establishing limits and schedules early helps to prepare children for the real world, and to keep them from becoming "spoiled" and "entitled." Advocates point out, however, that training does not equal tyranny. Most extol a gentle brand of discipline undertaken in an environment of love and caring.

The important thing, according to this style, is that order and equilibrium rule, making the inevitable chaos of having a baby as manageable as possible. In order for the family as a whole to thrive, the baby must be a team player, children must be learning the rules rather than making them, and parents must be calling the shots.

IN PRACTICE: Following routines may sound more manageable than riding the waves of baby chaos, but scheduling an infant (not to mention the whole family) is not always easy. It can require an iron will and a strong stomach to organize a baby's time.

- Training often involves resistance, which for the baby usually means a lot of crying. Some parents find it more difficult than others to tolerate the sounds of their babies' cries without responding. → See Crying It Out, page 347.

- Parent-led routines hinge on regular structure. Many manuals emphasize "sticking to the plan" when they pitch a particular scheduling strategy, and warn that slipups could cause the whole project to crumble. This kind of rigor can be stressful and time consuming.

- You may find that a routine that works well at home may be hard to translate to changing circumstances. Your baby may sleep like a log in his crib from 7 P.M. to 7 A.M. every night after his bath but might not be able to doze in his stroller in the spare room at a dinner party like your friend's "disorganized" baby. So while you are likely to gain some kinds of independence with this kind of parenting, realize that schedules may create dependencies of their own.

- The notion that the baby should be *a part of* the mother's life, rather than her whole focus, can be appealing, especially to working mothers. A scheduled baby may be easier to fit into a scheduled workweek, which can help make limited time together more predictable (though iron-clad routines don't always allow for unexpected late nights at the office).

- It's wise to be wary of plans that suggest they work equally well for everyone. This kind of attitude can make you feel like a failure if you can't get your baby to fit the mold.

- Schedules can impact some of the other choices you make for your baby, like whether or not to breastfeed. → See Scheduling, page 291.

child-led parenting

IN THEORY: Generally speaking, most child-led parenting advocates believe that being attuned and responsive to the needs of babies and children is a crucial aspect of their healthy development. Children are fundamentally different from adults, and proponents of this style assert that a child's unique point of view should be respected.

Child-led methods often focus on honing your "natural instincts" and letting your baby's needs guide you. From the very beginning of their lives, babies use nonverbal cues such as rooting, noises, body positions, and facial expressions to indicate their needs. Child-led parenting experts urge parents to become fluent in their baby's codes and to meet their pleas promptly and with love. They believe infants should be soothed by their parents, rather than being left to "self-soothe," and reject the notion that you can spoil a baby by responding to its cries. Many experts in this field suggest that ignoring a baby's signals can be damaging to the baby/parent relationship, if not the baby's psychological state.

To develop good baby-listening skills, parents need to spend a lot of time with their children. Some experts prescribe a lot of focused playtime. Others argue for as much physical contact as possible and suggest wearing the baby in a sling throughout the day and sleeping with the baby at night. This particular child-led style is often called Attachment Parenting. Some are adamant about the presence of one primary caregiver who is with the baby most (or all) of the time so that there is a consistent bond. Breastfeeding is encouraged to strengthen the mother-child connection. Child-led parenting advocates don't worry about overindulging a baby or young child with love and affection. They maintain it can't be done. Trust building is crucial to child-centered parenting. Parental attentiveness is the number one priority, for as long as a baby feels "heard" and trusts that she has someone she can count on, she will develop the secure attachment upon which a future of self-confidence and healthy relationships depends.

IN PRACTICE: The idea of parenting simply by reading your child's cues and responding according to instinct seems easy enough, but the reality is sometimes a little more complicated.

- In the chaos of new parenthood, it can be hard to even hear your own voice, much less trust it. A child-led parent must have the confidence to tune out all the experts promising easy answers and to delve into the sometimes confusing world of infant interpretation.

- Putting the baby's needs first can be hard on the mother's sense of self, as well as on other members of the family. It can be a real effort to find time for intimacy between partners as well as personal time in a parenting style that solicits maximum contact with your baby.

- The child-led approach can require redefining of expectations about things like sleep and personal space. Interrupted sleep is often seen as the norm rather than a problem to be solved. While gentle measures may be suggested to coax a baby to sleep longer, quick-fix formulas are frowned upon.

- Parents who like to go out and travel with their baby may find that this style gives them more flexibility. A baby who is not used to a strict schedule or routine is more likely to accept irregularities into the flow of her life. This approach can also be convenient for working parents with erratic schedules.

- Some types of child-led parenting, Attachment Parenting in particular, can be challenging for working mothers (or others who can't be with their babies for long stretches). Working moms who choose to parent in this way, however, often find that the emphasis on bonding helps to refuel their connections after a separation. Demand feeding while at home and during the night, for example, can help maintain a breastfeeding working mother's milk supply.

- Some people are drawn to this style of parenting for the seeming lack of structure and fuss. It can sound seductive to be able to continue a flexible lifestyle with a new baby. But the child-led approach isn't necessarily about "just going with the flow," despite the natural-parenting fantasy. Whether it's swaddling, baby wearing, rocking, nursing, or cosleeping, this style definitely requires technique and effort.

attachment parenting

Attachment Parenting (AP) is a parenting style based on the principles of attachment theory, which says that the caregiver/baby bond is crucially important to the child's well-being. Basic Attachment Theory suggests that being generally responsive to a baby's needs is enough to create a secure attachment. Attachment Parenting encourages specific behaviors to promote this connection. These methods include breastfeeding (ideally until the child weans himself) and minimizing separation between babies and parents throughout the day and night. Positive discipline and prompt attention to the baby's needs are also emphasized. Attachment Parenting discourages feeding schedules, sleep training, and anything else that interferes with parents responding instinctually to their baby's cries.

The real core of the philosophy is an emotional connection between babies and their caregivers—with as little interruption as possible. The principles of AP are partly inspired by anthropological research from other cultures, where babies and parents are in close physical contact all or most of the time. Believers in AP say parenting with these priorities helps children develop confidence in their relationships and themselves. Critics say that so much focus on babies' needs makes it difficult for parents to meet their own. The emphasis on constant closeness can make it difficult for working parents and can impact partner intimacy. Although "balance" is also part of the AP doctrine, parents are often encouraged to put their own needs on the back burner if they can. Some people can do this relatively easily. For others, this kind of parenting can create resentment. Attachment Parenting is not an all-or-nothing situation, and many would argue it's less about following rules than a state of mind.

➔ For more on the pros and cons of AP, see The Baby Gurus, page 371, on Dr. William and Martha Sears, the pediatrician and his wife credited with giving the movement its name.

resources
Anything from The Sears Parenting Library
The Continuum Concept by Jean Liedloff
Attachment Parenting: Instinctive Care for Your Baby and Young Child by Katie Alison Granju and Betsy Kennedy
Mothering magazine

finding your voice

How can you listen to your instincts when you don't know what they are yet? How can you do what's right for your family when your family's just forming? It takes time to understand everyone's changing needs, and the learning curve can be scary. For new parents who know nothing, the authority of experts can be especially intriguing. You may open a book because you desperately need to know whether nine poops a day is normal, and then get sucked into someone else's opinion on independence, family values, or working mothers. Becoming a parent is all about learning to process information in a way that works for you.

Some people find that a certain theory or doctrine feels right to them and let this govern most of their parenting decisions. Others see parenting as a series of independent decisions to be evaluated and considered in the moment. Parenting is all about making choices. Regardless of whether or not you identify your parenting style, you will need to develop some kind of strategy for making decisions about your baby and family's lifestyle, even if that strategy could be best described as "winging it."

Some things to think about:

flexibility

If there's one thing that's true about being a parent, it's that you never know what things will be like until you get there (or sometimes, in the case of the particularly fuzzy brained, until after you've gotten out of the baby woods altogether). What sounds appealing during pregnancy, for example, can seem absurd once there is a real-live (screaming, crying) baby in your life. You may come to the experience fully committed to Attachment Parenting and find that once you're in the thick of things, you're more stressed out by cosleeping than by letting your baby cry it out. Or you may plan your baby's schedule to mirror your own jam-packed date book, but find that once you've got the kid in your arms, you're much more inclined to follow his flow. There's a lot to consider, and so much of it can't be imagined before the fact.

reading between the lines

For every success story and glowing note of thanks you read, there are tales of people who found the theories or methods didn't work. Most of the time you won't hear these from the experts. They will all tell you that their technique is the best—and quite possibly the only— way to ensure the healthy, secure development of your baby. Some books are so convincing that readers may find they need to deprogram themselves a little afterward. New parents are easy targets for conversion, vulnerable from lack of sleep and lack of experience. But as much as we sometimes really wish there was, *there is no right way*. Whether a particular idea will work depends on who your baby is, who you are, and the circumstances of your family.

> When somebody asks me our parenting philosophy, I reply confidently: "It's parent-led but child-directed." We place a heavy emphasis on a strictly enforced schedule that changes daily. I guess we don't really have a philosophy. We have a child.
>
> **—anonydaddy**

> I know I was extremely lucky with him; however, I also believe that my researching and preparation during pregnancy helped a great deal. I don't believe that "Mother Nature" will tell you what to do. I believe it's an extremely hard "project" you need to get familiar with to manage or do a good job.
>
> **—anonymom**

plan b (c, d, e, f, and g)

Though experts frequently present a system to be followed every step of the way, it's far more common for people to look into one or two or ten philosophies and pick a few choice nuggets from each. A majority of parents don't stick to a single prescribed "parenting" technique. If a particular expert's strategy or plan or "approach" seems appealing, go for it. Just don't panic if it doesn't work—and if the next three things you try don't work, either. Don't be surprised if you find yourself throwing more than one "parenting bible" across the room . . . it happens more often than you think. Just aim it away from the baby.

filtering out the noise

Try not to freak out about every new "study" that makes the headlines. Whatever you do, it's likely that sooner or later some study will denounce it . . . followed by another one that says you were right all along.

> I get frustrated because I feel there are two extremes with little middle ground. It's either all-natural and if you have a C-section or don't breastfeed until the kid is three you're a bad mother. On the other hand, I feel most "mainstream" information gives too much power to the doctors and not enough to women.
> —anonymom

your baby isn't everybaby

When you have a baby, you enter into a relationship—it's not just parent acting upon baby. It's a dynamic. As you get to know each other, your baby will help you understand *her* world, just as you'll help her understand *the* world. As you get to know each other, you'll start to get a feel for how a particular parenting maneuver will go over. Thinking about your baby, not just "a baby," will help you sort out what's going to work and what's not.

conscious parenting

Whatever your style or circumstances, whether you're going primarily by the book or by the seat of your pants, one of the most valuable tools in any parent's pocket is the ability to make conscious and informed choices. We call this conscious parenting, but you can think of it as whatever you want: sensitivity, responsibility, attunement, common sense.

> Each time someone has a baby, they reinvent the wheel and for good reason. Every pregnancy, baby, and mother/child relationship is different. Read each labor and birth, child-rearing, sleep-training, breastfeeding book with one eye open. Don't be afraid to create your own routines and style.
> —anonymom

for us, conscious parenting means

- Being aware of the needs of your baby, yourself, and other family members
- Making informed decisions that take these needs into account
- Taking responsibility for the choices you make

We think these things are even more important than most of the individual choices along the way. Why? Well, the debates over parenting issues have been raging for ages and will probably rage on forever. And at this point, there's no real way of knowing what's "best," aside from figuring it out for yourself. You need to learn how to make decisions that honor your own values, not someone else's agenda. So how do you get to a place where you can make the best possible choices? Stop, look, and listen . . . and then think clearly to determine the path you want to take.

This is admittedly not as easy as it sounds. One thing that can help is giving yourself some leeway to think about how different solutions sit with you. Explore how you feel about ways of responding to and guiding your baby. If a particular path feels wrong to you, think about it. You might discover that your gut response reflects how you really feel, or realize that you're responding to something else in your psyche or experience. Once you've given it some thought, you can decide whether you want to change course, or if the goal is important enough to pursue this route even if the process is difficult.

The payoff can be enormous. Knowing you're taking the time to stop and think about your choices takes the pressure off each individual choice. Everyone makes mistakes . . . but most of the time, they don't matter. They'll blend into the backdrop for your baby unless they become a regular occurrence. But they may matter to you. When you've made a choice you regret, it's a huge relief to know that your own backdrop is one of care and consideration. And when you do take a wrong turn, learning to make educated choices will help you accurately assess the risks and impact, rather than let your anxiety run amok. A disruption in a baby's routine, for example, will be a lot less traumatic for everyone if you're not reverberating with the idea that you've made a horrible mistake and are therefore a horrible mother. If you know that you're making your decisions with the best interests of your baby and your family at heart, you can be confident that you're doing a good job as a parent—on a cumulative level, which is where it really counts.

GURU: PENELOPE LEACH
BIBLE: *Your Baby and Child: From Birth to Age Five*

British child-rearing expert and psychologist Penelope Leach has been a major force in bringing child-led parenting to the mainstream. When her first books, *Babyhood* and *Your Baby and Child: From Birth to Age Five*, hit the shelves in the 1970s, they were considered revolutionary. She was one of the first experts to present issues from the child's point of view. Parents and babies, she argued, are intertwined, so whatever's in the best interest of the baby benefits its parents as well. This child-centered viewpoint, which okayed demand feeding and denounced spanking, really changed the way many parents saw their children. They were allowed to stop worrying about controlling their babies, and assured that a little love and responsiveness wouldn't spoil them.

One of Penelope Leach's hallmarks is balancing compassion for the baby with sensible advice for the parents. She talks about the futility of "guilty soul-searching." By stressing the practical and giving voice to the unpleasant feelings that may come with parenting, Leach keeps things in the here and now. She favors pragmatic suggestions, not grand theories, in the midst of unraveling infant chaos: "Carrying him may not suit you very well right this minute, but it will suit you far better than that incessant hurting noise. And when, and only when, peace is restored you will have a chance of finding a more permanent solution."

Leach distinguishes between newborns, settled babies (3—6 months), and older babies (6—12 months) and suggests different tactics for dealing with common issues at each developmental stage. (This emphasis on development can make some parents worry if their baby's behavior doesn't match her descriptions.) While she definitely advocates putting your baby's needs first, Leach doesn't prescribe any particular means to that end. Cosleeping is no better or worse than crib-sleeping in her book—there are pros and cons to each, for her. There are a few subjects on which she comes down with a hard line (circumcision is one), but in general, she suggests that people make their own choices based on their own situations.

There have been some complaints from working mothers who feel that Leach would rather have them at home than on the job. Leach, however, claims that she strongly supports working mothers, that it's the lousy governmental policies she has a beef with. Though her ideas may not seem as radical now as they once were, Penelope Leach remains one of the world's most powerful advocates for children and parents.

GURU: GARY EZZO
BIBLE: *On Becoming Baby Wise* (cowritten with Dr. Robert Bucknam)

Gary Ezzo brings the ideology, and Dr. Robert Bucknam brings the medical muscle, to this hugely successful and controversial "infant management" bible, *On Becoming Baby Wise*. Their basic pitch is that a "parent-directed" family—with requisite feeding schedule and sleep training—will thrive and produce happy, well-adjusted, secure kids who sleep through the night, allowing Mom and Dad's marriage to remain strong and central. Ezzo's company, Growing Families International, uses a "church-based curriculum" to help promote his values and methodology. The ideas in *On Becoming Baby Wise* are at the core of that campaign. In the book, Ezzo and Bucknam almost obsessively pit their techniques against those of the child-led camp. The message is clear: Child-centered parenting is a pernicious threat to the family. Put the kids first, they warn, and the marriage "gets lost in space." Put the marriage first, and kids will bask in the glow of their parents' union, "happy beyond their own understanding." Ezzo and Bucknam's emphasis on protecting the marriage can be very appealing to new parents who suddenly see their time together slipping away. They do make assumptions about who works and who stays home with the kids: "When daddy gets home," they tell us, he should spend time with mommy first, then the kids. They repeat the credo "marriage comes first" like a mantra.

Meanwhile, the picture they paint of the child- or mother-led family is one of spoiling, tantrums, and the "emotionally crippling attitude of me-ism." Ezzo and Bucknam would rather see families who practice "we-ism," and babies who learn from day one that life is about giving as well as taking. Though it might be disturbing for some new parents to read such a partisan account of parenting, many readers are attracted to Ezzo's authoritative "parental" tone and value-laden message. The appeal of this book is strong, but the science behind it isn't the soundest. In 1998, the American Academy of Pediatrics spoke out against Ezzo and Bucknam's Parent-Directed Feeding (PDF) schedules citing evidence that PDF babies were failing to thrive. Although the authors have updated their book to address these concerns, some feel that the gist is the same.

GURUS: WILLIAM AND MARTHA SEARS
BIBLE: *The Baby Book*

The major mouthpieces of Attachment Parenting, pediatrician William Sears and his wife, Martha (a nurse, childbirth educator, lactation consultant, and self-defined "professional mother"), have produced a library of books addressing most phases and problems of young childhood. They've also raised a small army of kids of their own—including two coauthoring pediatricians, an adopted child, and a child with Down syndrome—and draw liberally from personal as well as professional experience. By referring to themselves and their kids in these firsthand tales, they drive home some of their major values: intimacy, warmth, and the superiority of parental instinct over culturally imposed ideas about how babies should behave.

The Sears philosophy is child-centered to the max. Distilling Attachment Parenting's tenets down to a set of seven core concepts, the book prescribes baby wearing, sleep sharing, breastfeeding, and responsiveness. The primary message of the Sears books is that young babies' wants *are* their needs, and those needs must be met. The more you give to your baby, say the Searses, the more you'll receive: in the short term, as love, affection, and connection, and in the long term as your child grows into a confident, secure kid.

The book takes parents from postpartum to toilet training and suggests ways of staying connected to your child through the challenges of each stage. Most problems, the Searses think, can be solved by turning up the volume on nurturing, whether it's through nursing, holding, or wearing your baby. What happens when parents question whether they can handle such a labor-intensive parenting style? The Searses say that the *real* hard parts of parenting are the feelings of disconnection from your child. Focusing on attachment in babyhood can help circumvent this problem when your child gets older. Although the refrain "If you don't like it change it" appears periodically throughout the pages of *The Baby Book,* there's not much practical advice given for parents who feel overwhelmed by the demands of Attachment Parenting. In cases of extreme burnout, mom could perhaps arrange for a few hours of "me time." Beyond that, the Sears strategy is usually to reinforce the positive impact of the right choices on a child's well-being.

This "accentuate the positive" attitude is a common feature throughout the Sears library, and it's surely a big part of what makes the books so appealing. Many people are won over by the loving image of seamless parent/baby bonding, so much kinder and gentler than the idea of leaving your beloved baby alone to cry. But the real world doesn't always live up to the fairy tale in *The Baby Book*. There are good and bad parts to parenting (attachment or otherwise), and the Sears style is not equally suited to everyone. By glossing over the negative stuff, they can leave struggling parents feeling inadequate and guilty.

Whatever your take on the AP ethos, *The Baby Book* offers excellent medical advice. The Searses' straightforward and relaxed style makes the book feel far less alarmist than most M.D. child-care books we've seen, and their information is clear and well researched. While some medical books tend to undermine parental confidence with an authoritative tone, the Searses place an encouraging amount of trust in parents' judgment in medical as well as emotional matters. The Searses' website, askdrsears.com, contains even more detailed information about things like medication dosage and common illnesses.

GURU: GINA FORD

BIBLE: *The New Contented Little Baby Book: The Secret to Calm and Confident Parenting*

Gina Ford is a hard-core British fantasy nanny, complete with all the benevolent dominatrix overtones. One quick glance at the feeding schedules in her best-selling *The New Contented Little Baby Book* and you can easily imagine her whisking into your nursery, drawing the curtains, rolling up her sleeves, and declaring "Hmph." She will not only tell you when your baby should bathe, eat, and sleep—"He must start his bath no later than 5:35 P.M., and be massaged and dressed no later than 6 P.M."— she will tell *you* when you should bathe, eat, and sleep: "You should have cereal, toast and a drink no later than 8 A.M." As for the dishes, you will be doing those at 6 P.M.: "Dim the lights and sit him in his chair for ten minutes while you tidy up." The sheer *force* of her nursery know-how could flatten a new mom's doubts like a steamroller. Who has time for second-guessing when you're scheduled to the minute, prodded gently on by Ford's fabulously British way with words? "Wash and dress baby, remembering to cream all his creases." Gina Ford offers a life of pure, simple organization: no confusion about naps and nursing, no guessing what the baby's thinking. Even the creases will be creamed on time.

If keeping track of what to do and when to do it makes you feel anxious, then Gina Ford is probably not your girl. Some people, however, really respond to the order a nanny expert like Ford promises. Ford says her techniques are a huge relief for mothers and a big confidence booster— once she knows exactly what to do, a mother will be cool, calm, and collected (and so will her baby).

Like many baby experts, Ford claims that infants establish strong associations from the very start. Because of this, she argues, it is essential that you establish good routines immediately to avoid having to reprogram later on. She believes in getting the baby in the big "cot" (crib) from day one, for example, so that he becomes familiar with the nursery environment and never gets the chance to perceive it as scary and foreign. Ford believes that breast milk is better for the baby than formula but states very clearly that the mother should do whatever makes her happiest.

Though many swear by her techniques for success, Gina Ford's ideas are controversial—partly because she is very quick to eliminate nighttime feedings, which, according to a number of other experts, can be bad for the newborn's physical and emotional well-being. → See Breastfeeding, page 282, and "Is He Sleeping Through the Night?," page 340.

more baby gurus

Dr. Marc Weissbluth, page 352
Dr. Richard Ferber, page 352
Tracy Hogg ("The Baby Whisperer"), page 351
Dr. Harvey Karp, page 259

more parenting resources

adoption and surrogacy

Assisted Reproduction: The Complete Guide to Having a Baby with the Help of a Third Party by Theresa Marie Erickson and MaryAnn Lathus

Beyond Infertility: The New Paths to Parenthood by Susan L. Cooper and Ellen S. Glazer

Cross Cultural Adoption: How to Answer Questions from Family, Friends & Community by Amy Coughlin and Caryn Abramowitz

Dim Sum, Bagels, and Grits: A Sourcebook for Multicultural Families by Myra Alperson

The Kid: What Happened After My Boyfriend and I Decided to Go Get Pregnant by Dan Savage

A Love Like No Other: Stories from Adoptive Parents by Pamela Kruger and Jill Smolowe (Editors)

A Matter of Trust: The Guide to Gestational Surrogacy by Gail Dutton

Mommies, Daddies, Donors, Surrogates: Answering Tough Questions and Building Strong Families by Diane Ehrensaft

The Post-Adoption Blues: Overcoming the Unforeseen Challenges of Adoption by Karen J. Foli and John R. Thompson

Raising Adopted Children, Revised Edition: Practical Reassuring Advice for Every Adoptive Parent by Lois Ruskai Melina

Real Parents Real Children by Holly Van Gulden

Secret Thoughts of an Adoptive Mother by Jana Wolff

Surrogacy Was the Way: Twenty Intended Mothers Tell Their Stories by Zara Griswold

aap.org/sections/adoption (the AAP nationwide directory for pediatricians with a special interest in adoption and foster care medicine)

adopting.org

theadoptionguide.com

adoptioninstitute.org

adoptivefamilies.com

The American Surrogacy Center: surrogacy.com

everythingsurrogacy.com

karensadoptionlinks.com

Surrogate Mothers Online: surromomsonline.com

single parenthood

The Complete Single Mother by Andrea Engber and Leah Klungness

Operating Instructions: A Journal of My Son's First Year by Anne Lamott

Raising Boys Without Men: How Maverick Moms Are Creating the Next Generation of Exceptional Men by Peggy Drexler and Linden Gross

The Single Mother's Book: A Practical Guide to Managing Your Children, Career, Home, Finances, and Everything Else by Joan Anderson

Single Mothers by Choice: A Guidebook for Single Women Who Are Considering or Have Chosen Motherhood by Jane Mattes

The Single Mother's Survival Guide by Patrice Karst

The Single Parent Resource by Brook Noel and Arthur C. Klein

Unsung Heroines: Single Mothers and the American Dream by Ruth Sidel

parentswithoutpartners.org

parenting multiples

The Art of Parenting Twins: The Unique Joys and Challenges of Raising Twins and Other Multiples by Patricia Malmstrom and Janet Poland

Double Duty: The Parents' Guide to Raising Twins, from Pregnancy Through the School Years by Christina Baglivi Tinglof

Mothering Multiples: Breastfeeding and Caring for Twins or More by Karen Kerkhoff Gromada

Raising Twins: What Parents Want to Know (And What Twins Want to Tell Them) by Eileen M. Pearlman and Jill Alison Ganon

Raising Twins After the First Year: Everything You Need to Know About Bringing Up Twins—from Toddlers to Preteens by Karen Gottesman

Ready or Not . . . Here We Come! The REAL Experts' Cannot-Live-Without Guide to the First Year with Twins by Elizabeth Lyons

thinking about parenthood

Mother Nature: Maternal Instincts and How They Shape the Human Species by Sarah Hrdy

Mother Reader: Essential Writings on Motherhood by Moyra Davey (Editor)

Mothers Who Think: Tales of Real Life Parenthood by Camille Peri and Kate Moses (Editors)

A Potent Spell by Janna Malamud Smith

Representations of Motherhood by Donna Bassin, Margaret Honey, and Meryle Mahrer Kaplan (Editors)

LGBT parenting

Buying Dad: One Woman's Search for the Perfect Sperm Donor by Harlyn Aizley

Confessions of the Other Mother: Non-Biological Lesbian Mothers Tell All by Harlyn Aizley (Editor)

The Lesbian Parenting Book: A Guide to Creating Families and Raising Children by D. Merilee Clunis, Ph.D., and G. Dorsey Green, Ph.D.

Mommies, Daddies, Donors, Surrogates: Answering Tough Questions and Building Strong Families by Diane Ehrensaft

The New Essential Guide to Lesbian Conception, Pregnancy, and Birth by Preston Sacks (Foreword) and Stephanie Brill

The Queer Parent's Primer: A Lesbian and Gay Families' Guide to Navigating Through a Straight World by Stephanie A. Brill

The Ultimate Guide to Pregnancy for Lesbians: How to Stay Sane and Care for Yourself from Pre-conception Through Birth, 2nd Edition, by Rachel Pepper

Human Rights Campaign Foundation: hrc.org

National Gay and Lesbian Task Force: thetaskforce.org

Our Family: ourfamily.org

parenting and disabilities

Bigger Than the Sky: Disabled Women on Parenting by Michele Wates and Rowen Jade (Editors)

The Disabled Mom: A Supplemental Guide for Mothers Who Are Ill, Disabled, or Have a Chronic Condition by Tonya Daughrity

Disabled Parents: Dispelling the Myths (National Childbirth Trust Guide) by Michele Wates

The Disabled Woman's Guide to Pregnancy and Birth by Judith Rogers

Parenting and Disability: Disabled Parents' Experiences of Raising Children by Richard Olsen and Harriet Clarke

Disabled Parents Online: disabledparents.net

Through the Looking Glass: lookingglass.org

babies with special needs

Breakthrough Parenting for Children with Special Needs: Raising the Bar of Expectations by Judy Winter

More Than a Mom: Living a Full and Balanced Life When Your Child Has Special Needs by Heather Fawcett and Amy Baskin

Nobody's Perfect: Living and Growing with Children Who Have Special Needs by Nancy B. Miller

Parenting Your Complex Child: Become a Powerful Advocate for the Autistic, Down Syndrome, PDD, Bipolar, or Other Special-Needs Child by Peggy Lou Morgan

Reflections from a Different Journey: What Adults with Disabilities Wish All Parents Knew by Stanley Klein and John Kemp

Voices from the Spectrum: Parents, Grandparents, Siblings, People with Autism, and Professionals Share Their Wisdom by Cindy N. Ariel and Robert A. Naseef (Editors)

You Will Dream New Dreams: Inspiring Personal Stories by Parents of Children with Disabilities by Kim Schive and Stanley D. Klein (Editors)

"Breastfeeding the Hospitalized Baby" by Cyndi Egbert (available at parentingweb.com/lounge/bf _hospital.htm and elsewhere online)

CLEFT PALATE
aboutfaceinternational.org

The Cleft Palate Foundation: cleftline.org or 800-24cleft

DOWN SYNDROME
American Academy of Family Physicians: aafp.org

Down Syndrome Educational Trust: downsed.org and downscity.org

Dr. Sears: askdrsears.com (parents of children with Down syndrome)

PREMATURE BABIES
The Early Birds: A Mother's Story for Our Times by Jenny Minton

Kangaroo Care: The Best You Can Do to Help Your Preterm Infant by Susan Ludington-Hoe

Parenting Your Premature Baby and Child: The Emotional Journey by Deborah L. Davis, Ph.D., and Mara Tesler Stein, Psy.D.

The Preemie Parents' Companion: The Essential Guide to Caring for Your Premature Baby in the Hospital, at Home and Through the First Years by Susan L. Madden, M.S.

Preemies: The Essential Guide for Parents of Premature Babies by Dana Wechsler Linden, Emma Trenti Paroli, and Mia Wechsler Doron, M.D.

The Premature Baby Book: Everything You Need to Know About Your Premature Baby from Birth to Age One by William Sears, et al.

Neonatology on the Web: neonatology.org

Parents of Premature Babies: preemie-l.org

preemieparents.com

preemieparentsupport.com

Premature Baby—Premature Child: Prematurity.org

premature-infant.com

prematurity.org

older parenthood
Baby B by Michael Ryan

The Essential Over 35 Pregnancy Guide by Ellen Lavin

Hot Flashes, Warm Bottles: First-Time Mothers Over Forty by Nancy London

Midlife Motherhood: A Woman-to-Woman Guide to Pregnancy and Parenting by Jann Blackstone-Ford

Older Mothers: Conception, Pregnancy and Birth After 35 by Julia Berryman, Karen Thorpe, Kate Windridge

You Make Me Feel Like an Unnatural Woman: Diary of a New (Older) Mother by Judith Newman

teen parents
Dear Diary, I'm Pregnant: Teenagers Talk About Their Pregnancy by Ann-renee Englander (Editor)

Life Interrupted : The Scoop on Being a Young Mom (Mothers of Preschoolers) by Tricia Goyer

Nurturing Your Newborn: Young Parents' Guide to Baby's First Month (Teen Pregnancy and Parenting series) by Jeanne Warren Lindsay and Jean Brunelli, P.H.N.

The Unplanned Pregnancy Book for Teens and College Students by Dorrie Williams-Wheeler

You Look Too Young to Be a Mom: Teen Mothers on Love, Learning, and Success by Deborah Davis (Editor)

Your Pregnancy and Newborn Journey: A Guide for Pregnant Teens (Teen Pregnancy and Parenting series) by Jeanne Warren Lindsay and Jean Brunelli, P.H.N.

creativity and parenthood

Big Purple Mommy: Nurturing Our Creative Work, Our Children, and Ourselves by Coleen Hubbard

The Fruits of Labor: Creativity, Motherhood and Self-Expression by Penny Summer

Literary Mama: Reading for the Maternally Inclined by Andrea J. Buchanan and Amy Hudock (Editors)

Mamaphonic: Balancing Motherhood and Other Creative Acts by Bee Lavender and Maia Rossini (Editors)

A Question of Balance: Artists and Writers on Motherhood by Judith Pierce Rosenberg

Strong Hearts, Inspired Minds: 21 Artists Who Are Mothers Tell Their Stories by Anne Mavor and Christine Eagon

artistmoms.com

literarymama.com

mamaphonic.com

motherswhowrite.com

resources

See fromthehips.com for more resources.

boys and girls

Between Mothers and Sons: Women Writers Talk About Having Sons and Raising Men by Patricia Stevens

It's a Boy: Women Writers on Raising Sons by Andrea J. Buchanan (Editor)

It's a Girl: Women Writers on Raising Daughters by Andrea J. Buchanan (Editor)

momsofboys.org

baby care

Mothers and Others for a Livable Planet Guide to Natural Baby Care: Nontoxic and Environmentally Friendly Ways to Take Care of Your New Child by Mindy Pennybacker and Aisha Ikramuddin

Naturally Healthy Babies and Children: A Commonsense Guide to Herbal Remedies, Nutrition, and Health by Aviva Jill Romm

The Vaccine Guide: Risks and Benefits for Children and Adults by Randall Neustaedter

What Your Doctor May Not Tell You About Children's Vaccinations by Stephanie Cave and Deborah Mitchell

memoir, fiction, and miscellaneous

Before: Short Stories About Pregnancy from Our Top Writers by Emily Franklin and Heather Swain (Editors)

Breeder: Real-Life Stories from the New Generation of Mothers by Ariel Gore and Bee Lavender (Editors)

Guarding the Moon: A Mother's First Year by Francesca Lia Block

The Imperfect Mom: Candid Confessions of Mothers Living in the Real World by Therese J. Borchard

Maybe Baby: 28 Writers Tell the Truth About Skepticism, Infertility, Baby Lust, Childlessness, Ambivalence, and How They Made the Biggest Decision of Their Lives by Lori Leibovich

What Do You Do All Day? A Novel by Amy Scheibe

parenting and race

Black Baby White Hands: A View from the Crib by Jaiya John and Charlene Maxwell (Editors)

Dim Sum, Bagels, and Grits: A Sourcebook for Multicultural Families by Myra Alperson

Does Anybody Else Look Like Me?: A Parent's Guide to Raising Multiracial Children by Donna Jackson Nakazawa

I'm Chocolate, You're Vanilla: Raising Healthy Black and Biracial Children in a Race-Conscious World by Marguerite Wright

Raising Biracial Children by Kerry Ann Rockquemore

Tripping on the Color Line: Blackwhite Multiracial Families in a Racially Divided World by Heather M. Dalmage

pregnancy and parenting after infertility

Adopting After Infertility by Patricia Irwin Johnston

A Few Good Eggs: Two Chicks Dish on Overcoming the Insanity of Infertility by Julie Vargo and Maureen Regan

A Little Pregnant: Our Memoir of Fertility, Infertility, and a Marriage by Linda Carbone and Ed Decker

The Long-Awaited Stork: A Guide to Parenting After Infertility by Ellen Sarasohn Glazer

infant development

Diary of a Baby by Daniel N. Stern

What's Going On in There: How the Brain and Mind Develop in the First Five Years of Life by Lise Eliot

references

pregnancy

In addition to the sources cited below, these books and websites were used for general information and statistics on pregnancy and prenatal health:

The Centers for Disease Control and Prevention, cdc.gov.

Harms, Roger W., M.D., E.I.C. *Mayo Clinic Guide to a Healthy Pregnancy.* New York: HarperResource, 2004.

Kitzinger, Sheila. *The Complete Book of Pregnancy and Childbirth.* New York: Alfred A. Knopf, 2000.

The March of Dimes, marchofdimes .com.

Nilsson, Lennart. *A Child Is Born.* New York: Delta, 2004.

DECISIONS, DECISIONS

Castellsagué et al. "Male Circumcision, Penile Human Papillomavirus Infection, and Cervical Cancer in Female Partners." *New England Journal of Medicine* 346:15 (April 11, 2002): 1105–12.

"Chorionic Villus Sampling and Amniocentesis: Recommendations for Prenatal Counseling." *Morbidity and Mortality Weekly Report* 44.RR-9 (July 21, 1995): 1–12, cdc.gov/mmwr/ preview/mmwrhtml/00038393.htm.

Eddleman, Keith E., M.D., et al. "Pregnancy Loss After Midtrimester Amniocentesis." *Obstetrics and Gynecology* 108 (November 2006): 1067–72.

FDA/Center for Food Safety and Applied Nutrition. "Draft Assessment of the Relative Risk to Public Health from Foodborne Listeria Monocytogenes Among Selected Categories of Ready-to-Eat Foods." USDA Food Safety and Inspection Service; Centers for Disease Control and Prevention, January 19, 2001, foodsafety .gov/~dms/lmrisk5.html.

Ferrara, Lauren A., M.D., and Joanne L. Stone, M.D. "The Evolution of Down Syndrome Screening and the FASTER Trial." *Frontiers in Women's Health,* obgyn.net/Frontiers_In_ Reproductive_Medicine/evolution.asp.

Hook, E. G., and A. Lindsjo. "Down Syndrome in Live Births by Single Year Maternal Age Interval in a Swedish Study: Comparison with Results from a New York State Study." *American Journal of Human Genetics* 30, no. 1 (Jan. 1978):19–27.

Rothman, Barbara Katz. *The Tentative Pregnancy.* New York: W. W. Norton and Co., 1993.

Sharp, Linda M. "Pink When You Wanted Blue." 2006, parenthood.com/ articles.html?article_id=2707.

Zepf, Bill, M.D. "Does Male Circumcision Prevent Cervical Cancer in Women?" *American Family Physician,* aafp.org/afp/20020701/tips/8.html (July 1, 2002).

THE PREGNANT BODY

American College of Obstetricians and Gynecologists. "Obesity in Pregnancy." *Obstetrics and Gynecology* 106, no. 3 (September 2005): 671–75.

Bell, E. M., I. Hertz-Picciotto, and J. J. Beaumont. "A Case-Control Study of Pesticides and Fetal Death Due to Congenital Anomalies." *Epidemiology* 12 (March 2001): 148–56.

"Body Burden—The Pollution in Newborns: A Benchmark Investigation of Industrial Chemicals, Pollutants and Pesticides in Umbilical Cord Blood." Environmental Working Group Executive Summary, July 14, 2005, ewg.org/ reports/bodyburden2/execsumm.php.

"Consumer Guide to Mercury in Fish: A Guide to Staying Healthy and Fighting Back." Natural Resources Defense Council, nrdc.org/health/effects/ mercury/guide.asp.

Daniel, Kaayla T. "Whole Soy Story: The Dark Side of America's Favorite Health Food." *Mothering Magazine* 124 (May/ June 2004).

Environmental Working Group, ewg.org.

Froen, J. F. "A Kick from Within—Fetal Movement Counting and the Cancelled Progress in Antenatal Care." *Journal of Perinatal Medicine* 32, no. 1 (2004): 13–24.

Meadows, Michelle. "Pregnancy and the Drug Dilemma." U.S. Food and Drug Administration, *FDA Consumer Magazine,* May–June 2001, fda.gov/fdac,

Motherisk, motherisk.org.

National Sleep Foundation, sleepfoundation.org.

Natural Resources Defense Council, nrdc.org.

"Nitrates in Drinking Water." Wilkes University Center for Environmental Quality, Environmental Engineering and Engineering Department, waterresearch.net/nitrate.htm.

Organization of Teratology Information Specialists, otispregnancy.org.

Pastore, L. M., I. Hertz-Picciotto, and J. J. Beaumont. "Risk of Stillbirth from Occupational and Residential Exposures." *Occupational and Environmental Medicine* 54 (1997): 511–18.

"Report Card: Pesticides in Produce." Foodnews, Environmental Working Group, Foodnews.org/reportcard.php.

Schreinemachers, Dina M. "Birth Malformations and Other Adverse Perinatal Outcomes in Four U.S. Wheat-Producing States." *Environmental Health Perspectives* 111 (July 2003): 1259–64.

Steingraber, Sandra. *Having Faith: An Ecologist's Journey to Motherhood.* New York: Berkley Books, 2003.

Strandberg, T. E., et al. "Birth Outcome in Relation to Licorice Consumption During Pregnancy." *American Journal of Epidemiology* 153 (2001): 1085–88.

THE PREGNANT BRAIN

BBCnews.com. "Pregnancy Stress 'Passed to Baby.'" September 27, 2005, news.bbc.co.uk/go/pr/fr/-/2/hi/health/4286512.stm.

Broder, Michael S. *The Panic-Free Pregnancy.* Matthews, N.C.: Perigee Trade, 2004.

Buitelaar, J. K., et al. "Prenatal Stress and Cognitive Development and Temperament in Infants." *Neurobiology and Aging* 24, no. S1 (2003): S53–S60.

Cohen, Lee S., M.D., et al. "Relapse of Major Depression During Pregnancy in Women Who Maintain or Discontinue Antidepressant Treatment." *Journal of the American Medical Association* 295, no. 5 (2006): 499–507.

Coker, A., et al. "Physical Health Consequences of Physical and Psychological Intimate Partner Violence." *Archives of Family Medicine* 9, no. 5 (2000): 451–57.

Davis, Jeanie Lerche. "Mother's Stress Affects Fetus: What Are the Long-Term Health Implications?" WebMD Medical News, February 12, 2003, webmd.com/content/article/60/67241.htm.

DiPietro, J. A., et al. "Maternal Psychological Distress During Pregnancy in Relation to Child Development at Age 2." *Child Development* 77 (2006): 573.

Dixon, L., K. Browne, and C. Hamilton-Giachritsis. "Risk Factors of Parents Abused as Children: A Mediational Analysis of the Intergenerational Continuity of Child Maltreatment (Part I)." *Journal of Child Psychology and Psychiatry* 46, no. 1 (January 2005): 47–57.

Ellison, Katherine. *The Mommy Brain: How Motherhood Makes Us Smarter.* New York: Perseus Books, 2006.

"The Facts on Reproductive Health and Violence Against Women." Family Violence Prevention Fund, endabuse.org/resources/facts/ReproductiveHealth.pdf.

Food and Drug Administration. "Advising of Risk of Birth Defects with Paxil Agency Requiring Updated Product Labeling." FDA Press Release, December 8, 2005, fda.gov/bbs/topics/NEWS/2005/NEW01270.html.

Gazmararian, J. A., et al. "Violence and Reproductive Health; Current Knowledge and Future Research Directions." *Maternal and Child Health Journal* 4, no. 2 (2000): 79–84.

Karla, Gavin. "Many Pregnant Women Show Signs of Depression, But Few Are Getting Treatment, U-M Study Finds." University of Michigan Health System News Release, May 20, 2003, med.umich.edu/opm/newspage/2003/pregdepression.htm.

Kaufman, J., and E. Zigler. "Do Abused Children Become Abusive Parents?" *American Journal of Orthopsychiatry* 57, no. 2 (April 1987): 186–92.

McFarlane, J., et al. "Abuse During Pregnancy: Association with Maternal Health and Infant Birthweight." *Nursing Research* 45 (1996): 32–37.

McFarlane, J., et al. "Physical Abuse, Smoking and Substance Abuse During Pregnancy: Prevalence, Interrelationships and Effects on Birthweight." *Journal of Obstetrical Gynecological and Neonatal Nursing* 25 (1996): 313–20.

"Nausea and Vomiting in Pregnancy (NVP)." Department of Psychology, University of Lincoln, UK, lincoln.ac.uk/psychology/study_of_sickness_in_pregnancy.htm.

Parker, B., J. McFarlane, and K. Soeken. "Abuse During Pregnancy: Effects on Maternal Complications and Infant Birthweight in Adult and Teen Women." *Obstetrics and Gynecology* 841 (1994): 323–28.

Parsons, L., et al. "Violence Against Women and Reproductive Health: Toward Defining a Role for Reproductive Health Care Services." *Maternal and Child Health Journal,* 4. no. 2 (2000): 135.

Richardson, P. "Women's Perceptions of Their Important Dyadic Relationships During Pregnancy." *Maternal Child Nursing Journal* 10, no. 3 (Fall 1981): 159–74.

"University Research Dispels Popular Myth," University Press Office Press Release, University of Sunderland, UK, March 13, 2003, sunderland.ac.uk/caffairs/203mar6.htm.

THE PREGNANT LIFE

Broder, Michael S. *The Panic-Free Pregnancy.* Matthews, N.C.: Perigee Trade, 2004.

Greenfield, Marjorie, M.D. "Air Travel in Pregnancy." September 5, 2006, drspock.com/article/0,1510,5773,00.html.

Mozurkewich, Ellen L., M.D., et al. "Working Conditions and Adverse Pregnancy Outcome: A Meta-Analysis." *Obstetrics and Gynecology* 95 (2000): 623–35.

WHEN THINGS GET COMPLICATED

American College of Obstetricians and Gynecologists. "External Cephalic Version." *ACOG Practice Bulletin* 13 (2000).

Beus, Tamara. "Fibroids." *Women's Health,* 2001, womenshealthlondon.org.uk/leaflets/fibroids/fibroids.html.

Coyle, M. E., C. A. Smith, and B. Pete. "Cephalic Version by Moxibustion for Breech Presentation." *Cochrane Database of Systematic Reviews* 3 (2006), cochrane.org/reviews/en/ab003928.html.

DES Action USA, desaction.org.

The Ectopic Pregnancy Trust, ectopic.org.

Fischer, Richard, M.D., "Breech Presentation." Department of Obstetrics and Gynecology, Section of Maternal-Fetal Medicine, Cooper Hospital/University Medical Center, July 10, 2006, emedicine.com/med/topic3272.htm.

Goldenberg, R. L., et al. "Bed Rest in Pregnancy." *Obstetrics and Gynecology* 84, no. 1 (July 1994): 131–36.

Hannah, M. E., et al. (Term Breech Trial Collaborative Group). "Planned Caesarean Section Versus Planned Vaginal Birth for Breech Presentation at Term: A Randomised Multicentre Trial." *Lancet* 356, no. 9239 (October 21, 2000):1375–83.

Henry J. Kaiser Family Foundation. "C-Section Rate in U.S. Reaches High of 1.2M in 2004 Despite Efforts to Lower Rate." November 16, 2005, kaisernetwork.org/daily_reports/rep_index.cfm?DR_ID=33758.

Hill, D. Ashley, M.D. "Molar Pregnancy." obgyn.net/women/articles/molarpreg dah.htm.

Hogge, W. A. "The Clinical Use of Karyotyping Spontaneous Abortions." *American Journal of Obstetrics and Gynecology* 189, no. 2 (August 2003): 397–402.

Mayo Clinic, ed. *Mayo Clinic Guide to a Healthy Pregnancy.* New York: Harper-Collins, 2004.

Mayo Clinic, ed. "Twin Pregnancy: What Multiples Mean for Mom." December 5, 2005, mayoclinic.com/health/twin-pregnancy/PR00120.

"Miscarriage: A Patient's Guide." *Medic8 Family Health Guide,* medic8.com/healthguide/articles/miscarriage.html.

The Miscarriage Association, miscarriageassociation.org.uk.

Nassar, N., et al. "Systematic Review of Adverse Outcomes of External Cephalic Version and Persisting Breech Presentation at Term." *Paediatric and Perinatal Epidemiology* 2 (March 20, 2006): 163–71.

National Center for Health Statistics, cdc.gov/nchs.

Raeburn, Daniel. "Vessels." *The New Yorker,* May 1, 2006, newyorker.com.

Rubin, Rita. "C-section Rate Hits Record High at 29%." *USA Today,* November 15, 2005.

The Stillbirth Alliance, stillbirthalliance.org.

"Uterine Fibroids Associated with Adverse Obstetric Outcomes." *Obstetrics and Gynecology* 107 (2006): 376–82.

Weismiller, David G., M.D., Sc.M. "Preterm Labor." *American Family Physician* 59, no. 3 (February 1, 1999): 593–602.

Wright, Victoria Clay, M.P.H., et al. (Division of Reproductive Health, National Center for Chronic Disease Prevention and Health Promotion). "Assisted Reproductive Technology Surveillance, United States," *Morbidity and Mortality Weekly Report* 54, no. SS02 (June 3, 2005): 1–24, cdc.gov/mmwr/preview/mmwrhtml/ss5402a1.htm.

birth

In addition to the sources cited below, these books and websites were used for general information and statistics on birth:

The Coalition for Improving Maternity Services, motherfriendly.org.

Kitzinger, Sheila. *The Complete Book of Pregnancy and Childbirth.* New York: Alfred A. Knopf, 2000.

The March of Dimes, marchofdimes.com.

BIRTH BASICS

Barclay, Laurie, M.D., C.M.E., and Charles Vega, M.D., F.A.A.F. "Practice Guidelines Issued for Use of Episiotomy." *Medscape Medical News,* April 6, 2006.

Bornstein, Myer S., M.D., and Don Shuwarger, M.D., F.A.C.O.G. "Controversy over Protocol: Misoprostol (Cytotec) for Cervical Ripening and Induction of Labor." *International Journal of Gynaecology and Obstetrics* 21, no. 43 (August 1983): 19–25.

Boulvain, M., C. Stan, and O. Irion, "Membrane Sweeping for Induction of Labour." *Cochrane Database of Systematic Reviews* 1 (2005): CD000451.

Bugg, G. J., et al. "Outcomes of Labours Augmented with Oxytocin." *European Journal of Obstetrics, Gynecology and Reproductive Biology* 124, no. 1 (January 2006): 37–41.

Dublin, Sascha, et al. "Maternal and Neonatal Outcomes After Induction of Labor Without an Identified Indication." *American Journal of Obstetrics and Gynecology* 183, no. 4 (October 2000): 986–94.

Greene, Alan, M.D., F.A.A.P. "Meconium Aspiration." August 31, 2002, drgreene.com/21_1138.html.

Hartmann, Katherine, M.D., Ph.D., et al. "Outcomes of Routine Episiotomy, A Systematic Review." *Journal of the American Medical Association* 293 (2005): 2141–48.

Howell, C. J. "Epidural Versus Nonepidural Analgesia for Pain Relief in Labour." Academic Department of Obstetrics and Gynaecology, North Staffordshire Hospital NHS Trust, Maternity Hospital, Staffordshire, UK, *Cochrane Database of Systematic Reviews* 4 (2005): CD000331.

Kripke, Clarissa C., M.D. "Why Are We Using Electronic Fetal Monitoring?" *American Family Physician* 59, no. 9 (May 1, 1999), aafp.org/afp/990501ap/editorials.html.

Laino, Charlene. "C-Section Rates: Obesity to Blame? Patient Requests May Not Be Major Factor in Growing Number of C-Sections." May 9, 2006, webmd.com/content/article/122/114508.htm.

Lieberman, E., and C. O'Donoghue. "Unintended Effects of Epidural Analgesia During Labor: A Systematic Review." *American Journal of Obstetrics and Gynecology* 86, no. 5 (2002 May): S78–80.

Lydon-Rochelle, Mona T., Ph.D., M.P.H., et al. "Delivery Method and Self-Reported Postpartum General Health Status Among Primiparous Women." *Paediatric and Perinatal Epidemiology* 15 (July 2001): 232–40.

Mayberry, et al. "Epidural Analgesia Side Effects, Co-interventions, and Care of Women During Childbirth: A Systematic Review." *American Journal of Obstetrics and Gynecology* 86, no. 5 (2002 May): S81–93.

Mittendorf, R., et al. "The Length of Uncomplicated Human Gestation." *Obstetrics and Gynecology* 75 (1990): 929–32.

Morabito, Christopher J., M.D., and Joseph V. DiCarlo, M.D. "Neonatal Respiratory Failure/Meconium Aspiration Syndrome." *All-Net Pediatric Critical Care Textbook.* Department of Pediatrics, Lucile Packard Children's Hospital, Stanford University, California, pedsccm.wustl.edu/all-net/english/pulmpage/neon/mecasp.html.

"NIH State-of-the-Science Conference: Cesarean Delivery on Maternal Request." National Institutes of Health, March 27–29, 2006, consensus.nih.gov/2006/2006 CesareanSOS027html.htm.

Putta, Lakshmidevi V., M.D., and Jeanne P. Spencer, M.D. "Assisted Vaginal Delivery Using the Vacuum Extractor." *American Family Physician Journal* 62, no. 6 (September 15, 2000): 1316–20.

Tenore, Josie, M.D., S.M. "Methods for Cervical Ripening and Induction of Labor." *American Family Physician,* May 5, 2003.

Wagner, Marsden, M.D., M.S.P.H. "Misoprostol (Cytotec) for Labor Induction: A Cautionary Tale." *Midwifery Today,* Spring 1999: 49. midwiferytoday.com/articles/cytotecwagner.asp.

Wong, Cynthia A., et al. "The Risk of Cesarean Delivery with Neuraxial Analgesia Given Early Versus Late in Labor." *New England Journal of Medicine* 7, no. 352 (February 17, 2005): 655–65.

Wong, S. F., et al. "Does Sweeping of Membranes Beyond 40 Weeks Reduce the Need for Formal Induction of Labour?"*An International Journal of Obstetrics and Gynaecology* 109 (June 2002): 632.

Yeast, John D., M.D., Angela Jones, M.S., Mary Poskin, M.S.N. "Induction of Labor and the Relationship to Cesarean Delivery: A Review of 7,001 Consecutive Inductions." *American Journal of Obstetrics and Gynecology* 180, no. 3 (March 1999): 628–33.

PREPARING YOURSELF

Brown, Petrina. *Eve: Sex, Childbirth and Motherhood Through the Ages.* (Chichester, West Sussex, UK: Summersdale Publishers, 2004.

Dick-Read, Grantly. *Dick-Read's Childbirth Without Fear: The Principles and Practice of Natural Childbirth,* fifth ed. Heinemann Medical, 1968.

Dunham, Carroll. *Mamatoto: A Celebration of Birth.* New York: Penguin, 1991.

Gaskin, Ina May. *Ina May's Guide to Childbirth.* New York: Bantam, 2003.

"Mortality for Complications of Pregnancy, Childbirth, and the Puerperium, According to Race, Hispanic Origin, and Age: United States, Selected Years 1950–2001." National Center for Health Statistics, cdc.gov/nchs/data/hus/tables/2003/03hus043.pdf.

Ness, Amen, M.D., Lisa Gould Rubin, and Jackie Frederick Berner. *The Birth That's Right for You.* New York: McGraw-Hill, 2005.

"Odds of Death Due to Injury, United States, 2002." National Safety Council, nsc.org/lrs/statinfo/odds.htm.

Wertz, Richard W., and Dorothy C. Wertz. *Lying-In: A History of Childbirth in America.* New Haven, Conn.: Yale University Press, 1999.

THE BIRTH ENVIRONMENT

"ACOG Statement of Policy as Issued by the ACOG Executive Board Home Delivery." American College of Obstetricians and Gynecologists, February 2006, collegeofmidwives.org/Political_Action_2006/ACOG_Mfry&PHB_Policies_Feb2006.htm.

Johnson, Kenneth C., and Betty-Anne Davis. "Outcomes of Planned Home Births with Certified Professional Midwives: Large Prospective Study in North America." *British Medical Journal* 330 (June 18, 2005): 1416.

AFTER THE BIRTH

Meikle, James. "One in 20 New Mothers May Suffer Post Traumatic Stress Disorder." *Guardian,* May 27, 2003.

Reynolds, J. L. "Post-traumatic Stress Disorder After Childbirth: The Phenomenon of Traumatic Birth." *Canadian Medical Association Journal/Journal de l'Association Medicale Canadienne* 156, no. 6 (March 15, 1997): 831–35.

becoming a parent

In addition to the sources cited below, these books and websites were used for general information about becoming a parent:

Bassin, Donna, Margaret Honey, and Meryle Mahrer Kaplan, eds. *Representations of Motherhood.* New Haven, Conn.: Yale University Press, 1996.

Davey, Moyra, ed. *Mother Reader: Essential Writings on Motherhood.* New York: Seven Stories Press, 2001.

Davis, Laura, and Janis Keyser. *Becoming the Parent You Want to Be: A Sourcebook of Strategies for the First Five Years.* New York: Broadway Books, 1997.

DelliQuadri, Lyn, M.S.W., and Kati Breckenridge, Ph.D. *Mother Care.* New York: Pocket Books, 1978.

Raffelock, Dean, D.C., Dipl. Ac., C.C.N., and Robert Rountree, M.D., et al. *A Natural Guide to Pregnancy and Postpartum Health.* Vonore, Tenn.: Avery, 2002.

THE POSTBABY BODY
Brown, Sylvia, and Mary Dowd Struck. *The Post-Pregnancy Handbook: The Only Book That Tells What the First Year After Childbirth Is Really All About—Physically, Emotionally, Sexually.* New York: St. Martin's Press, 2003.

Lim, Robin. *After the Baby's Birth: A Woman's Way to Wellness: A Complete Guide for Postpartum Women.* Berkeley, Calif.: Ten Speed Press, 2001.

THE POSTBABY BRAIN
Bennett, Shoshana S., Ph.D., and Pec Indman, Ed.D., M.F.T. *Beyond the Blues: A Guide to Understanding and Treating Prenatal and Postpartum Depression.* San Jose, Calif.: Moodswings Press, 2003.

Bruer, John. *The Myth of the First Three Years.* New York: Free Press, 1999.

Colino, Stacey. "Scary Thoughts." *Washington Post,* March 7, 2006.

Cusk, Rachel. *A Life's Work: On Becoming a Mother.* New York: Picador, 2003.

Douglas, Susan, and Meredith Michael. *The Mommy Myth: The Idealization of Motherhood and How It Has Undermined All Women.* New York: Free Press, 2005.

Figes, Kate, and Jean Zimmerman. *Life After Birth: What Even Your Friends Won't Tell You about Motherhood.* New York: St. Martin's Press, 2002.

Gladwell, Malcolm. "Baby Steps." *The New Yorker,* January 10, 2000.

Hanauer, Cathi, ed. *The Bitch in the House: 26 Women Tell the Truth About Sex, Solitude, Work, Motherhood, and Marriage.* New York: Harper Paperbacks, 2003.

Hrdy, Sarah. *Mother Nature: Maternal Instincts and How They Shape the Human Species.* New York: Ballantine Books, 2000.

Ingman, Marrit. *Inconsolable: How I Threw My Mental Health Out with the Diapers.* Emeryville, Calif.: Seal Press, 2005.

Lazarre, Jane. *The Mother Knot.* Durham, N.C.: Duke University Press, 1997.

Smith, Janna Malamud. *A Potent Spell.* Boston, Mass.: Mariner Books, 2004.

Swigart, Jane, Ph.D. *The Myth of the Perfect Mother.* New York: Contemporary Books, 1991.

Winnicott, D. W. *The Child, the Family and the Outside World,* 2d ed. Reading, Mass.: Addison-Wesley, 1992.

THE POSTBABY LIFE
Belsky, Jay, and John Kelly. *The Transition to Parenthood: How a First Child Changes a Marriage.* New York: Delacorte Press, 1994.

Crittenden, Ann. *The Price of Motherhood: Why the Most Important Job in the World Is Still the Least Valued.* New York: Henry Holt , 2001.

Greenspan, Stanley I., and Jacqueline Salmon. *The Four-Thirds Solution: Solving the Childcare Crisis in America Today.* New York: Perseus Publishing, 2002.

Moms Rising, momsrising.org.

Morris, Bob. "We Are Family: The Age of Dissonance." *New York Times,* May 22, 2005.

Mothers and More: The Network for Sequencing Women, mothersandmore.org.

The Mothers Movement Online, mothersmovement.org.

Oxenhandler, Noelle. *The Eros of Parenthood: Explorations in Light and Dark.* New York: St. Martin's Press, 2001.

Peskowitz, Miriam. *The Truth Behind the Mommy Wars: Who Decides What Makes a Good Mother?* Emeryville, Calif.: Seal Press, 2005.

Warner, Judith. *Perfect Madness: Motherhood in the Age of Anxiety.* New York: Riverhead, 2005.

baby

In addition to the sources cited below, these books and websites were used for general information on infant health and baby care:

The American Academy of Pediatrics. *Caring for Your Baby and Young Child.* New York: Random House, 2004.

askdrsears.com.

The Centers for Disease Control and Prevention, cdc.gov.

drgreene.com.

drspock.com.

Klaus, Marshall H., and Phyllis H. Klaus. *Your Amazing Newborn.* New York: Perseus Books, 2000.

Leach, Penelope. *Your Baby and Child, Birth to Age 5.* New York: Alfred A. Knopf, 1997.

The March of Dimes, marchofdimes.com.

Sears, Dr. William, M.D. *The Baby Book.* New York: Little, Brown and Company, 2003.

Small, Meredith. *Our Babies, Ourselves: How Biology and Culture Shape the Way We Parent.* New York: Anchor, 1999.

BABY CARE BASICS
Brazelton, T. B., et al. *Neonatal Behavioral Assessment Scale,* 2nd ed. Ames, Iowa: Blackwell, 1984.

Brazelton, T. Berry, M.D., *Touchpoints: Birth to 3.* New York: Perseus Books, 1992.

Karp, Harvey. *The Happiest Baby on the Block.* New York: Bantam, 2003.

Niemela, M., M. Uhari, M. Mottonen. "A Pacifier Increases the Risk of Recurrent Acute Otitis Media in Children in Day Care Centers." *Pediatrics* 96 (1995): 884–88.

Pector, Elizabeth A., M.D. "Premature Birth: Coping Tips for Parents." November 2000, synspectrum.com/preemiebirth.htm.

FEEDING YOUR BABY

American Academy of Pediatrics, ed. *Caring for Your Baby and Young Child: Birth to Age 5.* New York: Bantam, 1998.

Angier, Natalie. *Woman: An Intimate Geography.* Boston: Houghton Mifflin, 1999. pp. 144–62.

Becker, Allan B., M.D., et al. "Breast-feeding and Environmental Tobacco Smoke Exposure." *Archives of Pediatric Adolescent Medicine* 153 (1999): 689–91.

Berlin, Cheston M., et al. "Conclusions and Recommendations of the Expert Panel: Technical Workshop on Human Milk Surveillance and Biomonitoring for Environmental Chemicals in the United States." *Journal of Toxicology and Environmental Health* 68, no. 20 (September 2005).

Blum, Linda M. *At the Breast: Ideologies of Breastfeeding and Motherhood in the Contemporary United States.* Boston, Mass.: Beacon Press, 2000.

"Breastfeeding and the Use of Human Milk." *Pediatrics* 115, no. 2 (February 2005): 496–506.

Buehler-Stranges, Amy. "Breast-feeding Still Ideal for Infants, Despite Presence of Environmental Chemicals in Human Breast-milk." Medical News Today, September 23, 2005, medicalnewstoday.com/medicalnews.php?newsid=31069.

Dreher, Melanie C., Ph.D., et al., American Academy of Pediatrics. "Prenatal Marijuana Exposure and Neonatal Outcomes in Jamaica: An Ethnographic Study." *Pediatrics* 93, no. 2 (February 1994): 254–60.

Eliot, Lise. *What's Going On in There: How the Brain and Mind Develop in the First Five Years of Life.* New York: Bantam, 2000, pp. 192–93.

Hausman, Bernice L. *Mother's Milk: Breastfeeding Controversies in American Culture.* Boston, Mass.: Routledge, 2003.

Ito, S. "Drug Therapy for Breast-feeding Women." *New England Journal of Medicine* 343, no. 2 (2000): 118–26.

Kellymom breastfeeding and parenting site, kellymom.com.

Koren, Gideon. *The Complete Guide to Everyday Risks in Pregnancy and Breastfeeding.* Toronto: Robert Rose, 2004.

Kozer, Eran, M.D. and Gideon Koren, M.D., F.R.C.P.C. "Effects of Prenatal Exposure to Marijuana." *Canadian Family Physician* 47 (February 2001): 263–64.

La Leche League International, lalecheleague.org or LLLI.org.

Smith, Linda J., B.S.E., F.A.C.C.E., I.B.C.L.C. "Don't Shake the Milk." Bright Future Lactation Resource Centre, BFLRC.com.

Villamagna, Dana. "Smoking and Breastfeeding." *Leaven* 40, no. 4 (August–September 2004): 75–78.

Wilson-Clay, Barbara, B.S., I.B.C.L.C., and Kay Hoover, M. Ed., I.B.C.L.C. *The Breastfeeding Atlas.* Austin, Tex.: LactNews Press.

Yaron, Ruth. *Super Baby Food.* Archbald, Penn.: F. J. Roberts, 1998.

SLEEP

Ferber, Richard, M.D. *Solve Your Child's Sleep Problems.* New York: Fireside, 1986.

First Candle: The SIDS Alliance, sidsalliance.com.

Pantley, Elizabeth. *The No-Cry Sleep Solution.* New York: McGraw-Hill, 2002.

Small, Meredith. *Our Babies, Ourselves: How Biology and Culture Shape the Way We Parent.* New York: Anchor Books, 1999.

Walls, Susan. "Tears Before Bedtime? Not Any More." *Junior Magazine* 67 (March 2005).

Weissbluth, Marc, M.D. *Healthy Sleep Habits, Happy Child.* New York: Ballantine Books, 1999.

NUTS AND BOLTS: BABY LOGISTICS, HOME AND AWAY

Bass, Joel L., M.D. "Oxygen Desaturation in Term Infants in Car Safety Seats." *Pediatrics* 110, no. 2 (August 2002): 401–2.

Saunders, Jennifer. *Absolutely Fabulous 2: The Complete Second Season.* New York: Pocket Books, 1996.

SORTING THROUGH THE VOICES: EVERYBODY'S GOT AN OPINION

Aney, Matthew, M.D. " 'Babywise' Advice Linked to Dehydration, Failure to Thrive." *AAP News* 14, no. 4 (April 1998): 21.

Bowlby, Richard. *Fifty Years of Attachment Theory: The Donald Winnicott Memorial Lecture.* London: Karnac Books, 2004.

Ezzo, Gary, M.A., and Robert Bucknam, M.D. *On Becoming Baby Wise.* Missouri: Parent-Wise Solutions, Inc., 2001.

Ford, Gina. *The New Contented Little Baby Book: The Secret to Calm and Confident Parenting.* London: Vermilion, 2002.

Hulbert, Ann. *Raising America: Experts, Parents, and a Century of Advice About Children.* New York: Alfred A. Knopf, 2003.

Leach, Penelope. *Your Baby and Child: From Birth to Age 5.* New York: Alfred A. Knopf, 1997.

Sears, Dr. William, M.D. *The Baby Book.* New York: Little, Brown and Company, 2003.

Stearns, Peter N. *Anxious Parents: A History of Modern Childrearing in America.* New York: New York University Press, 2004.

index

about
the authors

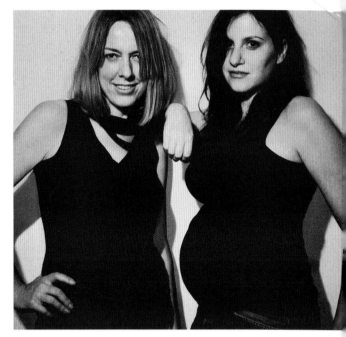

L: ceridwen, **R:** rebecca, photo by alexandra valenti

rebecca odes is the coauthor and illustrator of three books for young women, including the bestselling sex/life guide *Deal with It!* Rebecca cofounded the popular teen website gURL.com and has made numerous media appearances discussing issues relevant to teens and parents. She lives in New York with her husband, son, and daughter.

ceridwen morris is a writer living in New York City with her husband and son.

Visit their website fromthehips.com.